Introduction to Health Services

For N. Williams, the memory of D. Williams,
and J., C., J.C., and N. Torrens

Introduction to Health Services

Seventh Edition

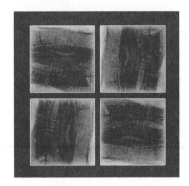

Edited by

Stephen J. Williams, Sc.D.

Associate Dean
College of Health and Human Services
San Diego State University
San Diego, California

Paul R. Torrens, M.D., M.P.H.

Professor of Health Services
School of Public Health
University of California, Los Angeles
Los Angeles, California

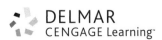

DELMAR
CENGAGE Learning

Australia • Brazil • Japan • Korea • Mexico • Singapore • Spain • United Kingdom • United States

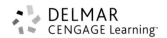

DELMAR
CENGAGE Learning™

Introduction to Health Services, Seventh Edition
Edited by Stephen J. Williams, Paul R. Torrens,

Vice President, Health Care Business Unit: William Brottmiller

Director of Learning Solutions: Matthew Kane

Acquisitions Editor: Kalen Conerly

Product Manager: Natalie Pashoukos

Editorial Assistant: Meaghan O'Brien

Marketing Director: Jennifer McAvey

Marketing Manager: Michele McTighe

Marketing Coordinator: Chelsey Iaquinta

Technology Director: Laurie Davis

Production Director: Carolyn Miller

Senior Art Director: Jack Pendleton

Senior Content Project Manager: James Zayicek

Technology Project Manager: Carolyn Fox

For product information and technology assistance, contact us at
Cengage Learning Customer & Sales Support, 1-800-354-9706

For permission to use material from this text or product, submit all requests online at **www.cengage.com/permissions**
Further permissions questions can be emailed to
permissionrequest@cengage.com

Library of Congress Control Number: 2007028380

ISBN-13: 978-1-4180-1289-2

ISBN-10: 1-4180-1289-0

Delmar
Executive Woods
5 Maxwell Drive
Clifton Park, NY 12065
USA

Cengage Learning is a leading provider of customized learning solutions with office locations around the globe, including Singapore, the United Kingdom, Australia, Mexico, Brazil, and Japan. Locate your local office at **international.cengage.com/region**

Cengage Learning products are represented in Canada by Nelson Education, Ltd.

For your course and learning solutions, visit **delmar.cengage.com**

Visit our corporate website at **www.cengage.com**

Printed in the United States of America
2 3 4 5 6 7 11 10 09 08

CONTENTS

PART ONE

Overview of the Health Services System / 1

PART TWO

Financing and Structuring Health Care / 75

PART
THREE
Providers of Health Services / 141

PART
FOUR
Nonfinancial Resources for Health Care / 245

PART
FIVE
Assessing and Regulating Health Services / 295

CONTRIBUTORS

Lester Breslow, M.D., M.P.H.
Professor and Dean Emeritus
School of Public Health
University of California, Los Angeles
Los Angeles, California

Connie J. Evashwick, Sc.D., F.A.C.H.E.
Dean
School of Public Health
St. Louis University
St. Louis, Missouri

Alma L. Koch, Ph.D.
Professor of Public Health
Graduate Program in Health Services
    Administration
Graduate School of Public Health
San Diego State University
San Diego, California

Stephen S. Mick, Ph.D.
Arthur Graham Glasgow Professor of
    Health Administration
Chair, Department of Health Administration
School of Allied Health Professions
Virginia Commonwealth University
Richmond, Virginia

Ruth Roemer, J.D. (Deceased)
Professor of Health Services Emerita
School of Public Health
University of California, Los Angeles
Los Angeles, California

Paul R. Torrens, M.D., M.P.H.
Professor of Health Services
School of Public Health
University of California, Los Angeles
Los Angeles, California

Pauline Vaillancourt Rosenau, Ph.D.
Professor, Management and Policy
    Sciences
Center for Society and Population Health
UT-Houston School of Public Health
The University of Texas
Houston Health Science Center
Houston, Texas

Kenneth R. White, Ph.D., F.A.C.H.E
Charles P. Cardwell, Jr., Professor
Director, Graduate Program in Health
    Administration
School of Allied Health Professions
Virginia Commonwealth University
Richmond, Virginia

Stephen J. Williams, Sc.D.
Associate Dean
College of Health and Human Services
San Diego State University
San Diego, California

PREFACE

The nation's health care system has increasingly moved to center stage, drawing the attention of many Americans and our nation's politicians. The long-predicted alignment of the stars for health services, including national costs, quality expectations and concerns, and payer pressures, has arrived. The recognition that the cost of health care and the increasing needs of an aging population would drain national finances and create tremendous political pressure for change in the health care system has occurred. At the same time, revolutionary changes in the practice of clinical medicine, in large part the result of the biomedical revolution of the past quarter century, has upped the ante in terms of public expectations and the potential achievements of health care in prolonging and improving life. And, of course, that achievement in and of itself creates added costs, pressures, and expectations as our functional status and longevity improve.

Improving the quality and quantity of life is what the nation's health care system is all about. It is ironic that our successes in these areas have also led us to question the extent to which we, as a nation, can provide an adequate level of health care for all Americans. As a result, increasing pressure to improve the effectiveness and efficiency of the health care system to utilize information, technology, and quality improvement matrixes and to address issues of rationing and consumer responsibility, have all moved to the forefront of the national debate. This seventh edition of *Introduction to Health Services* reflects these mounting opportunities and challenges as we seek to better understand, evaluate, and control the nation's health care system.

This new edition has streamlined and consolidated some content, although the successful overall design and format of previous recent editions has been maintained. This new edition is modernized, but familiar to our audiences. Information has been updated and a number of new features have been added, including study questions at the end of each chapter.

As in the previous editions, Part One presents an overview and background information to set the stage for assessing the organization, structure, and operation of the nation's health care system. Chapter 1 presents a historical overview of the system, which sets the stage for all the chapters that follow. Chapter 2 discusses the now fundamental technological basis upon which clinical medicine firmly rests. Chapter 3 describes the primary patterns of disease experienced in the twentieth and early twenty-first centuries in the United States. Because disease patterns are a principal determinant of health care utilization, understanding these trends is a particularly important core theme for the book. This chapter also includes consideration of the issues related to the differential access to health care services.

Part Two focuses on financing and financial management of health care systems and services. The chapters on this topic from the previous edition have been consolidated and streamlined to improve readability due to the complexity of this material. The first of the financial chapters focuses on overall trends and issues in financing and health services, including public programs and especially Medicare, while the second chapter, Chapter 5, discusses private health insurance and managed care and related health financing policy issues.

Part Three examines health care provider organizations and settings. The focus in this part of the book is on the major provider settings and organizations that form the distribution network for health care services. Chapter 6 addresses aspects of public health services in the United States. Public health and preventive services have played a key role in the reduction of illness and disease throughout our nation's history. The challenges from global epidemics and terrorism have heightened the importance of these services in recent years. Our commitment to public health services must be paramount to protect the nation's health in the future.

Chapter 7 focuses on noninstitutional services that are delivered through ambulatory care channels. Ambulatory care has assumed an increasingly important role in the nation's health care system, both with a shift of services from inpatient to outpatient settings, and in controlling patient utilization of services, particularly under managed-care plans.

Chapter 8 focuses on inpatient and related hospital and health systems. The hospital as an institution has undergone tremendous change over past decades and will likely continue to do so in the future. The hospital's role within the nation's health care system and the internal operation of hospitals are constantly in motion, responding to parameters of financing, politics, quality, and consumer expectations. Changing relationships between hospitals and other players in the system are also addressed in this chapter.

Chapters 9 and 10 address two other key areas of the nation's health care system: long-term care and mental health services. Both these areas have changed dramatically over the past few decades and will likely continue to do so in the future. Long-

term care services face the challenge of an aging American population while mental health services reflect both continuing financial constraints and dramatic changes in the technology of clinical medicine as it relates to mental illness.

Part Four deals with critical nonfinancial resources used in providing health care services. Chapter 11 examines the role of the pharmaceutical industry in meeting health care needs. The increasing delivery of pharmaceutical-based therapies is particularly important in the current evolution of clinical medicine and health care services in the United States. Chapter 12 examines the human resource side of health care, discussing the professionals who provide services within the system and without whose expertise the system would not function. Many complex issues relate to health care personnel and they are discussed in this chapter.

Finally, Part Five examines how our health care system can be evaluated, regulated, monitored, and assessed. Chapter 13 looks at the historical evolution and current status of health care policy in the United States, including the critical issue of the role of government in the system. Chapter 14 addresses assessing and ensuring the quality of the health care that is provided within the system, a key metric in overall system design. Chapter 15, a revised and updated performance of a very successful previous version, discusses the importance of the role of ethics in the operation of the health care system. Ethical issues are complex, but important as the evolution of clinical practice, cost pressures, managed care, and assessment of the uninsured and underinsured have challenged those who design, manage, and operate the health care system's components.

Chapter 16 serves to assess and, in some instances, critically analyze many of the issues discussed in the previous chapters of the book. This chapter also provides a platform for the reader to further think about the nation's health care system and the challenges that we all face.

The Committee on the Costs of Medical Care in the 1930s issued a report suggesting that cost pressures and demands for care would present a serious challenge to our nation. Perhaps they didn't realize how right they would be and how long this challenge would last. Indeed, there is no end in sight yet. We must continue to confront these issues and design a health care system that is efficient, but one that meets the expectations of all Americans.

Improving and rationalizing the nation's health care system remain great challenges for our nation and indeed for all nations worldwide in the future. Health care services interact with many aspects of our society, including economic, environmental, social, and psychological concerns. Health care is fundamental to a free nation and to the pursuit of life, liberty, and happiness.

Solving the problems of our nation's health care system, ensuring access to care, figuring out financial viability, and making fundamental decisions about what services will be available to all Americans and under what conditions comprise the ultimate health policy decision matrix that we must finally address and solve. Health care services utilize a huge amount of our nation's resources and we have the right to expect great things from those efforts. We can all agree that the nation's health care system is a critical aspect of our overall well-being, and it is in our best interests to have it run as smoothly as possible for the benefit of all our citizens.

This edition of the book continues the tradition of a multidisciplinary and empirical approach. The overall emphasis is on the practical application of sophisticated knowledge about the nation's health and health care system. Our objective is to explain the structure and function of the system so that all participants can better conduct their duties within the system itself.

We regret to report the death of one of our distinguished contributors, Dr. Ruth Roemer, of the University of California, Los Angeles. Her great contributions to the field continue to be incorporated in the book through the ethics chapter.

We also continue to acknowledge the contributions of our students and those practitioners who have also provided us with guidance and suggestions for continually improving this book. We appreciate our contributors and colleagues for all their contributions as well. And, we continue to have faith that this book, in some small measure, helps to contribute to a better health care system for all Americans.

Stephen J. Williams
Paul R. Torrens

ACKNOWLEDGMENTS

Data tables presented throughout this book for which specific sources are not contained within the table or figure were obtained from the National Center for Health Statistics, *Health, United States 2004, 2005,* or *2006,* Hyattsville, Maryland 2004, 2005, and 2006, respectively. U.S. government websites, particularly those at the National Center for Health Statistics, also provide current data for many tables.

The authors wish to thank Debbie Doan for her assistance in the preparation of this manuscript. Corinne D'Arco had the primary responsibility for assembling the online companion, including the Instructor's Manual and PowerPoint presentation, and her contributions are also greatly appreciated.

PART ONE

Overview of the Health Services System

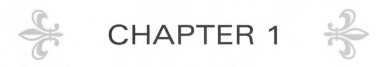

CHAPTER 1

Understanding Health Systems: The Organization of Health Care in the United States

Paul R. Torrens

CHAPTER TOPICS

🜚 Historical Evolution of Health Services in the United States

🜚 Involvement of the People in their Health and Health Care

🜚 The Structure and Organization of Health Care in the United States

🜚 A Management Strategy Perspective of the U.S. Health Care System

🜚 A Clinical Perspective on the U.S. Health Care System

🜚 The Basic Service Components of a Health Care System

🜚 Factors Affecting the Provision and Receipt of Basic Service Components in Health Care

LEARNING OBJECTIVES

Upon completing this chapter, the reader should be able to

1. Understand the major stages in the development of the nation's health care system.

2. Appreciate the many forces affecting the development of health services in the United States.

3. Understand the social, political, and economic forces affecting health care.

4. Follow the government's involvement in health services.

5. Describe a larger health care system in terms of the various subsystems that comprise it and serve different subsections of the population.

6. Explain how all parts of a health care system are related to each other and have a major impact on each other.

There are two ways to look at health systems, both of them useful and both somewhat flawed. On the one hand, individuals trying to understand health care in the United States can examine individual units (the "trees") and then try putting them together to get an idea of the system that contains them (the "forest"). On the other hand, individuals can look first at the broad collection of individual health services (the "forest") and then spend time examining the individual services (the "trees") that make up that system.

In this book, we take both approaches and try to explain to the reader that the informed health care professional must understand both health care systems and the individual services that comprise them—if one wants to have a fully workable understanding of health care. In this chapter, we focus our attention on the concepts of health systems and how to understand them in a broad sense; later chapters focus on the component parts of our system and why they are individually worthy of attention. This chapter also has two parts: One focuses on the historical development of health services in the United States, and the second focuses on analytical models for understanding those health services in the broad systemic context.

HISTORICAL EVOLUTION OF HEALTH SERVICES IN THE UNITED STATES

In trying to understand the present status of any country's health system, it is important to understand the evolution of that system over time. Each country's health services system is the result of that country's social, political, and economic history; it is also a reflection of that country's values, culture, and shared beliefs about itself. Each country generally gets the type of health services system most of its people want; each country generally gets the kind of health services system it deserves. Knowing how and why a health services system has developed

in a particular fashion can go a long way to explaining why a present system is organized and functions the way it does. Knowing how and why a country's health services system has developed may also give an observer significant clues as to how it is likely to develop and perform in the future.

Table 1.1 describes how the American health care system has evolved with regard to four important issues over four consecutive time periods: the major health problems upon which the existing system focused at the time (the "targets"); the resources that were available to the system to bring to bear on these "targets"; the vehicles of social organization that could bring the resources to bear on the disease "targets"; and the involvement of people in the health care system as it was evolving toward its present shape and form.

Four consecutive time periods are listed in Table 1.1 as significant eras or epochs in the development of health care in the United States: 1850–1900; 1900 to World War II; World War II to 1980; and 1980 to the present. Each of these time periods has been used because they signify important developmental eras for health care in the United States.

The year 1850 marked the development of the first hospitals in the United States and marked the beginning of formal organization of health care in this country. The year 1900 roughly coincides with the movement of health care in the United States into an era of scientific medicine. World War II and the years following it until 1980 was a period of major social and political development in health care here, while the years 1980 (approximately) to the present represented the change of health care from a primarily clinically driven system to one that was increasingly economically driven.

Primary Disease Targets for the Health Care System

With regard to the disease targets for the health care system from 1850 to 1900, the system focused its efforts mostly on public health problems (i.e., epidemics of acute infections, affecting large

Table 1.1. **Major Issues in the Development of Health Care in the United States, 1850 to Present**

Issues	1850–1900	1900 to World War II	World War II to 1980	1980 to Present
Predominant "targets" of the health system at the time	Epidemics of acute infections related to food, water, housing, and conditions of life	Acute events, trauma, or infections affecting individuals, not groups	Chronic diseases such as heart disease, cancer, and stroke	Chronic diseases, particularly emotional and behaviorally related conditions, as well as conditions related to workplace, environment, genetic inheritance, and terror threats
Technology to handle predominant health problems	Virtually none	Beginning and rapid growth of basic medical sciences and technology	Explosive growth of medical science; technology captures the health care system	Continued explosive growth and expansion of technology, with parallel rise in costs of health care
Social organization for health care	None; individuals left to their own resources or charity	Beginning societal and governmental efforts to care for those who could not care for themselves	Development of health insurance as the primary vehicle of social organization of health care in the United States	Increasing power of financial organizations to shape the health care system; increasing influence of governmental financial systems (e.g., Medicare and Medicaid)
Involvement of people in their health care	People actively involved in giving care to family; little factual knowledge	Beginning availability of medical knowledge to the general public	Increasing awareness of health care as a social and political issue by the public	Well-informed public, but increasing frustration with the complexity and expense of the system

numbers of people at the same time, caused by poor conditions of food, water, housing, and conditions of life in general). By 1900, many of these epidemic problems had begun to come under control and the system turned its attention toward disease targets of acute events, primarily acute infections and situations of trauma and disease that called for surgical intervention. The classical illness targets of this period could be said to have been acute appendicitis or bacterial lobar pneumonia.

By World War II, the discovery and the wide use of antibiotics and generally improved medical and surgical treatment of acute events allowed the health services system to turn its attention to chronic illnesses as its major target for the first time. The classic disease targets for these people were chronic illnesses such as cancer, heart disease, stroke, and renal failure—illnesses that had previously not been fully expressed because of the greater threat of acute infections and trauma. By 1980, the physical chronic illness targets were joined by chronic mental and emotional illnesses, including alcoholism and substance abuse, and increasingly the disease targets were understood to be closely related to such factors as stress, occupational and environmental concerns, genetic inheritance, and people's lifestyles.

It should be noted that while the disease targets of the health care system have evolved from acute to chronic illnesses, the system must still work with a form and a shape that appeared in the early 1900s to deal with acute illnesses. Although the targets have changed to long-term continuous chronic conditions, the basic structure of the delivery system continues to function as if its targets are short-term, discontinuous, and acute in nature.

Resources Available to the U.S. Health Care System

With regard to the resources available to affect the system's disease targets in the period 1850–1900, there really were very few. There was very little in the way of definite scientific knowledge, the professions were relatively primitive in training and practice, very little money was spent on health care, and hospitals were places of simple shelter—and little else. By 1900, the scientific revolution in medicine had begun in the United States, the professions began to have stronger training and standards, and hospitals began to be built in great numbers. The costs of care and the amount of money spent on health care were still very small, especially by today's standards.

Following World War II, all of this began to change at an explosive rate. The growth and expansion of the National Institutes of Health led to a parallel growth and expansion of the health care technology available to the health care system. The numbers of health care professionals, particularly physicians, also grew at a rate that hugely outpaced population growth. Hospitals increased in numbers, size, and technology, at least partially due to the federal Hill-Burton program that for the first time provided tax funds for the construction of health care facilities. Not

surprisingly, the explosive growth in technology, coupled with the rapid growth in the numbers of physicians and hospitals, led to rapidly rising health care costs and expenditures. Although previous periods could be described by shortages, early development of new resources, and gradual growth, the period after World War II could be described by explosive growth of everything. The challenges were no longer created by shortages, but by abundance.

In the period from 1980 to the present, the scientific and technological resources have continued to expand enormously, as have the costs and financial resources needed to sustain the system. The professions are no longer expanding in numbers and in the case of nursing at least, have actually been contracting in availability compared to need. Nursing has been experiencing a period of enhanced professionalism, credentialing, specialty training, and clinical responsibility. Very few new hospitals have been started, although the array of services provided by hospitals and the way they provide them has changed considerably. In this period, all other issues become somewhat insignificant next to the challenges of dealing with the continuing rapid growth of health care costs. Although the period immediately preceding this one was faced with the problems arising from abundance of technology and the great costs needed to sustain it, the present period is the first one to face the reality of containing growth—the first one to discuss the possible reality of reducing resources and constraining access to care.

Social Organization for Health Care in the United Sates

While the disease targets were changing over the years and while the resources of science, personnel, and finance for health care were expanding, how was the United States as a country developing its system of social organization of health care? What were the structures and broad organizations that emerged to provide a structure for planning and integrating services throughout the country?

In the period from 1850 to 1900, there was virtually no formal structure for health care in the United States and when individuals fell ill, they had to rely on the resources of their families and friends, as well as their churches or ethnic societies. Aside from some local efforts at quarantine and sanitary protection, government at all levels was almost entirely uninvolved in health care protection or provision of care. Health care was seen as a personal, family, and locality issue—not something with which state or national governments should necessarily become involved; indeed, it would be 1953 before there would be a cabinet-level Department of Health, Education, and Welfare in the federal government structure.

By 1900, some changes in thinking had begun and some significant developments did start to occur. In the early 1900s, various progressive candidates for national political office talked about national health insurance coverage for all, a position that was briefly supported by the American Medical Association. In a much more significant development, local governments began to build and maintain general hospitals, often the best in their communities and usually free of charge to all users. In a sense, this made local governments the guarantors of hospital care to the people of their immediate areas.

Although Franklin Roosevelt's New Deal was aggressively active in many areas of economic and social life in the United States, very little was done in health care except to provide some federal funds to individual states for programs for children and mothers.

In probably the most important development of all, local nonprofit hospitals and state medical societies began to develop nonprofit local hospitals and medical insurance plans under the generic titles of Blue Cross and Blue Shield.

During World War II, a freeze on wages and prices prevented any collective bargaining for increases in salary. Fringe benefits could be improved, however, and as a result there was considerable expansion of employer-provided health insurance. Indeed, employer-provided health insurance was virtually the only form of health insurance until the passage and implementation of Medicare in the mid-1960s, and it has remained the main source of health insurance for approximately two-thirds of the American people. While local governments continued to build and operate city and county hospitals for the poor in their areas, state and federal government involvement in either the financing or the direct provision of care was minimal.

This lack of involvement in health care financing by the state and federal governments changed abruptly and hugely with the passage and implementation of the Medicare and Medicaid insurance programs in the mid-1960s. Medicare provided health insurance to virtually everyone in the United States over the age of 65 through a single national insurance system managed by the federal government. Medicaid provided health insurance to virtually everyone in the United States receiving social welfare support through a joint federal-state system of fifty state-managed health insurance programs. In one sweeping set of political decisions, federal and state governments suddenly became the guarantors of care for the elderly and the poorest of the country's people.

The passage and subsequent implementation of Medicare and Medicaid strongly reenforced one aspect of social organization of health care in the United States and markedly changed another aspect. With regard to the way in which the United States wanted to approach the social organization and support of health care, the passage of Medicare and Medicaid reenforced the idea that health care financing (i.e., health insurance) was the vehicle for social organization and support; this country was not going to be directly involved in the delivery of care to individual citizens (with the exception of the Veterans Administration and Military and Prison Systems).

While reaffirming health insurance as the vehicle for social organization of health care in the United States, the passage of Medicare and Medicaid totally changed the role of government in the provision and management of this insurance. Previously, private employers and individual citizens were responsible for obtaining and paying for health insurance and government was not involved at all. After the passage of Medicare and Medicaid, the federal government and the individual state governments were active providers and managers of the health insurance programs themselves, making them equally responsible for the social organization and support of health care financing in the entire country.

In the period of 1980 to the present, the central role of the federal and state governments in the social direction and supervision of health care in the United States has only been further strengthened, largely as the result of the rapid expansion of funds now passing through these two programs. In 2005, Medicare contributed nearly one-quarter of all the funds spent on health care in the United States, while Medicaid contributed approximately another 20 percent. This expansion of total volume of federal government financing has been accompanied by an ever-increasing set of regulatory guidelines and rules for compliance governing the provision of those funds by government and the use of those funds by physicians and hospitals throughout the United States.

INVOLVEMENT OF THE PEOPLE IN THEIR HEALTH AND HEALTH CARE

While all the other changes were taking place with regard to health care in the United States, the involvement of people was also undergoing significant change. Indeed, all the previously mentioned changes in the health care system cannot be fully understood unless there is also consideration of how people understood the system and involved themselves in it.

Surprisingly, the period from 1850 to 1900 may have been the time when the people themselves were most involved in health care and how it worked. They did this, not because their efforts were elaborate or effective, but rather because they knew that they were all that their families and friends had to rely on. Although the public's general level of education was low and their understanding of health care even lower, their acceptance of personal responsibil-

ity for obtaining health services was perhaps the highest it has ever been. There simply was little public understanding of health and little confidence in the system itself, so the public had to count on its own resources—and it did to a degree understood only in terms of its necessity.

By 1900, the picture of health care had begun to change for the American public in many ways. The science of medicine and the abilities of physicians to actually treat and sometimes cure illness were advancing, and the public began to rely more and more on the health care system's effectiveness. Also, many new hospitals were being built across the country and there seemed to be a great expansion of the technology available in hospitals. Finally, the training of physicians was moving into universities, the standards for participation were becoming more stringent, and specialization of medicine was creating a new class of "experts." All these trends led the public to put more faith into the health care system itself. That the public itself was virtually excluded from participation in how care was provided or how the system was run was not obvious at this point.

World War II changed many American's understandings and perceptions of health care. First of all, the many thousands of people drafted into military service now had well-organized health services as part of their employment in the military, and they appreciated what it could do for them. Also, military personnel now received basic education about health and illness, as part of their basic training, and for the first time felt better informed about these matters. Finally, many members of the military were given the option of actually becoming part of the health care system by opting for training as hospital and medical corpsmen, something previously unthinkable for them and something that probably attracted many of them into health care after the war was over.

On the home front, the public's involvement in health care underwent some changes as well. For one thing, the public was provided with more direct education about health and illness and allowed for the first time to receive information about the functioning of their own bodies that had previously been denied to them. For another, members of the public were encouraged to volunteer their services in one way or another in the health care system, as substitutes for health workers who had been called away to military service. Finally, as mentioned previously, health insurance became a much more available benefit during the war years and individuals and their families began to gain experience in its use and operations.

After World War II, two significant factors moved the public's awareness and understanding of health care even further: One was the rapid growth and presence of television and the other was the political ferment about health insurance, particularly coverage for the elderly. With regard to television, the public now began to regularly receive increased information on topics of health and health care in their own homes, information ranging from the relatively informal to entire programs focusing on in-depth coverage of a single issue. With regard to increased political involvement around health care, the arrival of health care for the elderly as a political issue in the national campaigns of the early 1960s brought people forcibly face to face with the political aspects of care. This allowed them to play an important direct part in the decision to create a national health insurance plan for people over the age of 65.

Before 1980, there were also three other elements that brought people more directly in touch with their own health and the health care system that was supposed to serve their needs. One of these was President Lyndon Johnson' self-declared War on Poverty that had as one of its slogans, "Maximum feasible participation of the poor" in the social systems that were supposed to serve them. In the case of health care, this effort included the creation of a national network of community health centers and programs that continue to this day, bolstered by the additional slogan, "Health care as a right, not a privilege."

Also on the political side was an attempt at the creation of a national health planning system, an elaborate complex of local, state, and national attempts to rationally assess the country's needs for

service and to distribute new services and facilities in a way to meet those needs. It was an important first attempt in organized priority setting for health care and involved a broad spectrum of public participation in its efforts. Its inherent complexity, bureaucracy, and ineffectiveness led to its elimination when its enabling legislation expired.

Perhaps a more far-reaching development involving the participation of the public before 1980 was the explosion of the personal fitness, aerobics, cosmetic surgery, weight loss, and related programs for the general public. These programs encouraged people to take charge of their own fitness, their own weight and bodily appearance, and in many instances, their own mental health. This has empowered people to become more directly involved in aspects of their lives that are ultimately directly connected to their health. Previously, people had been passive participants in their own health care, but now they were encouraged to take their health into their own hands, on a long-term continuing basis.

In the period from 1980 to the present, this movement toward more involvement of people in their own health and health care has increased greatly, the result of several further important developments. The widespread presence of the Internet and various web-based sources of information about all aspects of health care has allowed individuals to inform and educate themselves about the complexities of health care in ways that were available only to health care professionals a few years ago. The public now has vastly more information readily available to them about their health and their health care system than they have ever had before, and it shows in their active participation in all aspects of the health services system. Wider access to information and other trends has also spurred interest in alternative and complementary health care, holistic services, and other services and products.

With the rising costs of health care and with the attempts to develop consumer-driven health care, individual men and women are being drawn into important decisions about their use of health care services and efforts to contain health care costs. Participation in new programs such as the Medicare drug benefit is calling for public understanding of complex questions of costs and benefits and is requiring public participation in decision making on a scale never before considered. Increasingly, people are understanding that programs of these two types are driven by political and policy decisions in which it is vital that the public express its preferences in ways never considered or allowed before.

An increasingly educated consumer is rapidly being expected to participate in complex decision processes related to health care services and clinical medicine. The shift of responsibility from insurers and clinicians to consumers has yet to be proven to yield better outcomes at more moderated costs. This issue remains one of the key challenges for the future as policy makers continue to seek effective approaches to intervening in the function of the health care system.

In summary, the health care system in the United States has evolved in many important ways over the last 150 years, an evolution that is important to document and understand if today's system is to be fully understood. Its disease targets have moved from acute illnesses to chronic illnesses (including chronic mental illnesses) although the system basically remains an acute care system in its actual design and function. Its resources have expanded vastly in terms of technology, people, and finances, from scarcity to abundance, but today its challenges are not about scarcity of resources, but rather about control of costs, optimal use of available resources, and avoidance of rationing and other constraints on access. In terms of social organization, the country has moved to the use of health insurance as its most important source of social support and direction, and the most important focus of that health insurance effort has been in the federal Medicare and Medicaid programs; in essence, the social direction of health care has moved, albeit unofficially, to the federal government as the guarantor of health care for the American people. Finally, those people are better informed, more directly involved, and more politically aware than ever before and want to

be more directly involved in all aspects of their health care system.

THE STRUCTURE AND ORGANIZATION OF HEALTH CARE IN THE UNITED STATES

In trying to understand and describe the American health care system, it should first be understood that different people with different backgrounds and different interests can look at the same object and come up with different interpretations. An economist looking at health care in the United States might likely come up with the system as an economic model. A sociologist, on the other hand, might focus more the interactions of people in the system and less on the economic implications. A management expert might look at the system and see issues of organizational efficiency and effectiveness. In other words, what one sees is often determined by how one looks; indeed, what one sees may actually be determined by what one wants to see.

In this section, three different ways of looking at the American health care system will be presented: (a) first, from a public policy perspective; (b) second, from a management strategy perspective; and (c) third, from a clinical/patient perspective. The three ways of looking will produce different results, each of which is valuable individually; all of them taken together provide an array of powerful analytical tools that can be used to analyze any health care system in the world.

A Public Policy Perspective on the U.S. Health Care System

One of the first things that strikes a foreign observer of the U.S. health care "system" is that there really is no formal and organized "system," at least in the sense of such systems in other countries of the world. There is no national health insurance covering everyone in the country as exists in Canada, and there is no national health service that provides care to everyone in the country as exists in England. If one tries to find any type of central coordinating body or group—either locally or nationally—there is simply no such entity in the United States.

Instead, what one finds in looking at the U.S. health care system from a policy perspective is a series of subsystems of financing and services, each of which is designed to serve the needs of one particular subsection of the American population or another. In other words, to understand the organization of health care in the United States one must first identify the individual subsystems of care and then examine them separately in terms of how they are financed and how health care is delivered to people served by that subsystem of care.

The individual subsystems that make up the larger U.S. health care system are as follows: (a) the "subsystem" that serves those people and their dependents who are regularly employed and have health insurance available to them from their employer; (b) the "subsystem" that serves those people who are not regularly employed or who are impoverished to some degree, and who (most important) do not receive sustained health insurance coverage from an employer; (c) the "subsystem" that serves military veterans who are eligible to use the Veterans Administration hospitals; (d) the "subsystem" that covers injuries and illnesses related to the workplace, generally known as the worker's compensation system; (e) the "subsystem" that serves active-duty military and their families. Many of these "subsystems" also have subsections within their particular "subsystem," making the situation even more complicated.

Employment-Related Subsystem

This first subsystem covers approximately two-thirds to three-quarters of the total American population and depends on insurance provided by an employer as a fringe benefit as its major source of financing. It involves two-thirds to three-quarters of the U.S. population but provides only one-third of the total financing of U.S. health care, since most of the

people covered are young and healthy enough to be employed and therefore at lower risk for illness.

The availability of health insurance coverage from employment (most commonly provided by private, nongovernmental insurance companies) allows the people in this subsystem to seek care from private health care providers, such as physicians in private practice or private, nongovernmental community hospitals. In other words, this subsystem is basically a nongovernmental collection of private employers providing private insurance that allows beneficiaries to seek care in the private sector. This is the most common system of financing and provision of care in the United States (at least in terms of numbers of people covered) and is often called *the* U.S. health care system, as if all others are somehow secondary to this one.

This all-private set of arrangements changes, however, when the employed beneficiary reaches age 65 and retires from formal employment. At that time, the primary source of coverage may change to the federal Medicare program, the national health insurance system for the older population and for some people with certain chronic and disabling conditions. At this time, the financing for the care comes primarily from a governmental insurance program that is supported by payroll taxes paid during one's working life; the funding, therefore, no longer comes from private sources but now comes from public sources. The provision of services, however, does not change and remains the same collection of physicians in private practice and nongovernmental community hospitals. While the system for people under the age of 65 is totally private and nongovernmental in nature, the system for people over the age of 65 becomes a mixture of public financing and private provision of care.

The System Serving the Poor and the Uninsured

For the members of the U.S. population who either do not have regular employment and have limited incomes, or who may be employed but do not receive health insurance as a fringe benefit from their employers, an entirely different subsystem serves their needs. With this population, their limited incomes and their lack of health insurance are the defining characteristics that determine how their subsystem is financed and how care is provided.

For most of the people in this subset of the population, the financing of their care comes either from their own use of whatever funds they have or from programs of care provided by local government hospitals that are operated with local and state governmental tax support. This group of the population is very dependent on their own limited financial resources and on the use of health services provided by safety-net providers who either do not charge any fees or charge fees that are only a fraction of the cost. These safety-net providers may be a loose collection of voluntary nonprofit hospitals, academic medical centers, and local government hospitals, with local government hospitals being the greatest source of care and support. In other words, both the financial support and the provision of care are public in nature, with local and state government funds being the prime source of that public support.

This subsystem of local government public financing and provision of care changes, however, if the individual person is poor enough to qualify for social welfare financial support. If the person is poor enough, they will qualify for the Medicaid program, a federal- and state-government-sponsored insurance program that gives them many of the advantages of private insurance. In particular, it allows them to seek and receive care in the private sector, if private physicians and hospitals will accept the Medicaid insurance as payment for care. For those people who are poor enough to qualify for Medicaid, the financing for their care moves from the local government tax base to the state and federal government one; it also allows them to move out of the local government hospitals into the private sector of health care provision. What starts as a totally public system of financing and provision of care now becomes a publicly financed system that uses private providers.

This system for the poor may also change significantly when the poor person becomes 65 years of age, because this may make him or her eligible for coverage by the federal Medicare program. Theoretically at least, the elderly poor person who has worked enough time in his or her past life to qualify for Medicare can now leave the local government hospital system and move to the private sector physicians and hospitals just like the person who was previously covered by health insurance from employment and then becomes 65. There are a number of reasons why this frequently doesn't happen as easily or completely as that, but the poor person with Medicare can possibly have a health system that is publicly funded by the federal Medicare program and is privately provided care by the community's private practitioners.

Veterans Administration Health System

For military veterans who are eligible for care in the Veterans Administration (VA) system by reason of length of service or service-connected disability, there is a totally separate subsystem of care made up of 155 (as of 2007) VA hospitals and more than 1,000 clinics and support services. This is a national system operated by the federal government and funded by federal taxes, and the physicians and other health care personnel working in these institutions are federal government employees. Entry into this system is governed by various VA eligibility criteria and is not available to dependents or other family members.

Interestingly, people who would otherwise be included in either of the previous two subsystems (the employer-insured system and the poor-uninsured one) can use the VA subsystem if they otherwise meet the criteria of eligibility. Although the VA system is entirely a publicly financed and publicly provided system of care, the people eligible to use it come from all walks of life, all ages, and all income levels. It is as close to a national health service as this country has ever seen but serves only a particular subset of the population. In recent years, the war in Iraq and Afghanistan has strained VA and military medicine resources.

The Worker's Compensation Health System

There is yet another subsystem of care that deals with people who have suffered injuries or illnesses related to their work situation. These people are covered by a separate set of insurance benefits that includes both financing for health care and direct financial support for living expenses. Employers are usually required by law to provide worker's compensation insurance, which can be obtained from either private or public insurance organizations. The employer and the employee share the cost of the insurance, which is usually selected and managed by the employer. The insurance is provided under a governmental regulatory mandate but financed by private funds for the most part, an unusual mixture of public mandate and private funding.

The services provided under worker's compensation insurance can only be used to cover illness or injury directly related to the work situation and only as long as the effects of the job-related illness or injury are evident; the insurance does not generally assume responsibility for other health or illness conditions that might exist outside the work situation. The services are often provided by a specific subset of private physicians and hospitals that specialize in the problems of workers and their injuries.

Active-duty Military and Their Families

Members of the military services on active duty receive their care within the military system that is financed by the military and provided by other members of the military and by civilians in hospitals and clinics operated by the military. It is a totally integrated system of health care operated for its members only and integrated completely into the other activities of the military.

Dependents of active-duty military personnel are covered by private insurance provided to them by the military. This private insurance allows them to use private sources of medical care and hospitalization for the most part, although dependents are often allowed to use specific services provided by military physicians and personnel at military out-patient facilities, if space is available. In this way, dependents often obtain services in two very different ways: one provided directly by the military itself in some circumstances and the other provided by physicians and hospitals in the private sector, financed by private health insurance.

Why Multiple Systems?

Why is it important to understand that there is a myriad of subsystems in what has previously been thought to be a single entity? From a policy analyst's point of view, there are a number of compelling reasons to think through carefully the various implications of this mixed bag of services and financing.

First of all, understanding the complex structure of the many health care subsystems in the United States goes a long way to explaining why it is often so hard to get anything done or to create change; a system this complicated does not move quickly or easily—or sometimes, at all. Second, understanding that the system is made up of multiple separate and unconnected collections of financing and provision of care reveals how difficult it is to carry out any reasonable system-wide planning for the entire system and the entire population; we are forced to microplan because there is no one place or organization that has responsibility for the entire collection of services and finances. Third, the existence of these multiple separate and non-integrated subsystems increases the administrative and managerial cost for the entire system, driving up the costs of care overall for everyone. At a time when efficient use of all resources—financial and otherwise—becomes increasingly important, this complex and complicated maze of organizations and structures often makes reasonable efficiency impossible.

A MANAGEMENT STRATEGY PERSPECTIVE OF THE U.S. HEALTH CARE SYSTEM

For a manager within the U.S. health care system, what type of organizational framework analysis will help him or her understand how the system works and what managers must do to effectively lead their organizations? The public policy model is instructive in general, but a more dynamic management-oriented model might better serve the manager's pragmatic day-to-day needs.

The interests and the interactions among the major participants in the health care system are continuously changing. There is a constantly shifting balance of power between and among the groups involved in the system; the U.S. health care system is constantly changing, reshaping interactions, and in flux.

The six major participants are (1) patients/customers; (2) providers of health services; (3) suppliers of services and goods, including pharmaceuticals; (4) insurance intermediaries, including Medicare and Medicaid; (5) primary sources of funds to pay for health care insurance, including employers, Medicare, and Medicaid; and (6) government (as regulator, planner, financier for research and training, etc.).

For many years, the dynamic strategy model of health care worked in a very simple fashion and the roles of the various players *vis-à-vis* one another were very straightforward and well understood by all the various participants in the health care system. In the 1980s, that dynamic was replaced by a newer, more market-dominated one—one that reversed much of the way things had been done before.

Before 1980, the health system's activities were initiated by an insured person deciding that he or she was sick and needed care. That person usually had a wide-open choice of providers—all licensed physicians and hospitals—and could proceed directly to primary care physicians and specialists alike. They could also go as often as they chose, confident that their health insurance policies would pay for much of the cost of the visits. There were no incentives to the patients to use certain providers and not others, and absolutely no incentives to constrain their visits or use of services.

For their part, providers knew that all the individual visits and services they provided and all the individual days in the hospital would be reimbursed on a fee-for-service basis, without question or restraint. In this way, there were no real incentives for physicians or hospitals to constrain their provision of care to their patients, and there were, perhaps, incentives to actually do more rather than less.

When the physicians and hospitals had provided their services, they sent the bills on to the insurance plans which promptly paid them without question. The plans then determined how much a particular group of employees had used in the way of services and how much those services cost in total. The next year's premiums were then increased to cover the increased costs of increased services and no incentives were placed on the insurance plan to constrain or contain health care costs in any effective way.

Unfortunately, when next year's health insurance premium increases became apparent, the employers felt trapped and had no place to go. They had no way to pass on the costs to someone else and so they paid the premiums and watched them increase every year. The dynamics of power were very clear and the employers had no choice.

This pre-1980 dynamic could be described as "patient initiated," since the patient was the one who put the system into action. It could also be called "provider controlled," since the physicians and hospitals controlled the way in which services were offered and paid for. In economic terms, it could be described as a "sellers'" market, since the sellers really controlled the shape and structure of the transaction. From a power point of view, the power in this dynamic seemed to be clearly on the side of the providers and to a certain extent, patients.

From the point of view of the patients, the providers, and the insurance companies, this dynamic seemed to work very well and they were happy to have it continue in just the manner that it had always followed. Unfortunately, the dynamics of power did not suit the employers who were ultimately paying the bill, and around 1980 they started to turn the picture around. By the time they had finished, they had turned it around almost completely in terms of system power and control.

Beginning in the 1980s, employers began demanding that the insurance companies develop new products to better constrain the rapidly rising costs of health care to employers. Although there had been a somewhat limited use of health maintenance organizations (HMOs) before 1980 and other types of prepaid health care dating back to the early twentieth century, employers began to move strongly to use them and other aspects of what was now being called "managed care" in the policies being offered employees. Some of these managed care principles included paying providers on a capitated rather than fee-for-service basis and providing incentives to use fewer services rather than more. Other aspects of managed care included the use of bulk purchasing power by the insurance companies to obtain greater discounts in prices from hospitals and other providers. Finally, the employers allowed insurance plans to reduce the numbers of providers who could serve the plans' beneficiaries, in a way forcing the providers to accept lower reimbursement from the plans in return for being included on "preferred provider" lists.

Before 1980, the employers had passively accepted the way the system was organized and worked, and they accepted the fact that they were relatively powerless to change things in any significant way. After 1980, employers (and the insurance plans that followed their clients' directions) accepted the fact that they had to be more aggressive in changing the incentives and the behaviors of both providers and patients. Rather than being passive premium payers at the end of a long process that denied them a role, they now proceeded to turn the dynamics of power around to put themselves in a more active role.

After 1980, the system was still a "patient-initiated" one, but patients no longer had wide-open access to whichever generalists and specialists they wanted; physicians and hospitals were now given incentives to control utilization and they did so. What had been a provider-controlled health system before 1980 now became a payor-controlled system after 1980. What had been a sellers' market before 1980, now became a buyers' market after 1980. Although power to shape and control the dynamics of the system had rested with patients and providers before 1980, after 1980 it shifted to the insurance plans and the employers who were the main source of funds to purchase insurance.

It is interesting to note that government in its regulatory and directing roles played a comparatively minor role in most of these changes. The federal government, as the sponsor of Medicare and Medicaid (i.e., insurance programs and a source of funds to purchase care), played an important role, but more like the one that other large purchasers of health insurance were playing, and not the more typical governmental controlling and directing role. These dynamic changes were primarily initiated by the private sector—particularly by private employers—not by government in any sort of authority role.

In more recent years, the balance of power between and among patients, providers, and insurance plans and the purchases of health insurance has become more balanced and represents more of a continuous bargaining relationship rather than one in which one side tells the other what to do. It is doubtful that the situation among all the players will ever again be one where any one participant can dictate to all the others how things should be.

In summary, the second analytical perspective on the health care system in the United States is a management strategy one. In this framework, there is a continuous interaction and relationship between and among the major participants, with the balance of power continually shifting back and forth among them. In this model, the relative position of each of the players changes over time, but the entire system must find some equilibrium among its parts—or the system will fail. In this model, the individual managers in each of the participating sectors of the system must understand their relative strengths and weaknesses in relation to the other players, and they must manage their interactions accordingly to preserve the broader system of which they are all a part.

A CLINICAL PERSPECTIVE ON THE U.S. HEALTH CARE SYSTEM

The third perspective for analyzing health care in the United States is that of the patient/consumer who is seeking services of various types from the system. In this perspective, the basic service components of a health care system can be reviewed to determine how a particular patient or group of patients obtain that type of care and how satisfied they are with the services provided. It can also include a review of the factors that affect the way in which those services are provided and received. The combination of the two approaches—how patients receive health services of certain kinds and the factors that influence the delivery and receipt of that care—can provide a powerful analytical tool for understanding the health care system.

THE BASIC SERVICE COMPONENTS OF A HEALTH CARE SYSTEM

The basic service components of a complete health care system are listed in Table 1.2 and range from care for simple uncomplicated events that require relatively low levels of technology, personnel, and

Table 1.2. Basic Service Components of a Health Care System

- Health promotion and disease prevention services
- Emergency medical services (including transportation)
- Ambulatory care for simple/limited conditions
- Ambulatory care for complex/continuing conditions
- Inpatient care for single/limited inpatient conditions
- Inpatient care for complex/multiple inpatient conditions
- Long-term care (either in-home or institutional services)
- Services for social/psychological conditions (both inpatient and ambulatory)
- Rehabilitation services (both inpatient and ambulatory)
- Dental services
- Pharmaceutical services

facilities, to care for complex events that require high and intense levels of specialized personnel, hospitals, and equipment. By reviewing the pattern of obtaining care for each of these services, an overall pattern of organization for all services can be identified and the boundaries of a system—formal or informal—understood.

For example, one could examine one person's pattern of obtaining care and find that most preventive services, simple ambulatory care, and complex ambulatory care are obtained from a long-time family physician in private practice in the person's neighborhood; it may also be found that this physician has a strong relationship with a local community hospital and its specialists, as well as with several mental health practitioners who have offices nearby. Dental care may be obtained from local dental practitioners, and there may be a convenient local pharmacy nearby. Nursing home care may come from facilities located nearby with which the family physician has some connection or relationship. The pattern that emerges is one of stability and continuity within the local community, with access and availability not a major difficulty.

By contrast, examining the pattern of another person may reveal that there is no single source of continuing care and coordination, significant dependence on the public hospital emergency room, and limited access to specialists through the clinics of that same public hospital. Dentists may not be available at all (at least to this person) and pharmaceuticals are available only in limited fashion because of a lack of funds or health insurance to pay for them. Long-term care may not be available at all to this person and he or she may be totally dependent on family members for care if chronic illness services are needed. The pattern that emerges here is one of instability and uncertainty in obtaining care, with great dependence on already-crowded public hospitals and clinics.

A third person's pattern of care may involve the use of private family practitioners for simple and routine care, but also the use of the Veterans Administration hospital clinics for specialist services and inpatient care; the VA may also be the source of long-term care when it is needed. This person may obtain dental services from a private practitioner but may need to obtain prescriptions from the VA pharmacy. The pattern here may be one of some basic stability for minor problems combined with a less certain or well-coordinated use of specialist services at a more distant facility.

These three patterns might be contrasted by the pattern of care of someone who is obtaining care through an integrated delivery system such as the Kaiser Permanente system in California. In this system, the system itself assumes responsibility for providing and coordinating care within its own system, using its own physicians and hospitals. With this pattern, the individual patient does not have to figure out where to go for each service and how to make contact, since the system itself provides that connection. The individual patient may not have a choice in terms of one individual physician specialist or another, but there is assurance that some specialist of appropriate training and experience will certainly be available. The pattern here has significant certainty and continuity, even if it has less choice than some of the other patterns.

By using this system of pattern analysis, the observer quickly realizes that most people are forced to put together an informal system of their own, unless they belong to an intentionally organized and integrated system like Kaiser Permanente or

the military, whether they have significant financial and health insurance resources or not.

The person who is employed and has employer-provided health insurance may appear to have more resources than a poor, unemployed, or uninsured person, but each of them has to put together a network of services for themselves, providing the connection, coordination, and communication themselves. The only difference is that the employed/insured person has a much wider range of choices, while the poorer person is forced to use only those limited resources that may be available to him or her. For most people, except those in an intentionally organized and coordinated system, health care in the United States is usually a disconnected, uncoordinated, poorly communicating cottage industry, sorely in need of organizational reform.

FACTORS AFFECTING THE PROVISION AND RECEIPT OF BASIC SERVICE COMPONENTS IN HEALTH CARE

For each of the individual basic service components, there is a set of factors that determines how well those services will be provided and utilized. Each basic service component, in each individual setting, will be affected by factors of finance, culture, geography, and other influences that will determine the availability and effectiveness of those services. The second part of the clinical pattern analysis involves identifying the most important factors that affect each of the basic services for a particular person or family. A short list of possible factors affecting the provision and utilization of health services is given in Table 1.3, although it should be pointed out that the list is by no means complete or all-inclusive.

For example, in analyzing one person's pattern for obtaining specialist medical services, the

Table 1.3. Illustrative Factors Affecting Utilization

Consumer
- Signs and symptoms
- Beliefs
- Insurance coverage
- Income and wealth
- Information access and knowledge

Provider
- Access mechanisms
- Provider incentives
- Operational systems (i.e., appointment scheduling)
- Technology and medical information
- Referral arrangements

System
- Contractual arrangements
- Payment mechanisms
- Legal considerations
- Networks and providers

deciding factors influencing the use of these services may be adequate insurance coverage, appropriate referral mechanisms, and a personal trust in medical science. For that same person, however, when the services of a psychiatric specialist may be needed for depression, the key factor influencing use of those services might well be a cultural skepticism about psychiatry, a belief that psychiatrists should be used only for serious psychoses, and a personal unwillingness to admit that the individual actually needs help. Understanding the factors affecting each of the various basic service components may change or influence the pattern of care in significant (and different) ways.

In another situation, a particular person may not have good access to specialist medical care because of a lack of health insurance and a dependence on a local government public hospital with very long waits and delays in obtaining an appointment, let alone care. The situation may also be compounded by the geographic location of that public hospital at some distance from the patient's home and the complicated public transportation system needed to get from home to the clinic. A final factor affecting the use of specialist medical services may be a cultural belief or disbelief that may either enhance or detract from the personal value placed on that service component by the patient.

In a completely different situation, for a person in a developing country the factors affecting the provision of specialist care may be a lack of specialist with particular training and a lack of technology to support the provision of that type of care. An individual patient may wish to use that type of service and may be willing to pay for it, but there may simply be no capacity at all to provide it. The individual may have to travel away from his or her own country to another place, if he or she wishes to obtain those services from an appropriate specialist. A service cannot be provided if there aren't the appropriate personnel or technology to support that service.

Summing up this portion of the chapter, a third way in which to better understand health care systems is to identify how various people obtain individual services and how they organize their individual services into a system of some kind, formal or informal. Add to this an analysis of the various factors that affect the provision or utilization of each service and a powerful analytical tool emerges, one that can provide valuable insights into the workings of any collection of health services.

SUMMARY

It is essential that each health care professional take a systems approach to understanding health care and develop for themselves a working model of the entire system before they spend time trying to understand one individual part of the system. It is also important that health care professionals understand that all systems have histories and patterns of development that not only tell where they came from but also where they are going. Finally, it is important that health care professionals develop analytical models of health care systems, so that they are better equipped to create change and improvement in those systems over the years. Promoting that goal is an intrinsic objective of this book.

REVIEW QUESTIONS

1. Describe the major trends in the evolution of health care services in the United States over the past 100 years.
2. How has the role of government changed in the U.S. health care system, and what future trends in government involvement do you anticipate?
3. Describe the differences in health care systems for the middle class, the poor, and the military.
4. How is health affected by behaviors, economics, and social structure?
5. Describe your view of the role of health care services in the nation's success and survival as a coherent democracy.

REFERENCES & ADDITIONAL READINGS

Andersen, R., Rich, T. H., & Kominski, G. F. (2001). *Changing the U.S. health care system: Key issues in health services, policy, and management.* San Francisco: Jossey-Bass.

Committee on Quality of Health Care in America, Institute of Medicine. (2001). *Crossing the quality chasm: A new health system for the 21st century.* Washington, DC: National Academies Press.

Havlicek, P. L. (1999). *Medical groups in the U.S., Vital and Health Statistics, 13*(159). Chicago: American Medical Association.

Herzlinger, R. E. (1997). *Market driven health care.* Reading, MA: Addison-Wesley.

Herzlinger, R. E. (2004). *Consumer-driven health care: Implications for providers, players, and policymakers.* San Francisco: Jossey-Bass.

Keagy, B. A., & Thomas, M. S. (Eds.). (2004). *Essentials of physician practice management.* San Francisco: John Wiley.

Lee, P. R., Estes, C. L., & Rodriguez, F. M. (Eds.). (2003). *The nation's health,* 7th ed., Sudbury, MA: Jones & Bartlett.

Rorem, R. (1931). *Private group clinics.* Chicago: University of Chicago Press.

Starr, P. (1982). *The social transformation of American medicine.* New York: Basic Books.

Schappert, S. M., & Burt, C. W. (2006). Ambulatory care visits to physician offices, hospital outpatient departments, and emergency departments: United States, 2001–2002.

CHAPTER 2

Technology in the U.S. Health Care System*

Paul R. Torrens

CHAPTER TOPICS

- Types and Classifications of Health Care Technologies
- The Development, Diffusion, and Utilization of Health Care Technology
- Scientific Background and Development of the Idea for a Product
- Product Development and Distribution
- Diffusion, Adoption, and Utilization of New Products and Technology
- Specific Methods for Evaluating Medical Technologies
- Differential Impacts of Technology on Health Care

LEARNING OBJECTIVES

Upon completing this chapter, the reader should be able to

1. Appreciate the importance of technology in health care.
2. Classify health care technologies.
3. Understand product development and diffusion.
4. Assess the impact of technology on various health care parties.
5. Understand how technology assessment is conducted.

*Many of the ideas expressed in this chapter have been sharpened by reference to an excellent text, *Technology in American Health Care: Policy Directions for Effective Evaluation and Management,* edited by Alan Cohen and Ruth Hanft, 2004, Ann Arbor: University of Michigan Press.

In an earlier edition of this textbook, the author of a chapter on technology in American health care summarized the important issues very well.

> Technology is credited with the benefits of American medicine as well as what ails it. It is the hope for a long, productive life for millions of people, a primary reason for the spiraling costs of care, and the source of many social and ethical dilemmas such as rationing of health care and the harvesting of human organs for transplants. It has even given rise to new definitions of death. At different times and places and by different policy makers and analysts, it has been accused of not being accessible to all members of the population, or by contrast, being overused, misused, and misunderstood by others. It has been said to have diffused too rapidly without adequate assessment or regulation, yet today some express a concern that innovation is being stifled, capital is unavailable for technology acquisition, and reimbursement is inadequate. (Luce, 1993)

As with the earlier edition of this text, this chapter is intended to shed light on many of these issues. It will attempt to explain how medical technology fits into the American health care system, how it impacts the various stakeholders in that system, and how the public policy issues affect these impacts. By the end of this chapter, it is hoped that the reader of this chapter will understand that "medical technology" is a broad and general term for a vast collection of issues, pressures, forces, and challenges, each and all of which must be understood separately as well as collectively if this remarkable expression of American science and industry is to have maximal good effect on health care as a whole.

The contents of this chapter are divided into several parts. In the first, the types, definitions, and classifications of technology are discussed, highlighting the great difficulties in developing standard descriptions that are agreed upon by all. Next, the general pattern of development, diffusion, and adoption of medical technologies is discussed, pointing out the similarities and the differences between and among the various types of technologies; included in this section is a discussion of the reasons various types of technologies appear and flourish while others do not. Third, the methods for evaluating medical technologies are described, pointing out that different assessment methods are appropriate for use in different settings, for different purposes, or for different types of technologies. Finally, the differential impacts of technology on the economics of health care, the practice of clinical medicine, the management of health care organizations, and the personal behavior of individual people are discussed.

TYPES AND CLASSIFICATIONS OF HEALTH CARE TECHNOLOGIES

In numerous current discussions about health care, particularly those focused on the rising costs of care, reference is often made to the influence of "technology," as if it were a single unitary force or presence that could be categorized and discussed as a whole. In fact, health care technology is made up of a myriad of subgroups, each with its own definition and existence, and each exerting its influence on health care in quite different ways and to quite different degrees. The former Congressional Office of Technology Assessment described health care technology as combining all the drugs, devices, and medical and surgical procedures used in patient care, and the organizational and supportive system with which such care was provided (Cohen & Hanft, 2004). While this is a useful generalization, it does not really help much in specific analysis and understanding of the individual subsegments.

Following this broad definition, health technologies can be seen to range from the simplest new variation on a previously standard medication to the development of an entirely new medication or device. The first is quite limited and represents a small improvement on a previously existing drug, while the second represents an entirely new breakthrough in the understanding and treatment of a particular disease process, utilizing scientific understanding that was not fully expressed before. Because they are so different, it is therefore important to classify and differentiate medical technology into its various subgroups so that each one can be understood in a more specific and detailed way.

Classification of Health Care Technology by Industrial Group

With regards to a typology of health care technology, one easy approach is to categorize the field by recognizing the industrial groups that develop the individual products. This has the advantage of providing a generally useful view of the major players in the field of medical technology and also of pointing out the difference between and among those players, how they are affected by quite different regulatory forces, and how they create different economic impacts. Using this framework, medical technology can be subdivided into pharmaceuticals, medical devices, medical equipment, medical procedures and processes, and information technology. Pharmaceuticals can be further subdivided into biological pharmaceuticals (sometimes labeled as "biopharma" or even "biotechnology") and chemical pharmaceuticals. The medical equipment segment can be divided into diagnostic and nondiagnostic technologies, while the diagnostic technologies can be even further subdivided into large-scale imaging devices such as MRIs and smaller-scale devices such as lab equipment and the like. The medical information sector can be subdivided into communication technologies on the one hand and those technologies more related to data storage, retrieval, and management on the other. Table 2.1 lists these different industrial groupings.

Table 2.1. Classification of Health Care Technology by Industrial Group

Pharmaceuticals
- Biological pharmaceuticals
- Chemical pharmaceuticals

Medical Devices

Medical Equipment
- Nondiagnostic equipment
- Diagnostic equipment
  - Large-scale imaging equipment
  - Small-scale imaging and diagnostic equipment

Medical Processes and Procedures

Health Care Information Technology
- Communication technologies
- Data storage, retrieval, and management technologies

Using this format, the two largest technology areas are pharmaceuticals and information technologies, both of which are heavily represented by large publicly traded corporations with significant financial assets; examples of these might be Merck and Pfizer in the pharmaceutical arena and IBM and General Electric in the information technologies area. The strategies of these companies are usually driven by a desire to satisfy the investment community's needs for stability and predictability, continuing short-term profitability, and financial risk aversion. Because of their generally strong financial positions, they are usually able to invest heavily in applied research and new product development, either by means of their own internal capacities or by the acquisition of smaller companies. Their industries are usually very competitive, which requires them to be quite heavily involved in major marketing efforts of their products in order to maintain their market position (Goldsmith, 2005; Northrop, 2005).

The biopharmaceutical subsection of the pharmaceutical industry, however, has characteristics that may be quite different from those of the larger and more general pharmaceutical industry in many of its aspects (Pfeffer, 2005). Biopharmaceutical companies tend to be much smaller, usually limited to a few very specialized products (perhaps even just one), and heavily invested as much in research and product development as they are in marketing. Their total financial assets tend to be much smaller than those of the larger general pharmaceutical companies with much of their financial support coming from venture capital sources rather than the more traditional equity community; more likely, they tend to be privately held corporations rather than the larger publicly traded ones more commonly associated with general pharmaceutical firms. If these companies are successful (or sometimes, just promising), they are often acquired by larger companies, often the large general multiproduct pharmaceutical companies mentioned earlier. The management strategies of the biopharmaceutical companies often focus on the early development of a product, obtaining regulatory approval, and demonstrating the product's effectiveness to a small group of specialized clinical leaders; the longer-term strategy may also include positioning these smaller companies for eventual acquisition by one of the larger general pharmaceutical giants.

In the information technologies subset, the two major groupings are those companies that focus on new methods of communication and those companies that focus more on the accumulation, storage, and use of data and information (as opposed to its transmission). The companies in this entire subset are usually large, multiproduct organizations that already have a wide range of technological products and capacities. Health care may be only a more recent area of expansion for them, but in all cases health care is generally seen as an important expanding market. In the past, many of these companies did not have great experience or knowledge about the intricacies of health care and spent more time getting health care to adapt to their existing products rather than the other way around. As these companies learn more about the unique characteristics of health care, this has changed a great

deal, with the new emphasis on the development of entirely new products that are tailored to the needs of this field.

Although these two major segments of the medical technology world—pharmaceuticals and information—may have significant similarities with regard to public financing, there are also major differences between them in terms of their operations. For one, all the products of the pharmaceutical sector must be approved by regulatory agencies for safety and efficacy, as well as by insurance carriers for payment as a covered benefit; the information systems segments do not have any requirement to satisfy regulators before their products can be sold. The costs of the pharmaceutical industry's products are tabulated separately and presented publicly in the usual national accountings and reporting of health care costs, while the costs of utilizing the products of the information industry are not so visible, are submerged in the total operating costs of hospitals and other organizations, and are not generally topics of public policy or public debate. Finally, the ultimate purchaser or user of pharmaceutical products will generally be a clinically or scientifically trained person, while the decision maker for information products will generally be a manager, a financial expert, or a board of directors.

In the medical device segment of the health care technology industry, the participating companies and organizations are quite different from both the pharmaceutical industry and the information industry (Kruger, 2005). These companies typically make devices to be used by clinicians in their direct contacts with patients and include such items as coronary artery stents, insulin pumps, or artificial hip and knee prostheses. These companies are often quite small and develop around a single product—often a product developed by a single creative physician-scientist. Their regulatory oversight involves the Food and Drug Administration in much the same way that pharmaceuticals do, but that oversight seems to be less rigorous, time-consuming, and dependent upon randomized clinical trials than drug development and regulation calls for.

As with the biopharmaceutical industry, the medical device industry must spend considerable time in clinical research, product development, and communication with a specialized set of medical leaders and technical experts. Once the product is developed and has gained some general acceptance, the original company may find itself the target of acquisition by larger companies, sometimes in the medical device field, but sometimes in the broader pharmaceutical field, depending on the product. The usual chart of national financial accounts does not specifically identify medical devices for separate tabulation, and the costs of medical devices are often hidden in the broader financial accounts of hospitals, clinics, and many physician practitioners. While the products of the pharmaceutical and information segments of the technology industry may have some significant effect on an individual physician's clinical options, the successful products of the medical device industry, by contrast, can have a major impact on the way an entire clinical field may be organized. For example, the arrival of a new drug for the treatment of congestive heart failure may add a new pharmaceutical treatment option to a physician's medication list, but the development of an implantable heart assistance device may completely change the way the entire field approaches the disease process itself.

The medical equipment segment of the larger health technology field is different again from either the pharmaceutical, the medical device, or the information segments. This industrial segment provides equipment and technical supplies for the health care system, and this equipment may range from relatively small, uncomplicated, and low-cost (in terms of unit price) items (such as intravenous fluid needles, tubing, and monitoring devices), all the way to relatively large, very complex, and extremely expensive equipment such as MRI or PET imaging systems. Their products may be used directly by patients themselves, by clinicians in their direct care of patients, and by nonclinicians in the performance of various support functions. In a general way, the medical equipment segment of

health technology can also be divided into diagnostic and nondiagnostic supplies, with the diagnostic being much more directly connected with clinical judgments and decisions, while the nondiagnostic is focused more on supportive functions and processes.

Most of these medical equipment companies are larger publicly traded, multiproduct organizations and very often may actually be subsidiaries of some of the larger pharmaceutical organizations, depending on the particular supply or equipment item. This arrangement allows the larger companies to market a wider range of pharmaceutical and nonpharmaceutical products to the large hospital-sponsored purchasing cooperatives that have developed in recent years. Like the medical device and information segments of health care technology, the total costs of medical equipment and supplies are difficult to measure accurately, since these costs are often not singled out for special notice in the broader budgets of hospitals, clinical organizations, and physicians' offices. They are, however, generally assumed to be quite large.

The final "industrial" segment of health care technology is actually not industrial or commercially sponsored at all; it is almost entirely clinical in nature and does not ordinarily have an organizational base. This segment of health care technology is related to new clinical procedures and processes, which are not necessarily new products that can easily be identified and labeled as such. New surgical procedures; new combinations of already-existing medications and therapies; and new uses of old products, instruments, and equipment would be included here. New approaches to spine surgery by orthopedic surgeons might also be included, as might new approaches by neurologists entering the cerebral blood vessels to remove blood clots that are blocking blood supply to the brain.

Often these new procedures (such as laparoscopic surgery for gall bladder disease) might simply use existing equipment, and in other cases the new procedures may utilize new medical devices to implement a new procedure (such as the new clot-snagging equipment used in the cerebral blood vessels of stroke patients). Very often, these innovative procedures are not initially well supported by randomized clinical trials or other appropriate research methods, sometimes resulting in later findings of no obvious clinical benefit (Grady, 2006). The use of autologous bone marrow transplants as an adjuvant therapy in the treatment of breast cancer is an example of a new procedure or process initially greeted with great enthusiasm, only to be discarded later as more rigorous clinical testing showed it to have limited value (Mello & Brennan, 2001; Rettig et al., 2007).

Aside from the obvious industrial group method of segmenting health care technology, a variety of other classification systems have been suggested, as well summarized by Cohen and Hanft (2004). Many of these attempts at classification took place in the 1970s when there was a significant surge of interest in the role of technology in health care policy, those efforts led by the Congressional Office of Technology Assessment on the one hand, and the Institute of Medicine of the National Academy of Sciences on the other (Table 2.2).

The Congressional Office of Technology Assessment used a two-dimensional classification of medical technology based on a combination of the physical nature of the technology and the medical purpose to which it was put (U.S. Congress, 1976). The Institute of Medicine's classification system was also two-dimensional, subdividing medical technologies by their functions in one group, and the stage in the medical care process in which it was used in the other. A similar early framework developed by Rosenthal suggested classifying technologies by the particular medical objectives of that technology (Rosenthal, 1979).

More informal technologies appeared from time to time and were somewhat helpful in dealing with the issues presented by health care technology. Lewis Thomas, a distinguished health care scholar suggested the use of the terms "halfway technologies" and "high technologies," meaning those that having a partial impact on illnesses or disease and those that having a major, substantive, and possibly

Table 2.2. Classification Schemes/Typologies for Medical Technology

Source	Major Dimension	Category/Class
OTA, 1976	Physical nature	Technique Drug Equipment Procedure
	Medical purpose	Diagnostic Preventive Therapeutic Rehabilitative Organizational Supportive
Committee on Technology and Health Care, National Academy of Sciences, 1979	Function	Clinical Ancillary Coordinative
	Stage in the medical care process	Preventive Diagnostic Therapeutic Rehabilitative
Rosenthal, 1979	Medical objectives	Diagnostic Survival Illness management Cure Prevention System management

SOURCE: From *Technology in American Health Care: Policy Directions for Effective Evaluation and Management,* by A. B. Cohen and R. S. Hanft, 2004, Ann Arbor: University of Michigan Press.

transforming impact on the conditions under treatment (Thomas, 1977).

Other yet more informal methods of classifying health care technologies have included the use of the terms "big ticket" and "little ticket" technologies, roughly describing the investment needed to purchase them. Another approach suggested the use of the terms "high," "medium," and "low" technologies, depending on the resources necessary not only to purchase them but also to utilize them in practice. Another typology suggested dividing medical technologies into "substitutive" and "additive" categories, with substitutive technologies those that simply replaced existing technologies to one degree or another and the additive technologies being those bringing something entirely new to the diagnostic or treatment situation. Finally, there have frequently been suggestions that an informal classification system be developed based on the impact a technology has on its particular target or objective, utilizing the terms "high," "medium," and "low" impact. Cohen and Hanft (2004) summarize the situation very well when they say, "Not surprisingly, there is a lack of consensus regarding the best way to classify technology and none of these systems has been adopted universally."

Why is it important to understand that "medical technology" is actually a collection of very specific subgroupings, each of which is quite different and distinct from the others?

The first and most obvious answer is an awareness of the necessity to separate the various technologies one from the other, so that the unique dynamics and impacts of each subsection can be understood in a more specific and detailed way. Perhaps more important and more urgent is that a greater knowledge of the different types of technologies can lead to more focused, effective, and relevant solutions to the problems and challenges presented by some, but not all, medical technologies in general. More specifically, as the efforts to contain health care costs increase in intensity and scope, it will be important to have more detailed knowledge of the various individual types of medical technologies and their characteristics, so that more focused and effective cost-containment strategies can be developed for those technologies needing those interventions while avoiding damage to those that do not.

THE DEVELOPMENT, DIFFUSION, AND UTILIZATION OF HEALTH CARE TECHNOLOGY

The development, diffusion, and eventual widespread utilization of a particular health care technology is a three-phase process that moves from the birth of a scientific concept, through the development of a specific product, and on to acceptance and use by physicians and their patients (Table 2.3). For each of the various industrial subgroupings mentioned earlier, the process may vary widely, but overall, the process is similar for all innovations that eventually become viable technologies.

SCIENTIFIC BACKGROUND AND DEVELOPMENT OF THE IDEA FOR A PRODUCT

In the first phase, a significant amount of individual basic science research is carried out that eventually comes together in the development of an idea for a treatment, a drug, a medical device, or piece of medical equipment. Depending on the subject, the background work can take many years or even

Table 2.3. Stages in the Development of Medical Technologies

- Scientific background and development of the idea for a product
- Product development, approval, and distribution
- Diffusion, adoption, and utilization of the product

several generations to get to the point where a product can be visualized or even imagined. The fact that the last step of conceptualizing a new product may seem to happen very quickly should not obscure the fact that a huge amount of basic science research and development must precede that final step out of the lab and into the world of implementation. Nor should it obscure the fact that an enormous corps of skilled scientists must be educated and trained, an extensive array of basic science laboratories developed, and an effective means for communication of scientific findings constructed. It takes a very significant amount of time and money just to bring the scientific establishment to the point where it can begin to conceive the medical technologies that we have come to value so greatly.

There is general agreement that the ultimate engine fueling the growth and expansion of this massive basic science machine is the National Institutes of Health (NIH), a branch of the federal government. From its relatively humble size and scope immediately after the end of World War II, NIH has grown to the point where the 2006 budget reached approximately $29 billion (Research America, 2005). Over the years, the NIH has provided funds for the establishment of research institutes, the construction of laboratory facilities, the development of academic institutions and societies to sponsor and nurture these ambitious scientific efforts, and finally to educate and train people to staff them and provide leadership for the scientific explorations that take place in them. Without this sustained and massive public investment in the basic scientific efforts of this country, our medical technology development would not have advanced to its current status—an object of admiration throughout the world.

In recent years, there has been a parallel growth in the support of basic science research by private sources, although still small by comparison to the overall NIH investment in the development of the country's basic science infrastructure. Recently, the bulk of private sector investment in scientific research is more applied research targeting the second phase of technology development—the

product development phase—rather than in the more fundamental basic science phase.

The overwhelming dependence of the U.S. basic science effort on long-term public funding raises several important policy questions regarding technology development. First, if the basic science research establishment is so dependent on public support, it might seem possible that a governmentally determined set of priorities could take precedence over a broader set of mandates determined by the scientific community. Fortunately, NIH developed a broad set of advisory panels and consensus mechanisms to ensure that good science drives the direction of NIH and other federal government support. There appears to be general consensus that NIH has been quite wise and evenhanded in its support of basic scientific inquiry across a broad array of subjects.

A second policy-related question about such dominant public funding for basic science research centers on how best to evaluate the returns from this huge investment on a cost-benefit or cost-effectiveness basis. In this age of federal budget deficits and stringencies, the question can well be asked, "What is the country getting back for its investment in science and how do we know?" A similar question might also be, "Shouldn't we be spending a greater proportion of our investment in science on translational research in an effort to more quickly develop and deliver new products and treatments to the public who needs them?"

A third set of policy-related questions deals with the question of industrial and commercial benefit from the significant public investment in basic science in this country. In this set of inquiries, the questions arise from the fact that private industry benefits greatly from the immense amount of public funds spent to develop the trained scientists and the basic science discoveries that industrial organizations need to develop their commercial products. Without this enormous public support for basic science development, industrial companies would need to spend that money themselves before they could come anywhere near to the development of a commercial product. For the most part, the responses to these types of policy questions suggest that the massive investment of public funds in basic science support has significantly benefited both sectors—the public as well as the private—and that actually a very useful and productive partnership has emerged.

In summary, the first phase of the eventual production of useful medical technologies is a broad array of basic science discoveries that provide a fertile scientific environment from which useful products may eventually emerge. Without this broad-based, politically supported scientific establishment, the development of modern medical technology would be much more difficult and possibly much less productive.

PRODUCT DEVELOPMENT AND DISTRIBUTION

The second phase of turning a scientific idea into a deliverable technology involves product development; the process of moving from basic research to implementation. In this phase, the role of basic science research becomes somewhat less important than that of applied science and refinement of the original idea. In this phase, much of the network created with NIH support—the institutions, the laboratories, the network of communication of basic science results—becomes less important and the role of private sector companies and their research and development teams take on a more important role. Interestingly enough, while the basic science sectors of academic institutions may become slightly less important in this phase, their clinical departments become rather more important locations for conducting appropriate clinical trials.

In this phase, three basic questions must be answered. First, is there an obvious need and a viable market for this product? Second, can an appropriate product (i.e. drug, device, piece of equipment) be developed that accomplishes what the basic

science suggests it can? Third, can the necessary tests and clinical trials be carried out that will win the important regulatory approvals required for public sale and use of the product?

With regard to the first question, since the development and launch of a particular technology or pharmaceutical is an extremely expensive venture, private companies must spend considerable time verifying that there is a real need for the product in terms of a viable market, simply to confirm that a reasonable economic return can be generated. They must also spend considerable time examining their relative position in the appropriate marketplace to determine how likely it is that their efforts will succeed in competition with other manufacturers' products. It may benefit a company very little to have an excellent product for which there is not a sufficiently large market to sustain its development, just as it may not benefit a company very much if a competitor has dominant control of the market for that type of product.

Looking at the second question, the process of taking a scientific idea or discovery and transforming it into a useful product involves a great deal of applied research, which can be very expensive and time consuming. In this phase, the scientific work involves clarification and refinement of the original scientific idea, determining its safety and effectiveness, and developing the best design and package for the final product. Informal estimates have suggested that perhaps 95 percent of proposed new drugs never make it through the beginning stages of this development phase, and those that do face a complex, multiyear process of refinement, testing, and approval before ever being released for use. While there is considerable disagreement on the exact real costs of bringing a new technology, drug, or device to market, there is general consensus that it is a costly and risky enterprise at best, not one to be taken on lightly.

With regard to the third challenge, most of the new technologies and drugs will require several types of formal approvals before they are made available for general use, and success in obtaining those approvals governs whether the development process can go forward or not. For example, the usual first step in the development of a new product, drug, pharmaceutical, or device is obtaining a patent from the federal government for the central features of the product and its development. While this first approval step has nothing to do with the product's potential scientific benefit or effectiveness, it is necessary for the economic protection of any product that might be forthcoming; without this patent protection as first step, it is understood that most new product development would simply never go forward because the economic risk of infringement by competitors would be too great.

For health care technology, the most important regulatory approval comes from the federal Food and Drug Administration (FDA), which must approve all drugs and pharmaceuticals as well as all medical devices and some medical equipment. The FDA approval process is a lengthy and complex set of individual phases, each of which is focused on a different aspect of the new product—safety, efficacy, adverse reactions, and side effects. The clinical trials conducted in this phase are central to FDA regulatory approval, and they also serve the purpose of alerting the technical and clinical community that a new treatment or product is on the way. (The FDA approval process will be discussed in more detail later in this chapter.)

Although the FDA approval process is widely viewed as appropriately rigorous and well conducted, it has been criticized as being too lengthy and too complicated on the one hand, and not rigorous and protective enough on the other. Those who say that the process is too rigorous and cumbersome complain that the expense and delay involved in obtaining FDA approvals discourage the innovative energies of the drug industry, add undue delay in getting promising new drugs to market, and add substantially to the eventual cost of the drugs to patients and the public. Those who say the process is not rigorous enough point to recent examples in which pharmaceuticals have been approved that were later shown to have serious risks and side effects not identified during the standard FDA approval process. In general, the relationship

between the pharmaceutical industry and the Food and Drug Administration is a mixture of mutual dependence, mutual wariness, and mutual respect (Berndt et al., 2006).

DIFFUSION, ADOPTION, AND UTILIZATION OF NEW PRODUCTS AND TECHNOLOGY

In this phase of the technology development process, the emphasis is on taking the drug, device, or technology and making it generally accepted, available, and used by patients and clinicians. This phase involves private companies and private capital almost entirely and calls for a mixture of scientific promotion to the technical expert community and broader general marketing to the health care system that must ultimately approve it for purchase and clinical use.

In the product development phase, considerable time and money are spent on conducting the appropriate clinical trials that must be completed to eventually gain FDA approval. Such clinical trials also serve as the first introduction of the new drug or device to the medical community that will eventually use it. These clinical trials move through preliminary tests of the overall safety of the medication or device and then move on to more elaborate clinical trials to test the effectiveness of the drug or device.

In the process of these clinical trials, which are carried out by reputable clinicians using commonly accepted clinical research methodologies, the new drug or product undergoes close clinical scrutiny, has its results widely publicized in reputable peer-reviewed scientific or clinical journals, and acquires a set of clinical "champions" who become familiar with the details and advantages of its use. In some instances, the champions become so closely connected to the new drug, device, or technology that they may also assume an unofficial advocacy role for the new product they had a hand in testing. Whatever the degree of actual advocacy, the process of rigorous clinical trials, publication of the results of successful trials in appropriate scientific journals, and the appearance of general support for the new drug or device by well-known academic and research centers all lend considerable support in marketing campaigns to clinical practitioners which eventually occurs.

Once the appropriate regulatory approvals are obtained for a new device or drug, the development process moves into an active marketing phase designed to encourage the use of the product by individual clinicians and medical groups. For the pharmaceutical industry, the breadth and intensity of the marketing efforts to physicians have become legendary and the "drug rep" has become a well-accepted presence in the lives of clinicians and health care organizations alike In their one-to-one encounters, usually brief in time, the representative of the drug firm attempts to inform the physician of the benefits of the new drug or product and to encourage its use by that clinician; the provision of free samples of the product is also a part of the marketing effort, so that the clinician can easily test the effectiveness of the product on individual patients under care.

In the case of medical devices that require surgical intervention, the company representative may also provide appropriate training and education on the use of the device or intervention itself. These aggressive marketing efforts for drugs and devices are generally agreed to be widespread and expensive although the extent of the exact cost is difficult to determine.

In recent years, with the development of direct-to-consumer marketing of drugs and pharmaceuticals, a new type of marketing effort has emerged. It is now a well-accepted practice to advertise specific drugs directly to potential users and purchasers so that they might be more inclined to request that medication from their physicians or purchase it themselves if no prescription is required. The overall impact of direct-to-consumer advertising is not completely known yet, but it is clear that the impact

is significant enough for the drug firms to include it as a large part of their overall marketing strategies (Bradford et al., 2006).

Also in recent years, the traditional marketing patterns of drug firm representatives working with individual clinicians and pharmacists have been joined by efforts aimed at the large drug and equipment purchasing cooperatives and the larger health insurance companies. With regards to the large purchasing cooperatives, much of the individual hospital or clinic purchasing efforts have been overtaken by large multihospital, multiorganizational purchasing cooperatives. In these new organizations, smaller organizations that ordinarily might not have enough bulk buying power to negotiate better prices might now obtain many of their supplies, equipment, and drugs through the larger purchasing cooperatives. These new purchasing organizations are able to exert much greater leverage over price and service than their individual member organizations did previously, and as such the purchasing organizations themselves become the targets of very different types of marketing efforts from the technology firms that previously dealt only with individual institutions and organizations.

In the same vein, health insurance companies now become important targets of marketing efforts from pharmaceutical firms, since as part of their benefit packages the insurance organizations now have the power to approve or disapprove payments for the use of various pharmaceuticals, devices, or drugs. For example, whenever a health insurance plan provides coverage for drugs and pharmaceuticals, that company will usually have a formulary or list of drugs approved for coverage; the company may also have a policy of encouraging the use of generic drugs rather than brand name drugs and may contract with a pharmaceutical benefits company to manage its drug programs.

Pharmaceutical and technology companies currently have specific marketing efforts and systems in place to ensure maintenance of good relations with the health insurance companies to ensure that their products are present in the insurance companies' formularies or list of approved technologies.

The same holds true for new medical and surgical devices, as well as new medical and surgical procedures. Most health insurance companies will have coverage guidelines that outline which of these new devices and procedures will be covered for payment by the plans and which will not; they also outline the process of technology assessment that the plan uses to assist it in making coverage decisions. (The process of technology assessment by health insurance plans is described later in this chapter.)

Needless to say, the availability of health insurance coverage for new procedures and products is a major factor in the eventual diffusion and use of new technology; as such, insurance firms themselves are objects of a wide variety of high-level marketing approaches directed at inclusion of the new products as covered benefits for beneficiaries.

In summary, the creation of a new drug, product, or device is only the first step toward its eventual widespread diffusion and use. The critical next steps involve convincing the individual clinician of the effectiveness of the drug, product, or device, and convincing the appropriate hospitals and medical organizations to make it available. An equally important next step is to obtain health insurance coverage for the drug or device, so that it will be included in a health plan's standard benefit package. Finally, the ultimate acceptance may have to come from individual patients themselves, and the marketing efforts here may involve direct-to-consumer advertising and education on a scale unprecedented in health care up to this point in our history.

SPECIFIC METHODS FOR EVALUATING MEDICAL TECHNOLOGIES

A major issue in the overall understanding of health care technology is the process by which it is evaluated before coming into use. There are three primary realms of evaluation applied to medical technology: (a) review by regulatory agencies such as the Food and Drug Administration; (b) technology assessment methods used by health insurance carriers in payment determinations; (c) personal and individual appraisals by purchasers and consumers of specific technologies. Each evaluation methodology operates in a different way, applies different measures, and sometimes arrives at different conclusions.

Review by Regulatory Agencies

The most well-known regulatory review of medical technology is that carried out on pharmaceutical products by the Food and Drug Administration, an agency of the federal Department of Health and Human Services. In this process, pharmaceutical products and to some degree medical devices are subjected to detailed preliminary approvals, clinical trials, and postapproval surveillance protocols that are widely respected around the world.

Before a pharmaceutical can enter first-phase clinical testing, a sponsor of a new drug or biological must evaluate the product's safety and biological activity through *in vitro* and *in vivo* laboratory animal testing. The Food and Drug Administration generally asks, at a minimum, that the sponsor develop a pharmacologic profile of the product's effects, determine its acute toxicity in at least two species of animals, and conduct short-term toxicity studies that range from several weeks to several months in duration. In general, the preclinical studies take approximately six years to complete before a potential new drug or biological is ready for clinical testing on human subjects.

Once the sponsoring company has finished these preliminary tests, it then submits an application to the Food and Drug Administration for IND (Investigational New Drug) status for its potential product, so that formal clinical trials can begin. These trials are carried out in three phases, with a fourth phase of postmarket surveillance taking place if the drug is approved.

The first stage of the clinical tests on humans (Phase 1 trials) is carried out on a small number (usually less than 100) of usually healthy volunteer subjects to observe how the drug works in humans, to determine general safety, and to see if there are any unexpected side effects. The purpose of the Phase 1 trials is not to measure clinical effectiveness but rather to get an early reading on safety in human use.

The second stage of the clinical tests on humans (Phase 2 trials) involves a somewhat larger (perhaps 250 subjects or more) group of actual patients with the target disease or illness, not just healthy volunteer test subjects as was the case in Phase 1 tests. The purpose of this limited clinical testing is to obtain a first reading about the potential effectiveness of the proposed drug and to determine whether it is appropriate for the trials to progress to the next stage of definitive testing. Phase 2 trials provide additional information on safety and side effects, as well as information that is helpful in planning appropriate Phase 3 trials.

Phase 3 trials involve much larger groups of patients, frequently in the thousands, and are carried out with strict research protocols approved in advance by the FDA. The Phase 3 trials are designed to determine the proposed drug's effectiveness and also to see if there are significant side effects that will need to be considered by anyone using the drug in the future. The results of the Phase 3 trials are usually those that are eventually published in the scientific literature, thereby providing researchers and potential future users with scientific data about the proposed drug's effectiveness in clinical settings with real patients.

When Phase 3 clinical trials have been completed and the Food and Drug Administration is satisfied with the results, the sponsoring company must submit an application to the FDA for approval as a new drug (NDA); if approved by the FDA, this allows the sponsoring company to market the drug as a commercial product to clinicians and the public. In this step, the FDA involves outside advisory groups in reviewing the data from Phase 3 trials and may place limitations on how the drug can be produced, labeled, and marketed.

If new drug (NDA) status is granted, the Food and Drug Administration also mandates that the sponsoring company carry out monitoring of the actual patient experiences with the new drug and reporting adverse events to the FDA through one of several reporting mechanisms. The purpose of this process, sometimes labeled Phase 4 studies, is to pick up on previously unexpected adverse reactions that may only appear with longer term and more widespread use of the medication. It is generally felt that Phase 4 postmarketing studies are much looser and less effective than the previous three stages of study because the Phase 4 studies are not formally organized as research protocols, the accumulation of data is dependent on effective identification of adverse effects, and reporting is somewhat dependent on the sponsoring companies' willingness to share potentially adverse information until absolutely proven.

Various industry observers have suggested that preclinical trials take an average of six years to complete, that the three stages of clinical trials take an average of several years more, and that final NDA approval takes an additional one to two years to complete. This would suggest that the entire process from early nonclinical studies to final FDA approval as a commercial product takes an average of 14 to 15 years to complete. Recent efforts have been made to shorten this process in order to get promising products to market sooner, but the overall process still remains a lengthy, cumbersome, and expensive one. It is further complicated by the large number of potential medications to be reviewed by the FDA: A recent survey of biotechnology medicines in development, carried out by the Pharmaceutical Research and Manufacturers of America, showed 418 biological medications alone in development, 214 of which were for cancer and related conditions ("New Cancer-Related Biotechnology," 2006).

The Food and Drug Administration also has a somewhat similar review system for medical devices, but it is modified in many important aspects from the review system for drugs. These modifications usually depend on the type of medical device being considered, the conditions under which the device will be used, the disease for which it may be employed, and the previous history of similar devices with the FDA. In general, it is considered less cumbersome and less rigorous than the drug approval process, although it is by no means easy or rapid overall.

Technology Assessment by Insurance Carriers

A second stream of technology reviews takes place within health insurance organizations as part of their process for paying for health services rendered to the insurance plans' beneficiaries (Robinson, 2006). The challenge to the insurance organizations is to use their reimbursement dollars to pay only for services or products that are proven to be effective and beneficial to patients, and the process of review is generally called "technology assessment." The Medicare program has its own system of technology assessment as does the national Blue Cross and Blue Shield Association. Most individual insurance plans either have technology assessment processes of their own, use standards established by others, or contract out for technology assessment advice to private expert sources.

The California Technology Assessment Forum was originally the in-house technology assessment process for Blue Shield of California but recently became more of a free-standing independent organization service to various types of health care organizations. Its technology assessment process is generally accepted as a model program throughout the country and will serve as the model for discussion of this activity (California Technology Assessment Forum, 2006).

To start the process, when a new technology is developed, the insurance organization will be approached by the developers of a new technology and/or the clinicians who want to utilize it in order to have it included as a reimbursable service under the terms of the insurance policies. Without this approval for payment, providers may not be able to obtain payment for the technology, even though it may have received approval from the FDA or other

Table 2.4. California Technology Assessment Forum Criteria

- Technology has final approval from regulatory body.
- Scientific evidence demonstrates effectiveness of health outcomes.
- Technology improves net health outcomes.
- Technology is as beneficial as existing technologies.
- Health improvement can be achieved in actual clinical practice.

regulatory agencies. Once the request for inclusion on the list of reimbursable services is received, the health insurance organization will usually ask for a formal assessment of the technology by whatever technology assessment process the plan uses. The request for assessment of a technology focuses on the effectiveness of the technology and usually does not include any reference to the cost of the technology or its price to the insurance organization.

In its review process, the California Technology Assessment Forum uses five criteria to determine if a medical technology improves outcomes and is safe and effective (Table 2.4).

The initial review of the scientific evidence and peer-reviewed scientific literature is carried out by university faculty members skilled in the review and use of such literature. When they finish their review of the evidence from peer-reviewed publications, they file a formal report with a scientific advisory panel composed of technology experts drawn jointly from academia and the professional community. After open public hearings, the scientific advisory committee decides whether the technology has been proven to be effective and then reports its opinion to the health insurance plan requesting the technology assessment. The health insurance plan then makes its own coverage decision, utilizing the background review and opinion filed by the advisory committee. Decisions regarding level of payment for the technology are handled within the health insurance organization and are not included in the activities of the independent technology assessment process or organization.

The strengths of this type of independent technology assessment process are several. First, the technology assessment is based on a rigorous review of the published scientific evidence, carried out by independent expert reviewers; there is generally a high level of respect for the reviewers and the review process itself. Second, the technology assessment process is not involved with economic or financial details of the technology; this separation of the scientific review process and the final implications of the ultimate advisory committee recommendation are seen as an important aspect of the technology assessment process. Third, the California Technology Assessment Forum process is carried out in an open public forum, with all background information and advisory committee discussions being fully available to all interested parties; technology sponsors are invited to take part in the public forum discussions and to provide additional technical information and expertise as they wish.

As was mentioned earlier, the Medicare program has a technology assessment process of its own, as does the national Blue Cross-Blue Shield Association (which includes all the "Blue" plans in the country, both for profit and nonprofit. While information and technology assessment decisions are shared between and among the health insurance plans, each health insurance plan in the United States makes its own decisions and is under no obligation to follow the guidance of any regulatory or licensing body.

Personal and Individual Appraisals by Purchasers, Clinicians, and Consumers of Health Care Technology

Perhaps the ultimate review of medical technology is made by the ultimate purchaser, user, or consumer of that technology. Just because the FDA has approved a technology, and just because an insurance carrier has decided to include it as a covered benefit, does not necessarily mean that the ultimate end user will actually authorize, purchase, or utilize it. The purchasing and use decision is complex and many faceted and often involves a number of different players.

Probably the most important end user of medical technology is the clinician who must continually determine how patients will be treated. If the physician does not think a new technology is useful in the treatment of a specific clinical condition, that technology will not be recommended, ordered, or used; if it is thought that the technology is advantageous to the patient, it will be ordered and used. Therefore, the physician is usually the critical decision maker with regard to the adoption and actual use of new medical technologies.

The purchasing of large-scale technology, such as imaging systems and diagnostic equipment, is usually a joint clinician/organization decision since both are directly affected by its availability and use. In this case, physicians are again extremely important in the decision making because they usually bring to the attention of hospitals and medical groups the availability of new technologies of various kinds. Physician specialists have particular influence on purchasing decisions, since the technologies in question usually have direct connection with, and impact on, their specialized medical practices. In this instance, hospitals, clinics, and medical groups are continually aware of the necessity to make the latest technologies available to their specialist physicians and are particularly sensitive to the requirements of those specialists for technology support.

At the same time, hospitals and medical groups are responsible for the financial and economic viability and survival of their institutions, and they must balance their desire to provide physicians with the latest technology against the availability of the economic and financial resources to do so; in an era of tightening financial reimbursement of health care, the capital budgeting process of health care organizations for new technology is an area of increasing tension between physicians and their hospitals and medical groups. At the same time, hospitals and medical groups may actually want to purchase new health care technology and may actually encourage their physicians to use it, since the use of that technology may be a source of additional revenue to the hospital or group; while the purchase price of new technology may be a deterrent to the installation of new medical technology, the revenue generated from its use may be a strong financial stimulant for its purchase and use.

Relatively new entrants into the decision making with regard to health care technology are the individual patient and consumer. In the past, individual patients had relatively little knowledge of what technology or medications were available and as a result generally followed the guidance of their physicians in these matters. Although that is still usually the case, patients increasingly come to physicians with a much greater level of information about new technologies, new procedures, and new medications, either because they have read or seen information about them in the media or because they have been the subject of direct-to-consumer advertising themselves. It is not clear how much influence this type of advertising has on the use of large-scale technologies, but it does seem clear that it is having significant impact on the demand for certain specific medications and procedures. This trend will only further reinforce the trend toward so-called "consumer-driven" health insurance options in which consumers will be asked or required to make individual decisions with regard to the expenditures of health care dollars.

In summary, there are three major types of evaluations of technology regularly and continuously carried out in the United States, the first involving regulatory agencies (particularly the FDA); the second involving health insurance organizations (particularly the Medicare program); and the third involving individual clinician, organizational, and consumer decisions to prescribe, buy, or use. Each of these evaluations involves different aspects of the technology spectrum and different parts of the adoption, diffusion, and use process.

DIFFERENTIAL IMPACTS OF TECHNOLOGY ON HEALTH CARE

It is clear that technology is a powerful engine for change in the American health care system; it is also clear that it has major impacts on different aspects of that system, often in quite different ways. To better understand the differential impact of health care technology on the system, it is appropriate to identify and examine the major types of impacts, as well as to attempt to appraise the positive and negative natures of each impact. The major areas of impact to be examined are shown in Table 2.5.

Economic Impact

Depending on the methods used and the specific author, "technology" has been described as either the major driver in the rise of health care costs in the United States, or one of many influences—but not the sole influence. The evidence for the major driver theory is that identifiable expenditures for health care technologies have increased steadily over the years, most visible in the percentage of health care costs attributable to drugs and pharmaceuticals, as well as new surgical procedures and increased utilization of new imaging techniques. It seems to be clear that more technology of a higher cost is being used more widely, but it is not clear

Table 2.5. Major Technology Impact Areas

- Economic impact
- Clinical impact
- Organizational impact
- Industrial impact
- Impact on patients and insurance beneficiaries
- Societal and governmental policy impact

whether that use is the result of the existence of a wider array of new technologies or whether it is the result of improved availability and greater insurance coverage to pay for the use of the new products. Expressed another way, it is not clear whether a more prominent economic role for technology itself is the cause or the effect of greater use and financing.

Complicating the economic picture further, arguments have been made that while many technologies are cost-elevating, others are cost-reducing. As a result, the net effect of new health care technologies may have less total effect on the rising costs of care than frequently suggested. Further complicating the economic analysis of technology's impact on health care costs is the suggestion that while short-term use of new technologies may raise the immediate or short-term expenditures (as shown in a typical cost-benefit dollar-to-dollar analysis), a longer-term cost-effectiveness (dollar-to-outcome in health status) analysis may show a much more positive impact on health status and a lower total cost over a lifetime (Rosen et al., 2007).

What is clear is that the development and use of new health care technologies have significant economic impact on the American health care system. The exact degree and direction of that influence is currently not completely clear and is a matter for vigorous debate by the various stakeholders. Since these major points are not generally agreed upon by all concerned, it should come as no surprise that attempts to detail an overarching national policy on health care technology costs have not been very successful. As a result, each individual participant in the American health care system, whether a provider of care, a payer, or patient consumer, has developed his or her own short-term strategies for dealing with the economic impact of technology on his or her part of the American health system.

Clinical Impact

A less controversial impact of the rapidly developing health care technology in the United States is the positive effect that it has had on the clinical practice of medicine. In every single area of medicine, physicians now have available to them an increasingly impressive and effective clinical arsenal to bring to bear on patients' illnesses. Whether it be in cardiology, psychiatry, neurology, oncology, surgery, or any other major specialty area of medicine, the development of new technologies and pharmaceuticals has vastly improved what physicians can do for patients and the outcomes that can be obtained. Indeed, the progress has been so rapid and so extensive that it may be entirely inappropriate to try to compare today's clinical practice of medicine with that of only a few years ago, either in effectiveness or costs, because the underlying process and practice has changed so much.

This great impact and the rapidity with which the changes have taken place also put special stress on physicians in a variety of new ways, the first and most obvious being the necessity to keep informed of the latest developments and advances in the various fields of medicine, and the second and least obvious being the increasing necessity to follow expert clinical standards and guidelines in practice. Recent surveys of the degree to which the clinical care of patients in the United States meets generally acceptable standards of practice show that patient care meets generally acceptable standards only one-half to two-thirds of the time, a disappointingly low adherence rate (McGlynn et al., 2003).

A further impact of technology on physician's clinical behavior is the competitive pressure to be seen both by physician peers and patients as current and up-to-date on new technologies and pharmaceuticals. Since many of the new technologies are "halfway" technologies and produce only marginal improvements on already available products, the rush to use new techniques and approaches may not be justified by significant improved outcomes. Nevertheless, the clinician may feel that failure to use the newest products may result in negative impressions by peers with regard to competence and currency. Similarly, the physician clinician may pass this pressure along to hospitals and medical groups to immediately obtain the latest diagnostic and therapeutic technologies so that the impression of institutional competency and currency is maintained as well.

Organizational Impact

As is the case for the individual clinician, health care organizations such as hospitals, medical groups, and health insurance plans are continuously pressed to maintain the latest technological and pharmaceutical resources, often despite a lack of detailed evidence that the new technology is a substantial improvement over the old ones. Hospitals are particularly susceptible to pressure from their medical staffs not to fall behind other similar hospitals in the region, either in the nontechnological aspects of their facilities (such as attractiveness and personal service) or the clinically more important aspects of technological capacity. In many ways, this pressure from medical staffs for hospitals to keep abreast of the newest developments in technology is a good influence and has probably been one of the reasons American hospitals have been so well equipped and resourced with technology; at the same time, this influence can be overdone, with costly results for the hospital.

It should also be stressed that many of the requirements with regard to technology and pharmaceuticals may be set by accrediting and licensing agencies on the one hand and insurance, contracting, and legal pressures on the other. Quite aside from the influence of their medical staff, hospitals and clinics are faced with a growing array of regulatory, compliance, and legal issues affecting everything from quality of care, patient safety, laboratory management, privacy of information, and range of services available. Many of these pressures can only be met by increased use of newer technologies or approaches to patient care, each of which carry organizational impacts of their own.

One of the most interesting impacts on health care organizations is the use of new technology and products in a marketing and business development sense. Increasingly, hospitals are actively developing new products and service lines (i.e., new areas of organizational involvement) for the primary purpose of attracting new patients. Very often, these new services or opportunities are centered around or personified by a new technology and its use, further driving the technological imperative for organizational change.

Industrial Impact

Health care technology has given rise to major new industrial organizations and has expanded the range of many already-existing companies. It has been suggested that much of the recent gain in strength in the general U.S. economy is the result of job growth and industrial expansion in health care in general and health care technology in particular. The degree to which this is true could easily be debated, but the overall impression that health care technology and pharmaceuticals are growth industries would certainly be valid.

There are certain specific segments of the broader technology sector that appear to have expanded most. Biological pharmaceuticals likely lead the list of rapidly expanding groups within health care, resulting from the huge and rapid expansion of basic science discoveries in the areas of genetics and molecular biology. Information systems companies have also expanded their health care portfolios heavily, as hospitals, medical groups, health insurance plans, and the government require new types of information that can be accessed widely and rapidly by multiple parties. Finally, demand for new large imaging technologies has continued strong growth, making the diagnostic imaging area one of the most important areas of investment growth in health care.

Not only have new technologies spawned new industrial organizations, but the increasing complexity and expansion of the health care system has also provided major new areas for niche companies to come forward to serve specialized needs that did not previously exist. For example, the widening variety and increasing complexity of health insurance plans and programs, including Medicare, have been followed by the creation of new information support companies offering services to those who must deal with the changes in Medicare rules, regulations, and conditions of participation. New genetic discoveries have changed the way that female patients and their physicians approach major decisions in the treatment of breast and ovarian cancer, providing opportunities for new companies to provide new services to parties ("Test Predicts," 2006). The arrival of implantable devices for hearing loss on the one hand and for diabetes control and maintenance on the other has opened up a new vista for implantable devices to monitor and control multiple body systems.

The growth of the health care technology and pharmaceutical investment sector has also made these industrial groups a standard part of most investment portfolios, and it would be difficult to find a broadly balanced investment plan or strategy that did not include health care technology stocks. Venture capitalists looking for appropriate areas of new investment regularly scan the health care technology horizon for appropriate investment opportunities likely to yield rapid returns, while large endowment funds and trusts regularly include health care technology and pharmaceutical stocks in their long-term plans.

Impact on Individual Patients and Insurance Beneficiaries

Perhaps the most marked impact of the growth in health care technology has been on individual people in their varied roles as patients, customers, purchasers, and insurance beneficiaries. With the growth of online information sources, individual people now have much more direct access to information (whether accurate or inaccurate) about health and illness, as well as technologies and pharmaceuticals available to deal with them. For better or worse, more than ever before individual people are now much more directly informed about their illnesses and the treatments and technologies available to mitigate them.

Because of the Internet, it is now relatively easy for people to access technical information online about recent developments in health care—information primarily restricted to well-informed health professionals just a few years ago. Most of the national organizations advocating for individual disease or illness conditions now have readily accessible online information that provides potential or actual disease sufferers with overwhelming amounts of professional opinions and data about their conditions. Added to this are the efforts of health insurance carriers to educate and inform their beneficiaries about ways of avoiding specific diseases, managing them better if they have them, or seeking additional support if they need it. Virtually all insurance carriers in the country now spend considerable effort and funds to help their members be better utilizers of health services, including high-cost technologies and pharmaceuticals, both to improve the quality of their care and to reduce the rising costs of these services.

Perhaps the most interesting and controversial change in individual patient and consumer informer and behavior has been the growth of direct-to-consumer advertising by technology companies in general and the pharmaceutical industry in particular (Wolfberg, 2006). For example, the rapid growth of direct-to-consumer advertising with regard to bariatric surgery approaches for treatment of obesity, for example, as well as the increasing ease in obtaining these services have led to a remarkable increase in the number of these procedures being performed each year. The direct-to-consumer advertising of medication for male erectile dysfunction has made these medications some of the most widely prescribed pharmaceuticals in the country. The creation of hospital-sponsored "centers of excellence" for every condition from sweaty palms to cerebrovascular aneurysms and the accompanying advertisement of these centers have made many people aware of various conditions they may never previously have known about.

Societal and Governmental Policy Impact

The significant expansion of the technology and pharmaceutical sectors and the attendant rise in health care costs have not gone unnoticed in the public policy and public advocacy arenas. The increase in the number of people in the United States without health insurance and their possibly reduced access to the latest technology and drugs have raised significant questions of social equity and fairness. This same increase in the number of uninsured in the United States has also heightened the belief that much of the cost of the uninsured is borne by the remainder of the population through increased taxes or more costly private health insurance premiums.

The congressionally imposed prohibition against the Medicare program's ability to negotiate with national pharmaceutical companies for lower prices is a subject of significant public debate in Congress, in the media, and among individual people in society as well. In the same vein, the federal government prohibition against importing drugs and pharmaceuticals from countries with lower drug prices and the willingness of some state and local governments to encourage and enable such purchases have pitted one level of American government against others. The creation of a complicated three-tiered drug benefit in Part D of the Medicare program has heightened public awareness of the costs of pharmaceuticals and the need to have more rational public policy and programs in this important area.

At the same time, Congress, the media, and the public have been increasingly concerned about the Food and Drug Administration's system for regulating and controlling the development and use of pharmaceutical and medical devices. The issues here have been the time it takes to obtain approval for new drugs and medical devices on the one hand, and the discovery that the FDA approval process has sometimes not discovered long-term hazards to health on the other. Other FDA public policy issues include debates over the influence of the pharmaceutical industry in FDA science decisions and the implication that nontechnical political concerns have influenced FDA staffing appointments and policy decisions The point here is not whether the various allegations and comments are true, but rather that the FDA has been elevated to a very public and visible position in national policy discussions and debates, primarily because of its important role in the approval and control of the prescription and use of drugs and medical devices in the United States.

SUMMARY

In summary, modern medical technology is a complex, powerful, and costly set of services and products that have broad and deep impacts on all aspects of American health care—many of them contradictory in outcome and purpose. It is incumbent on all health care professionals to understand technology's powerful set of forces and pressures, so that these strengths can have a maximum positive impact on the health and health care of all Americans. To ensure that, there are three of concern that will need further thought, debate, and decision in the future.

The first area of deliberation centers on the future *costs* of medical technology, and more important, its *value*. As the focus of public debate shifts to more careful examination of how health care funds are being spent, increasing attention will be paid to the benefit gained—if any—by the added expenditure of increasingly sophisticated technology, and more attention will be paid to the potential added value to patients and payers (Cutler & McCellan, 2001). Porter has suggested that the road to health care reform in the future will succeed only if the system becomes more value driven, and that will be possible only if the relative value of health care technology become a more central issue (Porter & Teisberg, 2006). Finally, the arrival of increasingly expensive and lucrative medical technologies in the future will raise new ethical and regulatory issues—for clinical practitioners, hospital managers, insurance executives, and industry leaders. New issues such as the ownership of genetic materials used in the development of new biopharmaceuticals, the possible conflict of physician ownership of technology centers and the investment in technology manufacturers, worldwide differences in prices for the same pharmaceuticals, and more—all these will bring widespread public interest and policy debates to a degree of intensity and sophistication not seen up to this point (Abelson, 2006; Finegold, 2005). The future of medical technology will be exciting, challenging, and incredibly important.

REVIEW QUESTIONS

1. List the different classifications of health care technology (by industrial group).
2. Why is it important to understand the medical technology is a collection of very specific subgroupings?
3. Briefly describe the stages of medical technology development.
4. Describe the four phases of clinical testing in humans.
5. Discuss the technological assessment process carried out by health insurance plans.
6. How has medical technology affected clinicians and organizations?

REFERENCES & ADDITIONAL READINGS

Abelson, R. (2006, December 30). Spine as profit center: Surgeons invest in makers of hardware. *The New York Times*, p. C1.

Berndt, E., Gottschalk, A., & Strobeck, M. (2006). Opportunities for improving the drug development process: Results from a survey of industry and the FDA. *Innovation Policy and the Economy, 6,* 91.

Bradford, W. D., et al. (2006). How direct-to-consumer television advertising for osteoarthritis drugs affects physicians' prescribing behavior. *Health Affairs, 25,* 1371–1377.

California Technology Assessment Forum. (2006). Criteria for technology assessment [mimeo]. Retrieved April 13, 2007, from http://www.ctaf.org.

Cohen, A., & Hanft, R. (2004). *Technology in American health care: Policy directions for effective evaluation and management.* Ann Arbor: University of Michigan Press.

Cutler, D., & McCellan, M. (2001). Is technological change in medicine worth it? *Health Affairs, 20,* 11–29.

Finegold, D. (Ed.). (2005). *Bioindustry ethics,* Burlington, MA: Elsevier Academic Press.

Goldsmith, J. (2005). The healthcare information technology sector. In L. R. Burns (Ed.), *The business of healthcare innovation.* Cambridge: Cambridge University Press.

Grady, D. (2006, November 23). Oxygen monitor fails to help doctors detect birth risks. *The New York Times* (National), p. A32.

Kruger, K. (2005). The medical device sector. In L. R. Burns (Ed.), *The business of healthcare innovation.* Cambridge: Cambridge University Press.

Luce, B. (1993). Medical technology and its assessment. In S. Williams & P. Torrens, (Eds.), *Introduction to health services* (4th ed.). Albany, NY: Delmar.

McGlynn, E., et al. (2003). The quality of health care delivered to adults in the United States. *New England Journal of Medicine, 348,* 2635–2645.

Mello, M., & Brennan, T. (2001). The controversy over high-dose chemotherapy with autologous bone marrow transplant for breast cancer. *Health Affairs, 20*(5), 101–117.

New cancer-related biotechnology medicines in development. (2006, September 25). *Oncology Times,* p. 26.

Northrop, J. (2005). The pharmaceutical sector. In L. R. Burns (Ed.), *The Business of Healthcare Innovation.* Cambridge: Cambridge University Press.

Pfeffer, C. G. (2005). The biotechnology sector—therapeutics. In L. R. Burns (Ed.). *The Business of Healthcare Innovation.* Cambridge: Cambridge University Press.

Porter, M., & Teisberg, E. (2006). *Redefining health care: Creating value-based competition on results.* Boston: Harvard Business School Press.

Research America. (2005). 2004 Investment in U.S. health research. Retrieved April 13, 2007, from http://www.researchamerica.org/advocacy/healthresearchinvestment.html.

Rettig, R., Jacobson, P., Farquhar, C., & Aubry, W. (2007). *False hope: Bone marrow transplantation for breast cancer.* Oxford: Oxford University Press.

Robinson, J. (2006). Insurers' strategies for managing the use and cost of biopharmaceuticals. *Health Affairs, 25*(5), 1205–1217.

Rosen, A., Cutler, D., Norton, D., Hu, H. M., & Vijan, S. (2007). The value of coronary heart disease for the elderly, 1987–2002. *Health Affairs, 26*(1), 111–123.

Rosenthal, G. (1979). Anticipating the costs and benefits of new technology: A typology for policy. In S. H. Altman and R. J. Blendon (Eds.), *Medical technology: The culprit behind health care costs?* [DHEW Publication (PHS)79-3216]. Washington, DC: Department of Health, Education, and Welfare.

Test predicts which breast cancer patients will benefit from chemotherapy. (2006, October 25). *Oncology Times,* p. 35.

Thomas, L. (1977). On the science and technology of medicine. *Daedalus, 106,* 35–46.

U.S. Congress, OTA. (1976). *Development of medical technology opportunities for assessment* (Pub. No. OTA-H-34). Washington, DC: U.S. Government Printing Office.

Wolfberg, A. (2006). Genes on the web—direct-to-consumer marketing of genetic testing. *New England Journal of Medicine, 335,* 543–545.

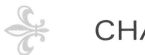

CHAPTER 3

Population and Disease Patterns and Trends

Stephen J. Williams

CHAPTER TOPICS

- Need, Demand, and Utilization
- The Underlying Demographic Determinants of Health Services Utilization
- Fertility Trends in the United States
- Mortality Trends in the United States
- Specific Causes of Death for the U.S. Population
- Incidence of Infectious Diseases
- Lifestyle Patterns and Disease
- Health, Lifestyle, and Social Structure
- Measuring the Impact of Illness on Society
- Access to Health Care Services

LEARNING OBJECTIVES

Upon completing this chapter, the reader should be able to

1. Trace U.S. demographic trends including births and deaths.
2. Understand correlates of mortality, especially with regard to the impact of population trends.
3. Understand disease patterns in the United States.
4. Relate lifestyle, behavior, and social patterns to health.
5. Appreciate cancer survival trends.
6. Understand issues of access to care.

Disease patterns throughout history and the underlying social and demographic characteristics of our population provide empirical evidence from which to view the need and demand for health care services in the United States. The principal purposes of this chapter include the review of fundamental demographic, social, and economic trends in our nation, principally throughout the past century, and of patterns of morbidity, mortality, and other aspects of the measurement of the incidence and prevalence of disease. Analytical, epidemiologic measurement of these patterns illuminate the underlying factors that define the nature of health care services required for our nation. The chapter also presents quantitative information that reflects the impact of illness and disease on our longevity and health status. Factoring in the impact of illness and disease further enhances our appreciation for the challenges and trade-offs faced by our nation's health care system.

An additional purpose of this chapter is to review population, disease, and illness trends and to relate these trends to issues of access to health care services. Access to care is a core theme throughout this book and a key health policy issue facing our nation. This chapter associates the various social, demographic, and disease patterns experienced by our nation with measures of access to health care and interpretation of these measures as a contributor to the national health policy debate.

The analysis presented here first focuses on the underlying demographic trends in our society during the twentieth century. Social and economic trends that define the character of our society and relate to the need and demand for health care services are also discussed.

The next section of the chapter focuses on disease patterns experienced in the past century. Differential mortality and morbidity are presented to emphasize the importance of such variables as age, race, and sex in defining population groups at particular risk for various diseases. Ultimately, identification of risk factors and their association with various personal, sociodemographic, and physiological characteristics, and genetic markers will greatly heighten our ability to target health services to individuals in the greatest need for each category of care.

All aspects of this chapter are integrally related to virtually every other section of this book. The nature of the delivery system itself, including the settings in which services are provided, the nature of services, the technology of our system, and even the financing of care are all directly related to the underlying disease patterns that we experience.

This chapter sets the stage and forms part of the foundation of knowledge necessary for critically assessing how the health care system is structured. Our ability to measure performance within the system itself, including access to and outcomes of care, and the costs of illness, is related to these fundamental trends as well. Ultimately, the success of the system should be measured against criteria that recognize the true needs of the population with regard to the physiological and psychological manifestations of injury, illness, and disease, and their ability to obtain needed care.

In purely quantitative terms the measurable impacts of disease and illness offer enticing avenues for measuring the success and failures of the health care system. Such measures as years of life lost and days of disability attributable to each illness and disease category provide an objective and comparative numerical assessment of the impact of these clinical and psychological problems on us individually and collectively as a society. Increasingly, the utilization of such quantitative measures facilitates the allocation of resources and priorities in decision making at various points within the health care system. As the system moves increasingly to objectively measure clinical care, disease impacts, and other aspects of its own operation, attention to such quantitative measures and objective indicators is paramount.

NEED, DEMAND, AND UTILIZATION

In discussions of disease patterns and their relation to the utilization of health care services, it is important to differentiate between the concepts of need, demand, and use of health care services. *Need* for health care services is defined as an interpretation of an individual's evaluated requirements for obtaining professional care through the health services system. *Demand* for health services is a function of an individual's actually seeking out, but not necessarily obtaining, health services. Demand may be a reflection of professional assessment of an individual's need for services or self-initiated desires for professional services, perhaps triggered by an individual's perceptions of potential illness. Finally, *utilization* is a measure of actual use of services, as discussed later in this chapter.

The extent to which there is a correlation between need, demand, and utilization is the central issue in addressing concerns of appropriateness of care, perceptions of when services should be obtained, and evaluation of access to health care services in our society. Many other issues related to these concepts are addressed throughout this book.

Data Sources and Quality

Morbidity, mortality, and other health status–related data are obtained from a variety of sources. Information presented throughout this chapter and elsewhere in this book is based on such sources as national vital statistics data. National vital statistics data are collected from birth, death, and marriage certificates. Mandatory data collection requirements in the United States provide the most consistent and generally highest quality data available for determining the health status of our population.

But even mandated vital statistics data collection produces information of inconsistent quality. All data should be viewed with a skeptical eye, recognizing the imperfections of the data collection effort. For primary demographic variables such as age, race, and sex, the quality of data recorded on the primary data source—the vital event certificate—is generally good. However, for more subjective data elements such as cause of death, the consistency and quality of data reported can vary appreciably, especially in past years, depending on the judgment of the individual, usually a physician, completing the certificate. Vital statistics data collected at the

local level are compiled by the states and the federal government, and efforts are directed toward improving quality at each level.

Data on health services utilization, health status, attitudes, and other variables are often collected through national probability surveys conducted by the federal government and some private organizations. The National Health Interview Survey, for example, collects data from a random probability sample of all Americans, asking questions regarding prior health services utilization, perceived health status, mobility, and other, often somewhat subjective, self-reported variables. Recall ability, response judgments, and other complex factors affect the quality of these types of data.

Primary data collection by the federal government has even included conducting physical examinations on a random sample of Americans. This research effort, the National Health and Nutrition Examination Survey, provides direct observation data on various health and disease indicators. This type of examination is very expensive to conduct but does provide considerable objective useful information to the extent that those randomly selected for participation reflect national patterns in our entire population.

A third category of data collection for health services use involves the compilation of data from other sources. An example of this is the National Hospital Discharge and Ambulatory Surgery Survey, conducted by the federal government, which compiles the data from a sampling of hospital discharges in the country. Another example is the National Ambulatory Medical Care Survey, also conducted by the federal government, which is based on a sample of physicians who report on the characteristics, diagnoses, and use of services for all patients seen during a 1-week interval of time.

Private data collection includes surveys of health services use, attitudes, and costs. National organizations such as the American Medical Association and the Medical Group Management Association conduct surveys on medical groups, physician practices, and hospital services. Various insurance companies, health care systems, and individual facilities also conduct surveys on patient satisfaction and other issues. Finally, data are collected by national voluntary accrediting agencies, health services researchers, and other organizations.

Health policy data analysis utilizes a variety of databases, producing more complex analyses that go beyond the descriptive nature of many of the surveys. Such analysis, by combining a variety of data and sources, allows for greater insight into the nature of health care services and population needs. For example, combining population data, longevity data, and data on the incidence and prevalence of disease allows for the analysis of the impact of various diseases on our population as measured by such variables as days lost from work, years of life lost due to mortality from specific diseases or behaviors such as smoking, and other analyses that provide a more in-depth reflection of the impact of illness and disease on our society.

It is important to recognize the sources, quality, and contingencies associated with the data that are analyzed and presented throughout this book. The book's analytical perspective on health services is dependent on the assessment of population-based data, and the best available information is utilized for discussion purposes. Even the relatively solid data available in the United States, however, are subject to numerous limitations. Needless to say, data from many other countries in the world often lag far behind our own in this regard.

THE UNDERLYING DEMOGRAPHIC DETERMINANTS OF HEALTH SERVICES UTILIZATION

The dynamics of population are the most fundamental determinants of the need, demand, and use of health care services. The size and age composition of a population have a tremendous impact on total health services use as well as on the distribution of the use of specific services. Therefore, trends in population dynamics, including population size and demographic characteristics as well as births and deaths, are a basic starting point for assessing the need for health services in a population.

Population Size and Composition

Population size, as reflected in the total number of people in a population, as well as the distribution of population by age group, defined as the population pyramid, is the appropriate starting point. Table 3.1 presents the age-specific distribution of the United States resident population since 1950. These data, obtained from the federal

Table 3.1. Resident Population: United States, Selected Years

Year	Total Resident Population (Population in Thousands)	Age Group (Population in Thousands)										
		Under 1 Year	1–4 Years	5–14 Years	15–24 Years	25–34 Years	35–44 Years	45–54 Years	55–64 Years	65–74 Years	75–84 Years	85 Years and Over
1950	150,697	3,147	13,017	24,319	22,098	23,759	21,450	17,343	13,370	8,340	3,278	577
1970	203,212	3,485	13,669	40,746	35,441	24,907	23,088	23,220	18,590	12,435	6,119	1,511
1990	248,710	3,946	14,812	35,095	37,013	43,161	37,435	25,057	21,113	18,045	10,012	3,021
2001	284,797	4,034	15,336	41,065	39,948	39,607	45,019	39,188	25,309	18,313	12,574	4,404
2003	290,811	4,004	15,766	40,969	41,206	39,873	44,371	40,805	27,900	18,337	12,869	4,713

government, are based on the national census of population data. The federal government is required by the United States Constitution to conduct a census count of the population once every ten years to compile as complete a count as possible of all citizens.

The United States Census of Population was most recently completed in 2000. Results of the 2000 census indicated an approximate United States population of 280 million individuals. Complete census results from the 2000 count are available in a variety of forms from the United States Bureau of the Census.

Population data between censuses and for future periods are determined through intracensual estimates and projections using prior data and adjusting for estimated population growth and migration. Intracensual data estimates are facilitated by using such available statistics as school enrollments, automobile registrations, and utility hookups. The original purpose of the census, of course, was to determine representation in the House of Representatives, although these data are now also used for an array of analytical, commercial, and social purposes.

The accuracy of the actual census count, of intracensual estimates, and of demographic projections into the future is a subject of considerable debate. The mobility of the population, the lack of tracking for internal migration, and illegal migration into the country complicate the picture. The cost of data collection, analysis, adjustment, and reporting has escalated greatly as the population has grown, as well.

The United States population has grown tremendously during the period presented in Table 3.1. This growth is a result of two principal factors. The first of these is the *rate of natural increase* attributable to the higher number of births as compared to deaths annually in the United States, leading to additions to the total population count. The second factor is the increase in population attributable to net in-migration, which historically has accounted for nearly all of the accumulated population of the country. The current United States population is more than 302,000,000 people, double the count in 1950.

A limited selection of the detailed demographic data available from the census is reflected in Table 3.2. This table presents age-specific total

Table 3.2. **Resident Population: Age, Sex, Race, United States, 2003**

Sex and Race	Total Population	Under 1 Year	1–4 Years	5–14 Years	15–24 Years	25–34 Years	35–44 Years	45–54 Years	55–64 Years	65–74 Years	75–84 Years	85 Years and Over
					Number in thousands							
Male	143,037	2,046	8,060	20,977	21,183	20,222	22,134	20,044	13,424	8,349	5,154	1,445
Female	147,773	1,958	7,706	19,992	20,024	19,650	22,237	20,761	14,475	9,988	7,714	3,269
White male	116,875	1,594	6,296	16,322	16,726	16,159	18,129	16,807	11,590	7,308	4,638	1,307
White female	119,474	1,525	5,999	15,488	15,658	15,310	17,813	17,034	12,263	8,576	6,859	2,950
Black or African American male	18,190	336	1,301	3,444	3,180	2,613	2,705	2,218	1,232	711	355	96
Black or African American female	19,958	323	1,260	3,337	3,140	2,862	3,052	2,579	1,531	999	627	247
Hispanic or Latino male	20,599	442	1,682	3,832	3,759	4,016	3,101	1,910	991	542	261	65
Hispanic or Latino female	19,300	424	1,611	3,659	3,235	3,363	2,815	1,908	1,097	680	380	128

population data for the country by sex, and by race and sex for whites, blacks, and Hispanics Careful observation of these data demonstrates, for example, the substantially higher number of individuals alive at age 85 and above who are female as compared to male, while showing a higher population of under 1-year-old males as compared to females.

The relative size of the race and sex-specific populations is also illustrated in Table 3.2. Such data are available for numerous subgroups within the population. This type of data is also available for various geographic regions within the country although the data presented in these tables are aggregate data for the entire nation.

Comparing data for various time periods allows for ready assessment of temporal changes. For example, the increasing minority count of population in comparison to total population over time is reflected in the data. The data present absolute numbers, but many of the numbers presented in the tables and other data from these sources are also used in calculating rates and ratios for more extensive analysis of demographic, disease, and other trends.

The age structure of the population is, as noted earlier, vitally important for health services purposes. The very young and the older population groups utilize considerably more health care services than other age groups. Table 3.1 also presents the age distribution, and hence the structure or pyramid of the population.

An important current trend is the aging of the population. On average, the typical American is getting older. This trend is the result of increased longevity and relatively lower fertility than was experienced earlier in the last century. The consequences of this trend are reflected in Table 3.3. Projections for the older population groups over the next half century suggest substantial increases in health services utilization, assuming current technology, access to care, and patterns of use. The population aged 65 and above currently uses, on average, approximately twice the health care services as the younger population. This trend in the age structure for the United States is the underlying

Table 3.3. Population Age Group Projections, Age 65 and Above

Age Group	Year (Population in Millions)			
	2000	2025	2050	2075
65 years and over	35.2	60.6	73.3	83.3
75 years and over	16.7	25.0	38.9	45.7
85 years and over	4.4	6.3	14.6	16.9

SOURCE: U.S. Social Security Administration Office of Programs: Office of the Actuary, 1993, Baltimore, MD.

demographic reason for concerns over the future financial viability of the Social Security system and the Medicare program.

Projections of the aging of the population as reflected in Table 3.3 are simple to perform since changes in mortality patterns by age typically do not vary drastically over relatively short periods of time. However, the implications of these fundamental demographic shifts are much more difficult to project. Our aging population of Baby Boomers appears to be healthier and more functional than predecessor generations. Their interest in an active lifestyle, social activities, and cosmetic medicines is clearly greater than that of previous generations. Preferences in housing, entertainment, behaviors, and politics are often difficult to predict. Changes in many of these parameters can have a significant impact on the scope, use, and nature of the health care system. Many dramatic changes that are now occurring in medicine and biomedical research further complicate any projections.

For example, although current demographic trends portend increases in the population of patients with Alzheimer's and related dementias, biomedical research may allow health care providers to prevent these diseases or to repair their damage. Such landmark advances would have a tremendous impact on the need for services and the cost of providing those services to an aging population.

Less invasive pharmacologically based interventions for various diseases might be significantly less expensive to implement than current alternative surgically based interventions. Then again, the high cost of many pharmacological products may narrow the cost gap.

The many longer-term implications of an aging population also extend to numerous economic concerns including labor force participation; the dependency ratio, which is the percentage of the population working to support the nonworking or dependent population; and impacts of economic growth rates from an aging population base. The challenge for the nation and its health care system is to create an environment that can adapt as the underlying parameters change over time with the aging of the population.

Parenthetically, many other countries in the world, especially in Europe, face an even more profound aging of their populations, so that future liabilities for social services, health care, and social security are even more serious than our own.

Enhanced longevity as a result of biomedical advances is a two-edged sword leading to longer periods of economic and social dependency, while at the same time enhancing quality of life. As the population ages, the burdens on the younger working groups increase. This can have significant long term impact on social policies, taxes, politics, and everyday life.

FERTILITY TRENDS IN THE UNITED STATES

A key determinant of population that affects health services utilization is fertility. Fertility is a key determinant of the population pyramid, as well as of the use of services for mothers, infants, and children. Fertility eventually influences total population size and has cohort effects in all age groups as a cohort ages.

Fertility behavior is also a socioeconomic characteristic of population. Developing nations, for example, are typically characterized by relatively high fertility rates, while developed, or postindustrial, societies usually experience low fertility rates.

Fertility is a measure of reproduction. Age-specific fertility rates are the primary indicator utilized in measuring this determinant of population. Age-specific fertility rates more accurately reflect differences in fertility patterns based on age groups of mothers than do birth rates, which are a cruder measure of reproduction. Birth rates are computed as the total number of births to total population. Age-specific fertility rates are computed as the number of births to women in a specific reproductive age group. The total fertility rate is the sum of all of the age-specific rates.

Table 3.4 presents age-specific fertility rates for the United States over the past half century. As for many of the other rates discussed in this chapter, age, race, sex, and other characteristics may be utilized to compute more specific rates than those presented.

Fertility, of course, differs greatly by age group, as reflected in Table 3.4. Fertility is highest for women in their twenties and generally declines thereafter as the age of the mother increases. Fertility rates drop off appreciably at the higher reproductive ages, with little fertility in the groups above 45 years of age.

Historically, and in most societies, the reproductive ages begin with the physiological marker of menarche. A variety of sociological determinants of reproductive behavior, such as marriage, combine with physiology to produce actual behavior. The reproductive ages usually end with menopause. Other physiological factors, such as voluntary sterilization and infertility, and sociological patterns, such as family dissolution, also have a substantial impact on reproduction. The interaction of these dynamics can be quite complex.

Technological change has impinged on our traditional concept of fertility behavior. Of course, natural and artificial means of birth control have long affected couples' actual fertility behaviors and outcomes. Few societies in history have not been affected by various natural patterns of birth control, mores, and societal behaviors and other influences

Table 3.4. Live Births and Birth Rates by Age of Mother: United States, Selected Years

Year	Total Fertility Rate*	Age of Mother (Live Births per 1,000 Women)							
		10–14 Years	15–19 Years	20–24 Years	25–29 Years	30–34 Years	35–39 Years	40–44 Years	45–54 Years
1950	106.2	1.0	81.6	196.6	166.1	103.7	52.9	15.1	1.2
1960	118.0	0.8	89.1	258.1	197.4	112.7	56.2	15.5	0.9
1970	87.9	1.2	68.3	167.8	145.1	73.3	31.7	8.1	0.5
1980	68.4	1.1	53.0	115.1	112.9	61.9	19.8	3.9	0.2
1990	70.9	1.4	59.9	116.5	120.2	80.8	31.7	5.5	0.2
2001	65.3	0.8	45.3	106.2	113.4	91.9	40.6	8.1	0.5
2003	66.1	0.6	41.6	102.6	115.6	95.1	43.8	8.7	0.5

*The sum of the age-specific rates.

on fertility outcomes. Demographers have searched for populations such as the Hutterites which strive for maximum fertility to provide a glimpse into reproduction potential in an uninhibited population. Many biological, economic, and social factors impact fertility behavior and outcomes as measured by live births.

Recent technological advances have also suggested the potential for significant impact on fertility behavior as a result of external interventions. Such technologies as in vitro fertilization, ovum freezing and storage, and enhanced infertility treatment have led to increases in birth rates for population groups, especially older women, and have also increased the number of multiple births. Although the actual impact of these technologies on total fertility rates has not been great, the longer-term impact of these and other yet to be discovered technologies could be significant. An increased ability to determine sex, to screen for genetic disorders, and to enhance and prolong fertility could eventually profoundly impact the demographic structure of our society. The cost and acceptability of many of these interventions, however, will limit their overall impact. Fertility patterns thus far clearly have not been hugely affected by these new techniques for the population overall.

Fertility has declined in most age groups over the past 40 years, as reflected in Table 3.4. Reductions in fertility have been rather dramatic in the United States since peak fertility occurred in the mid-1950s. Some uptake in fertility rates at the higher age levels is evident in Table 3.4 for the year 2001. This increase is primarily in the 30–44 age range and minimally so above that point. Further declines in the younger age groups are also evident from this table.

Data are available by various social demographic groups as collected on birth certificates. Table 3.5 presents differential fertility rates by age group for whites and blacks. Generally, dramatically higher fertility for most age groups is evident in this table for blacks as compared to whites. Differential fertility patterns combined with demographic trends in migration, population size, and other related information can provide useful data for projecting population trends in local communities and nationwide. The increasing diversity of our population is evident from these and other demographic data.

The dramatic decline in fertility that has occurred in the United States over the past 40 years is primarily the result of increases in female labor force participation, marital dissolutions, and other economic and social forces in our society. In recent years, our nation has also witnessed a delayed

Table 3.5. Live Births and Birth Rates by Race of Mother: United States, 2003

Race	Total Fertility Rate	Age of Mother							
		10–14 Years	15–19 Years	20–24 Years	25–29 Years	30–34 Years	35–39 Years	40–44 Years	45–54 Years
		Live births per 1,000 women							
Race of mother: White	66.1	0.5	38.3	100.6	119.5	99.3	44.8	8.7	0.5
Race of mother: Black or African American	66.3	1.6	63.8	126.1	100.4	66.5	33.2	7.7	0.5
Race of mother: Hispanic or Latino	96.9	1.3	82.3	163.4	144.4	102.0	50.8	12.2	0.7

average age of first marriage, reduced desired family size, delayed initiation of childbearing due to education and employment prospects, and a number of other important social and economic factors, all of which have further reinforced the primary underlying fertility trends.

Fertility data provide other useful insights into population behaviors as reflected in Table 3.6. In this table, percentage of women who have not had at least one live birth by attained age group is presented for selected years. Since virtually all fertility is complete by age 44, the column for ages 40–44 reflect lifetime childlessness for live births to individual women. Thus about 15 percent of women in the population have no lifetime live birth experience. These data do not specifically represent pregnancy

experience, however. Also evident is the increasing age of the typical mother. The percent of women who have not had at least one live birth has increased substantially from 1960 to the present for the younger age groups in this table. Since a woman's fertility time frame is finite, delays in live childbearing does contribute to reduced total fertility in the population. Indeed, the increasing recognition that fertility capacity, or what is termed fecundability, decreases significantly with age has been an impetus for much of the reproductive biology research on infertility that has been conducted in recent years.

Considerable other insight into reproductive patterns and behaviors is available from the fertility data collected from certificates of live birth. Another interesting component of these behaviors, nonmarital childbearing, is presented in Table 3.7. These data reflect live births to unmarried mothers based on birth certificate information. Differential patterns of nonmarital childbearing by race over time are reflected in this table. Nonmarital childbearing has increased substantially as a percentage of all live births from 1970 to 2003. Approximately one-third of all live births today are to unmarried mothers. Differential rates reflect substantially higher percentages of live births to unmarried mothers for blacks, American Indians or Alaskan Natives, and Hispanic populations, and significantly lower percentages for Asian populations. The

Table 3.6. Women Who Have Not Had at Least One Live Birth, Selected Ages: United States, Selected Years

Year	20–24 Years	25–29 Years	30–34 Years	40–44 Years
	Percent of women			
1960	47.5	20.0	14.2	15.1
1980	66.2	38.9	19.7	9.0
2002	66.5	41.3	24.8	15.8

Table 3.7. Nonmarital Childbearing According to Race of Mother: United States, Selected Years

Race of Mother	1970	1990	2003
	Percent of live births to unmarried mothers		
All races	10.7	28.0	34.6
White	5.5	20.4	29.4
Black or African American	37.5	66.5	68.2
American Indian or Alaska Native	22.4	53.6	61.3
Asian or Pacific Islander	—	13.2	15.0
Hispanic or Latino	—	36.7	45.0

implications of these data relate to family formation, social stability, issues of health insurance coverage and other economic concerns, and social and behavioral factors in child development. Generally, the poorest group within our population is single women with dependent children, so our concerns about the welfare of these mothers and their children are important considerations in the formation of health and social policies.

Other societies have experienced many of the same general changes in fertility experienced by the United States in the twentieth century. The change from a high-fertility, high-mortality environment to a low-fertility, low-mortality environment is typical of most developing countries. This change is termed the *demographic transition.* Countries that achieve low fertility and low mortality combined with relatively affluent economic conditions typically experience substantial social and economic change that results in permanent reversals of the underlying social factors associated with high fertility.

Abortion Trends in the United States

Reproduction may be more appropriately measured in terms of conceptions rather than live births. Conceptions include spontaneous and induced abortions as well as live and dead births. However, the empirical data to accurately count conceptions are considerably weaker than those for live births.

National data are available on therapeutically induced abortions. The United States experiences perhaps one million abortions annually at the current time, and an unknown number of conceptions result in spontaneous abortions, primarily in the first month of gestation. Abortion practices vary considerably from society to society and over time, and the current acceptance of abortion services in the United States dates back nationally to 1973 although some states and foreign nations had less restriction on access to such services before then.

National data on the number of medically or therapeutically induced abortions range from a little over 800,000 to approximately 1.2 million abortions per year depending on the source of the data. The availability of legal abortion services in the United States changed dramatically in 1973 with the Supreme Court decision to remove state barriers to access to care. Some erosion in access has occurred since that time, but these services are generally available in most communities. Thus far, the majority of such abortions are performed using suction curettage in the first trimester of gestation.

There is considerable controversy with regard to the availability of abortion services in the United States, although the relative safety of these procedures when performed in medical facilities is excellent. Abortion ratios, that is the number of abortions per 100 live births, is highest for the youngest group of women in the population and for those age 40 and over as well. Abortion ratios are substantially higher for black women than for Hispanic or white women. As might be expected, abortion ratios are substantially higher also for unmarried women as compared to married women. In addition to impacting patterns of fertility, abortion is also believed to affect the percent of births that occur to high-risk women and other aspects of reproductive health.

Technological change has affected the provision of abortion services in the United States and throughout the world. Less invasive pharmacologically based approaches to termination of very early term pregnancies is shifting the locus of abortion services to private physician offices and clinics without necessarily being associated with surgical procedures. Monitoring these services is extremely difficult. In addition, numerous political, economic, social, and psychological factors will continue to impact the provision of abortion services in the United States regardless of delivery mechanisms.

MORTALITY TRENDS IN THE UNITED STATES

Indicators of mortality are often used to measure a society's health status. Trends in mortality indicators over time also reflect a multitude of social, economic, health services, and other underlying trends in a society. Reasonably accurate mortality data are available for the United States population and for many other nations, although in some developing countries the quality of data may be limited.

Mortality data are collected at the time of death through the mechanics of the death certificate, a responsibility of local government. State and federal agencies compile data collected locally to produce the vital statistics for the entire country. Because various social and demographic variables are collected on the death certificate in addition to determinants of the cause of death, mortality data can be analyzed by selected characteristics of population.

Mortality Trends for the United States

This section of the chapter presents quantitative measures of mortality for the total United States population over time. Mortality data for infants and mothers and an analysis of specific causes of death are presented in later sections of this chapter as well. As for fertility, aggregate mortality data are generally age-adjusted to control for changes in the population age pyramid. Comparisons over time, in particular, require consideration of any substantial changes in the age structure of a population.

Life Expectancy

A common measure of mortality, particularly popular in the mass media, is life expectancy. Life expectancy is computed from mortality data and reflects a cohort effect for estimated years of life remaining.

The life table at birth reflects the entire expected mortality experience for a population. Life tables use current age-specific mortality experience so that if a population's mortality experience eventually improves or degenerates, the previously computed life table will be inaccurate. For this reason, life tables are periodically updated by insurance companies that use them to compute premiums for life insurance contracts. A life table presents a population's single best reflection of mortality expectation for the entire population, although for any one individual, the life table provides only an expectation.

Life expectancy can be computed for a population at any specific age, but it is most commonly presented at birth and at age 65. Table 3.8 presents such data for selected countries in the world. Mortality and life expectancy data are typically presented on a sex-specific basis due to the consistent and substantial differences in mortality experienced comparing males and females.

International life expectancy comparisons reveal that, for both males and females, life expectancy at birth is greatest in Japan. The United States falls somewhat short in these comparisons, which is a surprising finding for many people. However, the heterogeneity of our population and our complex social problems associated with violence, accidents, and infectious disease account for much of the cross-cultural deficiencies reflected in our mortality experience. Many Americans are surprised to

Table 3.8. Life Expectancy at Birth and at 65 Years of Age, According to Sex: Selected Countries, 1998

Country	Life Expectancy in Years		Country	Life Expectancy in Years	
	At Birth	At 65 Years		At Birth	At 65 Years
Male			*Female*		
Canada	76.0	16.3	Canada	81.5	20.1
Chile	72.3	15.1	Chile	78.3	18.4
Cuba	75.8	—	Denmark	78.8	18.1
Denmark	73.9	14.8	England and Wales	80.0	18.7
England and Wales	75.1	15.5	France	82.4	20.9
France	74.8	16.4	Germany	80.3	19.0
Germany	74.5	15.3	Greece	80.6	18.7
Greece	75.5	16.4	Italy	82.2	20.4
Italy	75.9	16.1	Japan	84.0	22.0
Japan	77.2	17.1	New Zealand	80.4	19.5
New Zealand	75.2	16.1	Norway	81.3	19.6
Norway	75.5	15.7	Portugal	78.9	17.9
Portugal	71.7	14.3	Puerto Rico	79.3	—
Sweden	76.9	16.3	Sweden	81.9	20.0
United States	73.8	16.0	United States	79.5	19.2

see that mortality experience measured by life expectancy at birth is lower in the United States than in such countries as Greece and France, perhaps owing a little to the value of red wine, paté, and olive oil!

Life expectancy at age 65 is also presented in Table 3.8 for selected countries. By age 65, past the highest-risk periods for mortality attributable to nonphysiological causes, the differences between sexes are much less, as are the differences between countries. Sex mortality differentials drop by about half by age 65, reflecting the higher risk from violent accidents and lifestyle causes for individuals younger than 65. The remaining differential is probably attributable to physiological factors such as hormones and genetics.

International differences are similarly moderated by age 65, as many of these same causes of mortality in the younger ages have been factored out of the equation. Even at 65, however, life expectancy is greatest in Japan, with females at age 65 expecting to live, on average, to about age 86, a truly impressive result.

United States Life Expectancy Data

Table 3.9 presents life expectancy data for selected subgroups of the United States population. Again, mortality experience differs by sociodemographic characteristics such as sex and race. Dramatic differences appear in these data at birth for males as compared to females and for blacks as compared to whites. As noted previously, data are available for numerous subgroups of the population, and only selected illustrative data are presented here.

At birth, females have a substantially higher life expectancy than males, a difference of more than five years of life. An equally dramatic differential is evident for whites as compared to blacks. These differences have been constant throughout modern

Table 3.9. Life Expectancy at Birth, at 65 Years of Age, and at 75 Years of Age, According to Race and Sex: United States, Selected Years.

Age and Year	White Male	White Female	Black Male	Black Female
	Remaining life expectancy in years			
At birth				
1900	46.6	48.7	32.5	33.5
1950	66.5	72.2	59.1	62.9
1970	68.0	75.6	60.0	68.3
1990	72.7	79.4	64.5	73.6
2003	75.3	80.5	69.0	76.1
At 65 years				
1950	12.8	15.1	12.9	14.9
1970	13.1	17.1	12.5	15.7
1990	15.2	19.1	13.2	17.2
2003	16.9	19.8	14.9	18.5
At 75 years				
1990	9.4	12.0	8.6	11.2
2003	10.5	12.6	9.8	12.4

Table 3.10. Death Rates for All Causes According to Sex: United States, Selected Years.

Sex and Age	1950	1990	2001
	Deaths per 100,000 resident population		
Male			
All ages, age adjusted	1,674.2	1,202.8	1,029.1
All ages, crude	1,106.1	918.4	846.4
Under 1 year	3,728.0	1,082.8	749.8
1–4 years	151.7	52.4	37.0
5–14 years	70.9	28.5	19.8
15–24 years	167.9	147.4	117.0
25–34 years	216.5	204.3	143.7
35–44 years	428.8	310.4	259.6
45–54 years	1,067.1	610.3	545.1
55–64 years	2,395.3	1,553.4	1,192.7
65–74 years	4,931.4	3,491.5	2,911.5
75–84 years	10,426.0	7,888.6	6,833.0
85 years and over	21,636.0	18,056.6	16,744.8
Female			
All ages, age adjusted	1,236.0	750.9	721.8
All ages, crude	823.5	812.0	850.4
Under 1 year	2,854.6	855.7	613.9
1–4 years	126.7	41.0	29.5
5–14 years	48.9	19.3	14.6
15–24 years	89.1	49.0	42.6
25–34 years	142.7	74.2	66.0
35–44 years	290.3	137.9	148.2
45–54 years	641.5	342.7	316.8
55–64 years	1,404.8	878.8	754.0
65–74 years	3,333.2	1,991.2	1,890.8
75–84 years	8,399.6	4,883.1	4,760.5
85 years and over	19,194.7	14,274.3	14,429.9

United States history, as reflected in Table 3.9. At age 65, the differentials continue to exist, but as for the international comparisons, the differences are much more moderate, indicating that on a biological basis sex differences may be on the order of two to three years. Black/white differentials are also quite moderate at this point.

United States Mortality Rates

Table 3.10 presents age-specific mortality rates for the United States by selected demographic characteristics. These data conform to the life expectancy numbers presented earlier. As expected, mortality rates increase with age. The United States age-specific mortality rates are relatively moderate until the older ages, although notable differentials occur by sex and race. The higher mortality rate for younger black males compared to same-age-group

white males is particularly startling; these data are discussed further later in this chapter in the discussion of specific causes of death.

Data on differential mortality help to identify problems in society with regard to causes of illness and disease and barriers to access to health care services. Trends over time reflect progress, or lack thereof, in achieving our goals for a greater quality and quantity of life.

Infant and Maternal Mortality

An oft-quoted set of data is mortality experience for infants and mothers. Table 3.11 presents international data on infant mortality. Infant mortality is measured as the number of infants who die in the first year of life per thousand live births. Related measures of mortality for infants include perinatal, postnatal, and other measures, all of which pertain to the time period before or after delivery in which the fetal or infant death occurs.

Once again, the United States falls short in international comparisons of infant mortality. Hong Kong leads all nations in having the lowest infant mortality rate. The relatively poor performance of the United States population is again a function of population heterogeneity and such factors as lack of access to prenatal care; high fertility among high-risk young women; poor maternal nutrition; genetic risks; and other complex social, economic, and physiological factors. Differential infant mortality among United States population subgroups indicates that rates are substantially higher for blacks than for whites due to differences in access to health care, nutrition, social factors, and other variables that affect infant viability. These differences reflect underlying social and economic concerns faced by our society. Poor gestational outcomes may result in huge social and economic costs. Implications of inadequate prenatal care, nutrition, and related factors also extend to serious concerns of child intellectual development, social adaptation, and physical maintenance.

Maternal mortality, reflected in Table 3.12, has declined dramatically in the United States since 1950. In addition to the overall decline in these rates, the reduction in maternal mortality for the higher age groups is quite notable.

Again, a very significant differential exists by race. Black women have experienced a significant decline in maternal mortality since 1950, but they still have rates that are much higher than those of

Table 3.11. Infant Mortality Rates and Rankings: Selected Countries, 2002

Country	Infant Deaths per 1,000 Live Births
Australia	5.0
Belgium	4.9
Bulgaria	13.3
Canada	5.4
Chile	7.8
Costa Rica	11.2
Cuba	6.5
Denmark	4.4
England and Wales	5.2
Finland	3.0
France	4.1
Germany	4.3
Greece	5.9
Hong Kong	2.3
Hungary	7.2
Ireland	5.1
Israel	5.4
Italy	4.7
Japan	3.0
Netherlands	5.0
New Zealand	6.2
Northern Ireland	4.7
Norway	3.5
Poland	7.5
Puerto Rico	9.8
Romania	18.6
Russia	17.3
Singapore	2.9
Spain	3.4
Sweden	2.8
Switzerland	4.5
United States	7.0

white women. The reductions in infant and maternal mortality discussed in this chapter represent a real success in our national efforts to improve the quality and quantity of life. But much remains to be done to achieve optimal results for all Americans and to fully invest in the future of our children.

Table 3.12. **Maternal Mortality Rates for Complications of Pregnancy, Childbirth, and the Puerperium, According to Race and Age: United States, Selected Years**

Race and Age	Year (Deaths per 100,000 Live Births)		
	1950	1970	2003
White			
All ages, age adjusted	53.1	14.4	6.9
Under 20 years	44.9	13.8	*
20–24 years	35.7	8.4	5.3
25–29 years	45.0	11.1	6.9
30–34 years	75.9	18.7	6.8
35 years and over	174.1	59.3	23.8
Black			
All ages, age adjusted	—	65.5	25.5
Under 20 years	—	32.3	*
20–24 years	—	41.9	15.8
25–29 years	—	65.2	20.7
30–34 years	—	117.8	46.1
35 years and over	—	207.5	104.1

*Rates based on fewer than 20 deaths are considered unreliable and are not shown.

SPECIFIC CAUSES OF DEATH FOR THE U.S. POPULATION

Age-adjusted death rates for selected causes of death for the U.S. population from 1950 to the present are presented in Table 3.13. Heart disease, cancer, and stroke are, of course, the three leading causes of death in the United States and have been for quite some time. Interestingly, examination of equivalent data at the turn of the twentieth century would reveal a much greater prevalence of infectious as opposed to chronic diseases for the leading causes of death. Mortality attributable to

such causes as nephritis and tuberculosis, which accounted for many deaths at the turn of the century, is far less common today. Influenza and pneumonia were also very important causes of death in the early 1900s. A dramatic outbreak of influenza occurred in 1918, causing considerable mortality.

Data on selected causes of death will be presented here in more detail. However, an examination of Table 3.13 reveals striking declines in mortality attributable to diseases of the heart, cerebralal vascular disease, and for some of the other major causes of death since 1950. Results for malignant neoplasms, however, are not comparable and reflect the greater challenge faced by biomedical researchers in controlling and curing the ramifications of the various types of cancer.

Stretching further back into history, among the most important trends in disease patterns and causes of mortality since the early 1900s has been the shift from the predominance of infectious disease to chronic disease. In approximately the early 1920s, mortality from chronic diseases, such as heart disease, cancer, and stroke, overtook mortality from infectious diseases, such as pneumonia and influenza, as the principal causes of mortality in the United States. Infectious disease mortality continued to decline throughout the remainder of the first two-thirds of the twentieth century, but the resurgence of some infectious diseases such as AIDS have created an awareness that infectious disease is still an important and challenging arena in mortality. While the control of infectious disease has been one of the most significant public health successes in the history of mankind, much of that success was attributable to improvements in living conditions and in the workplace as opposed to advances in biomedical research and clinical practice.

Although the predominant challenges for mortality are now focused on chronic diseases, our nation must remain vigilant against outbreaks of infectious disease. Morbidity and mortality associated with the epidemic of human immunodeficiency virus illustrate the constant threat of infectious disease that we face even today. In many

Table 3.13. Age-Adjusted Death Rates for Selected Causes of Death According to Sex: United States, Selected Years

Sex	1950	1980	2003
	Age-adjusted death rate per 100,000 population		
Male			
All causes	1,674.2	1,348.1	994.3
Diseases of heart	697.0	538.9	286.6
Ischemic heart disease	—	459.7	209.9
Cerebrovascular diseases	186.4	102.2	54.1
Malignant neoplasms	208.1	271.2	233.3
Trachea, bronchus, and lung	24.6	85.2	71.7
Colon, rectum, and anus	—	32.8	22.9
Prostate	28.6	32.8	26.5
Chronic lower respiratory diseases	—	49.9	52.3
Influenza and pneumonia	55.0	42.1	26.1
Chronic liver disease and cirrhosis	15.0	21.3	13.0
Diabetes mellitus	18.8	18.1	28.9
Human immunodeficiency virus (HIV) disease	—	—	7.1
Unintentional injuries	101.8	69.0	51.8
Motor vehicle-related injuries	38.5	33.6	21.6
Suicide	21.2	19.9	18.0
Homicide	7.9	16.6	9.4
Female			
All causes	1236.0	817.9	706.2
Diseases of heart	484.7	320.8	190.3
Ischemic heart disease	—	263.1	127.2
Cerebrovascular diseases	175.8	91.7	52.3
Malignant neoplasms	182.3	166.7	160.9
Trachea, bronchus, and lung	5.8	24.4	41.3
Colon, rectum, and anus	—	23.8	16.2
Breast	31.9	31.9	25.3
Chronic lower respiratory diseases	—	14.9	37.8
Influenza and pneumonia	41.9	25.1	19.4
Chronic liver disease and cirrhosis	7.8	9.9	6.0
Diabetes mellitus	27.0	18.0	22.5
Human immunodeficiency virus (HIV) disease	—	—	2.4
Unintentional injuries	54.0	26.1	24.1
Motor vehicle-related injuries	11.5	11.8	9.3
Suicide	5.6	5.7	4.2
Homicide	2.4	4.4	2.6

Table 3.14. Leading Causes of Death and Numbers of Deaths, Selected Ages: United States, 2003

Age and Rank Order	Cause of Death	Number of Deaths
Under 1 year	All causes	28,025
	Congenital malformations, deformations and chromosomal abnormalities	5,621
	Disorders related to short gestation and low birth weight, not elsewhere classified	4,849
	Sudden infant death syndrome	2,162
	Newborn affected by maternal complications of pregnancy	1,710
	Newborn affected by complications of placenta, cord, and membranes	1,099
	Respiratory distress of newborn	831
	Unintentional injuries	945
	Bacterial sepsis of newborn	772
	Diseases of circulatory system	591
	Neonatal hemorrhage	649
5–14 years	All causes	6,954
	Unintentional injuries	2,618
	Malignant neoplasms	1,076
	Congenital malformations, deformations, and chromosomal abnormalities	386
	Homicide	324
	Suicide	250
	Diseases of heart	264
	In situ neoplasms, benign neoplasms, and neoplasms of uncertain or unknown behavior	79
	Chronic lower respiratory diseases	118
	Influenza and pneumonia	147
	Septicemia	77
25–44 years	All causes	130,761
	Unintentional injuries	29,307
	Malignant neoplasms	19,250
	Diseases of heart	16,850
	Suicide	11,667
	Homicide	7,626
	Human immunodeficiency virus (HIV) disease	6,928
	Chronic liver disease and cirrhosis	3,378
	Cerebrovascular diseases	3,043
	Diabetes mellitus	2,706
	Influenza and pneumonia	1,365

(*continued*)

Table 3.14. (continued)

Age and Rank Order	Cause of Death	Number of Deaths
65 years and over	All causes	1,804,373
	Diseases of heart	563,390
	Malignant neoplasms	388,911
	Cerebrovascular diseases	138,134
	Chronic lower respiratory diseases	109,139
	Influenza and pneumonia	57,670
	Diabetes mellitus	54,919
	Alzheimer's disease	62,814
	Nephritis, nephritic syndrome and nephritis	35,254
	Unintentional injuries	34,335
	Septicemia	26,445

developing countries, infectious disease remains a principal cause of mortality, particularly among the very young and the very old. Such diseases as the Ebola virus and other startlingly virulent infectious diseases could become a threat to developed nations' populations at any time. Increased international mobility provides vectors of transmission for infectious disease that were not common years ago. And, as if the challenges of chronic and infectious disease were not enough, we now face the added threat of biological weapons in the war against terror. Fear of biological agents, which we had long considered conquered in the developed countries, are with us again.

Data for Specific Causes

Table 3.14 presents actual numbers of deaths for selected subgroups and causes for the United States population. The leading causes of death for each subgroup are listed. Although much more extensive analysis is available, these data sets dramatically demonstrate the tragic involvement of economic, social, and lifestyle factors in causing mortality in the United States. The high ranking for such causes as injuries and violence is quite striking in the younger age groups. Data for the older ages present a picture more common to our typical

characterization of mortality causes in the United States.

It should also be noted that the data presented in Table 3.14 are actual numbers of deaths rather than rates or ratios, which are generally more scientific. The presentation of absolute numbers provides a more dramatic illustration of the impact of specific causes of death in selected population subgroups.

Mortality rates attributable to selected causes are presented in the next few tables. Again, only limited data sets can be presented here; much more extensive statistical information is available from a variety of official governmental sources.

Table 3.15 presents data for cardiovascular mortality in the United States. The data illustrate the dramatic and generally consistent decline in mortality from this cause over time and across age groups. Data for various population subgroups based on age, sex, race, and certain other variables would reflect similar patterns. As is typical in illness and mortality data, declines have occurred for many population subgroups, but the results lead to numbers for blacks, American Indians, and some other population groups that are not nearly as low as for whites. This reduction in cardiovascular mortality is attributable to improvements in living conditions, diet, and health care services, particularly

Table 3.15. Death Rates for Diseases of the Heart, According to Sex and Age: United States, Selected Years

Sex and Age Group	Year (Deaths per 100,000 Resident Population)		
	1950	1970	2003
Male			
All ages, age adjusted	697.0	634.0	286.6
Under 1 year	4.0	15.1	12.1
1–4 years	1.4	1.9	1.1
5–14 years	2.0	0.9	0.7
15–24 years	6.8	3.7	3.4
25–34 years	22.9	15.2	10.5
35–44 years	118.4	103.2	42.8
45–54 years	440.5	376.4	136.2
55–64 years	1,104.5	987.2	331.7
65–74 years	2,292.3	2,170.3	785.3
75–84 years	4,825.0	4,534.8	2,030.3
85 years and over	9,659.8	8,426.2	5,621.5
Female			
All ages, age adjusted	484.7	381.6	190.3
Under 1 year	2.9	10.9	9.8
1–4 years	1.2	1.6	1.3
5–14 years	2.2	0.8	0.5
15–24 years	6.7	2.3	2.1
25–34 years	16.2	7.7	5.7
35–44 years	55.1	32.2	18.6
45–54 years	177.2	109.9	50.2
55–64 years	510.0	351.6	141.9
65–74 years	1,419.3	1,082.7	417.5
75–84 years	3,872.0	3,120.8	1,331.1
85 years and over	8,796.1	7,591.8	5,126.7

Table 3.16. Death Rates for Cerebrovascular Diseases, According to Age: United States, Selected Years

Age Group	Year (Deaths per 100,000 Resident Population)		
	1950	1970	2003
All ages, age adjusted	180.7	147.7	53.5
Under 1 year	5.1	5.0	2.5
1–4 years	0.9	1.0	0.3
5–14 years	0.5	0.7	0.2
15–24 years	1.6	1.6	0.5
25–34 years	4.2	4.5	1.5
35–44 years	18.7	15.6	5.5
45–54 years	70.4	41.6	15.0
55–64 years	195.3	115.8	35.6
65–74 years	549.7	384.1	112.9
75–84 years	1,499.6	1,254.2	410.7
85 years and over	2,990.1	3,014.3	1,370.1

interventions for such events as myocardial infarction and coronary occlusion, and for hypertension and high cholesterol.

Data for cerebrovascular disease-related mortality are presented in Table 3.16 and reflect a consistent decline over time and across age groups. Racial- and sex-specific data show similar declines as for cardiovascular mortality. Rates for whites are at lower levels at all points in time as compared to blacks.

Cancer Mortality in the United States

Among those disease categories where morbidity and mortality experience has been especially disappointing over the course of the last 50 years are various types of cancer. Mortality attributable to various cancers has remained fairly constant, in contrast to the dramatic declines experienced for cardiovascular and cerebrovascular disease. Furthermore, cancer survival rates after diagnosis generally have not improved dramatically thus far.

Table 3.17. Death Rates for Malignant Neoplasms, According to Age: United States, Selected Years

Sex and Age	Year (Deaths per 100,000 Resident Population)			Sex and Age	Year (Deaths per 100,000 Resident Population)		
	1950	1970	2003		1950	1970	2003
Male				*Female*			
All ages, age adjusted	208.1	247.6	233.3	All ages, age adjusted	182.3	163.2	160.9
Under 1 year	9.7	4.4	1.7	Under 1 year	7.6	5.0	2.1
1–4 years	12.5	8.3	2.8	1–4 years	10.8	6.7	2.1
5–14 years	7.4	6.7	2.8	5–14 years	6.0	5.2	2.4
15–24 years	9.7	10.4	4.6	15–24 years	7.6	6.2	3.4
25–34 years	17.7	16.3	8.9	25–34 years	22.2	16.7	9.9
35–44 years	45.6	53.0	30.8	35–44 years	79.3	65.6	39.1
45–54 years	156.2	183.5	127.4	45–54 years	194.0	181.5	117.1
55–64 years	413.1	511.8	386.8	55–64 years	368.2	343.2	302.3
65–74 years	791.5	1,006.8	931.7	65–74 years	612.3	557.9	635.3
75–84 years	1,332.6	1,588.3	1,695.4	75–84 years	1,000.7	891.9	1,040.1
85 years and over	1,668.3	1,720.8	2,413.8	85 years and over	1,299.7	1,096.7	1,381.9

Table 3.17 presents cancer mortality experience for the United States since 1950 by age group. As is evident from the data in this table, overall cancer mortality has actually increased over time. Increasing cancer mortality may be partially attributable to greater overall longevity, to genetic and environmental factors, to increased case-finding, to declines in other causes of death (leaving people more susceptible to cancer mortality), and to lifestyle issues.

Tables 3.18 and 3.19 present cancer mortality for two major categories of malignant neoplasms: breast cancer in women and lung cancer.

Breast cancer in women involves a complex array of diseases with environmental and genetic etiologies. Mortality attributable to this source of disease is significant and rises sharply with age. Even at younger ages, such mortality is important and suggests that for individuals with significant risk factors, preventive procedures and screening might be warranted. Breast cancer mortality in women is highest in the highest age groups although declining mortality from other causes, particularly diseases of the heart and cerebrovascular illness, at least in part, leads to higher mortality from various cancers.

Mortality attributable to malignant neoplasms of the lung and associated organs has risen sharply since 1950. Here again mortality rises with age, in this instance is significantly higher in general among males as compared to females, and has a multitude of etiologies, although the consumption of tobacco products and exposure to second-hand smoke are important risk factors in the epidemic of this form of cancer. Since the association between the consumption of tobacco products, and to a lesser extent, exposure to second-hand smoke, and the incidence and mortality attributable to lung

Table 3.18. Death Rates for Malignant Neoplasms of Breast for Females, According to Age: United States, Selected Years

Age Group	Year (Deaths per 100,000 Resident Population)		
	1950	1970	2003
All ages, age adjusted	31.9	32.1	25.3
25–34 years	3.8	3.9	2.1
35–44 years	20.8	20.4	12.2
45–54 years	46.9	52.6	30.4
55–64 years	70.4	77.6	56.6
65–74 years	94.0	93.8	82.6
75–84 years	139.8	127.4	123.7
85 years and over	195.5	157.1	189.4

Table 3.19. Death Rates for Malignant Neoplasms of Trachea, Bronchus, and Lung, According to Sex and Age: United States, Selected Years

Sex and Age	1950	1970	2003
	Deaths per 100,000 resident population		
Male			
All ages, age adjusted	24.6	67.5	71.7
All ages, crude	19.9	53.4	62.9
Under 25 years	0.0	0.1	*
25–34 years	1.1	1.3	0.4
35–44 years	7.1	16.1	6.1
45–54 years	35.0	67.5	36.5
55–64 years	83.8	189.7	136.7
65–74 years	98.7	320.8	346.6
75–84 years	82.6	330.8	525.1
85 years and over	62.5	194.0	475.1
Female			
All ages, age adjusted	5.8	13.1	41.3
All ages, crude	4.5	11.9	46.1
Under 25 years	0.1	0.0	*
25–34 years	0.5	0.5	0.4
35–44 years	1.9	6.1	5.1
45–54 years	5.8	21.0	24.4
55–64 years	13.6	36.8	87.1
65–74 years	23.3	43.1	204.8
75–84 years	32.9	52.4	279.4
85 years and over	28.2	50.0	221.0

*Rates based on fewer than 20 deaths are considered unreliable and are not shown.

cancer is so well established, public health efforts to intervene and reduce the impact of such risk factors is clearly warranted from a health care perspective.

Cancer Survival Rates

Cancer survival rates, presented in Table 3.20, are disturbing in that, for some categories of cancer, survival rates have not improved appreciably in recent years. Cancer survival is highly dependent on early detection and effective therapeutic intervention. Mass screening for various types of cancer, such as breast, cervical, testicular, and colorectal, can be beneficial for high-risk population subgroups. Population screening has complex cost-benefit trade-offs and other considerations such as test accuracy, identification of population subgroups appropriate for screening, and possible interventions.

Although cancer morbidity, mortality, and survival rate experience has thus far been disappointing, particularly in comparison with certain other disease categories such as coronary artery and cerebrovascular diseases, prospects for the future appear much brighter. Current biomedical research is successfully elucidating the underlying molecular and biological factors associated with the causes, development, and proliferation of various cancers. Many new pharmaceutical products are in clinical trials or have already been brought to market. An extensive commitment of our national research activity toward the development of additional interventions to address cancer in human populations is likely to lead to even greater successes in the coming years.

Table 3.20. Five-year Relative Cancer Survival Rates for Selected Sites, According to Race and Sex: Selected Geographic Areas, Selected Years

| | Percent of Patients Surviving More Than 5 Years | | | |
| | White | | Black or African American | |
Sex and Site	1974–1976	1995–2001	1974–1976	1995–2001
Male				
All sites	41.9	66.5	31.3	58.4
Oral cavity and pharynx	54.3	61.1	31.2	34.3
Esophagus	4.3	16.1	2.1	8.6
Stomach	13.2	19.9	15.5	21.5
Colon	49.8	66.1	44.1	56.3
Rectum	47.8	64.5	34.1	55.0
Pancreas	3.1	4.7	1.4	2.9
Lung, bronchus	11.0	13.7	11.0	11.6
Prostate gland	67.7	99.9	58.0	96.7
Urinary bladder	74.5	84.3	54.1	69.7
Non-Hodgkin's lymphoma	47.7	59.5	43.1	47.6
Leukemia	33.5	49.6	32.6	39.2
Female				
All sites	57.4	66.3	46.8	53.2
Colon	50.8	63.9	46.6	53.6
Rectum	49.7	65.9	49.3	57.0
Pancreas	2.1	4.2	3.1	5.6
Lung, bronchus	15.8	17.7	13.1	15.6
Melanoma of skin	84.8	93.5	—	78.2
Breast	74.9	89.5	62.9	75.9
Cervix uteri	69.2	74.6	63.5	66.1
Corpus uteri	88.6	86.2	60.4	61.8
Ovary	36.3	44.4	40.1	37.7
Non-Hodgkin's lymphoma	47.3	63.3	54.1	59.1

Data related to cancer morbidity, mortality, and survival rates are further complicated by the multitude of diseases that fall under this general category. Success has been and likely will continue to be uneven across different cancer sites and types. Success in treating cancer is often measured in terms of survival rates rather than outright cures, which are much more difficult to establish. Some cancers are increasingly being viewed by clinicians as chronic diseases and an increasing array of pharmaceutical products is being utilized to help avert recurrences after cancer treatment. Compared to the research and therapeutic environment thirty years ago, the prognosis for cancer detection, control, and even cure is greater today than ever before.

Because there is a substantial lag time in the collection, evaluation, and dissemination of morbidity and mortality data, particularly for cancer, it will take considerable time before the quantitative results of current biomedical research and clinical interventions become evident in the types of data presented here. Progress for certain types of cancers is already reflected in the results presented in these tables. However, most of these success stories focus on early detection and, in some cases, surgical intervention. A far greater impact from pharmaceutical progress and improvement in addressing more fundamental approaches to treating cancer based on an understanding of the biological causes of the disease is likely in the coming years. And, of course, as we conquer cancer as a cause of morbidity and mortality, we will see changes in the distribution of morbidity and mortality for other diseases.

Cancer Incidence Rates

Table 3.21 presents cancer incidence rates for selected sites for white males and white females in the United States over the latter part of the twentieth century. For many categories of cancer, particularly lung, prostate, and breast, incidence rates have increased, in some cases sharply. The extent to which increases in cancer incidence are the result of increased case-finding and greater patient awareness is difficult to elucidate. There is also controversy regarding the fundamental causes of cancer and the extent to which genetic, environmental, behavioral, and dietary factors trigger its development. Further clarification of the causation and biological mechanisms of various cancers will be a product of ongoing epidemiologic and biomedical research.

There is increasing recognition that even with likely further biomedical advances, cancer requires a multipronged approach. The first and perhaps the most critical component is to identify the etiology of various cancers and the risk factors for individuals. Doing so will allow for a potential reduction in the risk of developing cancer as well as identify those individuals at highest risk for various cancers as a result of their work environment, genetic composition, or other measurable risk factors.

Table 3.21. Age-adjusted Cancer Incidence Rates for Selected Cancer Sites, White Males and White Females, Selected Geographic Areas and Years

Race, Sex, and Site	Year (Number of New Cases per 100,000 Population)	
	1973	2000
White male		
All sites	364.3	561.2
Oral cavity and pharynx	17.6	15.6
Stomach	14.0	10.6
Colon and rectum	54.3	61.9
Pancreas	12.8	12.5
Lung and bronchus	72.4	75.9
Prostate gland	62.6	171.1
Urinary bladder	27.3	40.5
Non-Hodgkin's lymphoma	10.3	24.6
Leukemia	14.3	16.7
White female		
All sites	295.0	426.9
Colon and rectum	41.7	45.4
Pancreas	7.5	9.6
Lung and bronchus	17.8	50.6
Breast	84.4	140.1
Cervix uteri	12.8	8.8
Corpus uteri	29.5	25.5
Ovary	14.7	14.9
Non-Hodgkin's lymphoma	7.5	16.6

The second component for addressing cancer is the continued development of appropriate screening and diagnostic interventions. An emphasis on an increasingly personalized approach to cancer treatment will result in more efficient and meaningful results for patients. The third aspect of addressing the cancer threat to our society is effective interventions with measurable clinical success rates. This includes both surgical and medical interventions. Finally, the fourth aspect to addressing cancer concerns in our society is appropriate follow-up for patients and populations to assure that after patients are treated they receive continuing care to reduce the likelihood of recurrences and to provide a supportive environment for the physical, psychological, social, and economic ramifications of the disease. The movement toward an increasingly comprehensive approach to cancer not only encourages more effective interventions, but also a greater efficiency in the utilization of our technologies and eventually a much more positive long-term outlook for affected patients.

Cancer remains one of the most challenging categories of disease with respect to detection and successful therapeutic intervention. Biomedical researchers are successfully elucidating the causes and mechanisms of various cancers, although the challenges from this complex category of disease remain great. Future therapeutic interventions hold great promise. The biomedical research pipeline is producing discoveries daily. However, cancer incidence rates continue to climb, and survival rates remain little improved from earlier years, based on available historical data.

Human Immunodeficiency Virus Mortality

The epidemic of AIDS can be traced back to the late 1970s with rapid progression throughout the 1980s. Mortality attributable to AIDS is reflected in Table 3.22.

Mortality attributable to the human immunodeficiency virus began to decline with the introduction of a variety of new drugs for treatment of patients in the mid- to late-1990s. For many patients, this disease has evolved from a death sentence to a treatable chronic infectious disease requiring a lifetime of medical care and drug therapies. However, mortality attributable to this disease is still occurring and the epidemic still rages, particularly internationally. AIDS mortality is higher for males than for females, for the middle aged as compared to the very

Table 3.22. Death Rates for Human Immunodeficiency Virus (HIV) Infection, According to Age: United States, Selected Years

Age Group	Year (Deaths per 100,000 Resident Population)		
	1987	1995	2003
All ages, age adjusted	5.6	16.2	4.7
Under 1 year	2.3	1.5	*
1–4 years	0.7	1.3	*
5–14 years	0.1	0.5	0.1
15–24 years	1.3	1.7	0.4
25–34 years	11.7	28.3	4.0
35–44 years	14.0	44.2	12.0
45–54 years	8.0	26.0	10.9
55–64 years	3.5	10.9	5.4
65–74 years	1.3	3.6	2.4
75–84 years	0.8	0.7	0.7

*Too small numbers to compute.

young and the very old, for blacks and certain other minority groups as compared to whites and Asians, and is a particular threat to certain population subgroups such as intravenous drug users. Increases in incidence and mortality among women, heterosexuals, and especially black women are a growing concern. The dynamics of the AIDS epidemic in the United States has changed over time and is continuing to evolve.

Recent biomedical research has produced tremendous progress in treating individuals with this disease. Earlier and more aggressive intervention, primarily utilizing new drug therapies, has led to a tremendous reduction in mortality. Individuals diagnosed with this disease were, in the earlier stages of the epidemic, condemned to a shortened life expectancy. Today, many of the affected individuals can expect to live longer, although the epidemic still exacts a substantial toll from the nation. The cost and complexity of treatment combined with uncertainty regarding the long-term prospects for patients suggest that this is one of the more challenging health concerns our nation must face.

Other Causes of Mortality

Perhaps one of the most tragic causes of mortality and morbidity in our society is vehicular-related accidents. An estimated 40,000 people are killed and approximately 2,000,000 people are injured annually in vehicle-related accidents, a national tragedy. Safer roads and vehicles have led to reductions in vehicular mortality over the past twenty years. The tragic toll of motor vehicle accidents is reflected in Table 3.23. Those at highest risk are males, young adult drivers, and the oldest age groups.

Mortality attributable to firearms is another inexcusable national tragedy. Table 3.24 reflects mortality rates by age group due to firearms-related accidents and violence. This includes mortality associated with suicide, homicide, police intervention, and accidents. Approximately 20,000

Table 3.23. Death Rates for Motor Vehicle Crashes by Age: United States, Selected Years

| Age Group | Year (Deaths per 100,000 Resident Population) | |
	1950	2003
All ages, age adjusted	24.6	15.3
Under 1 year	8.4	3.6
1–4 years	11.5	3.9
5–14 years	8.8	4.0
15–24 years	34.4	26.6
25–34 years	24.6	17.1
35–44 years	20.3	15.7
45–54 years	22.2	14.9
55–64 years	29.0	14.2
65–74 years	39.1	16.2
75–84 years	52.7	24.9
85 years and over	45.1	28.8

Table 3.24. Death Rates for Firearm-related Injuries, According to Selected Sex, Race, and Age: United States, 2003

| Sex, Race, and Age | (Deaths per 100,000 Resident Population) | |
	White Male	Black Male
All ages, age adjusted	16.0	35.6
1–14 years	0.7	2.1
15–24 years	19.2	87.6
25–44 years	18.1	60.5
45–64 years	19.0	18.1
65 years and over	27.4	12.1

Americans are killed annually in firearms-related situations, with numerous others sustaining various injuries.

Violence in our society is also reflected in Table 3.25, which presents selected data on mortality attributable to homicide and legal intervention. These data partially overlap with firearms mortality when firearms are involved in the homicide or legal intervention.

Table 3.25. Death Rates for Homicide and Legal Intervention, According to Selected Sex, Race, and Age: United States, 2003

| Sex, Race, and Age | (Deaths per 100,000 Resident Population) | |
	White Male	Black Male
All ages, age adjusted	5.3	36.7
Under 1 year	8.1	17.8
1–14 years	0.9	4.1
15–24 years	10.6	84.6
25–44 years	7.7	61.0
45–64 years	4.2	22.2
65 years and over	2.7	10.9

Table 3.26. **Death Rates for Suicide, According to Sex and Age: United States, 2003**

Sex and Age	2003
Male	
All ages, age adjusted	18.0
5–14 years	0.9
15–24 years	16.0
25–44 years	21.9
45–64 years	23.5
65 years and over	29.8
85 years and over	47.8
Female	
All ages, age adjusted	4.2
5–14 years	0.3
15–24 years	3.0
25–44 years	5.7
45–64 years	7.0
65 years and over	3.8
85 years and over	3.3

Another disturbing source of mortality in our society is suicide. Table 3.26 presents mortality attributable to suicide for males and females by age group. As is evident from the data in this table, males have a much higher suicide rate than females, and suicide is not an infrequent source of mortality from the teens on upward in age, especially for males. The data are particularly striking for the oldest age group of males, age 85 and above. Some of these individuals are despondent, or they themselves or their spouses face serious illness.

As we seek to improve the quality and quantity of life in this country, we have to constantly appreciate the considerable morbidity and mortality attributable to social, economic, lifestyle, and other nonphysiological causes. Finding answers to problems of unhealthy diets and personal practices, consumption of alcohol, cigarettes, drugs, and other unhealthy substances, and the prevalence of social problems leading to violence in our society must be a high priority as we also seek biomedical solutions

to our physiological problems. At the same time, we also face a wide range of psychological and mental health problems that cause tremendous disruption in our lives and our society; these, too, must be addressed from both biomedical and social perspectives.

INCIDENCE OF INFECTIOUS DISEASES

Our nation is now largely spared the tragedies of many of the infectious diseases that are still prevalent throughout the world. However, not all infectious disease has been eradicated in this nation, and new challenges continue to surface.

Table 3.27 presents the incidence of infectious disease over the latter half of the twentieth century for the United States. The decline of many infectious diseases that are now avoidable through immunization and vaccination is evident in this table. At the same time, the table illustrates the continuing challenge of

Table 3.27. **Selected Notifiable Disease Cases: United States, Selected Years**

Disease	Year (Number of Cases)	
	1950	2003
Diphtheria	5,796	1
Hepatitis A	—	7,653
Hepatitis B	—	7,526
Mumps	—	231
Pertussis (whooping cough)	120,718	11,647
Poliomyelitis, total	33,300	—
Rubella (German measles)	—	7
Rubeola (measles)	319,124	56
Tuberculosis	121,742	14,874
Syphilis	217,558	34,270
Gonorrhea	286,746	335,104

many infectious diseases that remain, especially those associated with sexual activity.

Although not reflected in this table, the threat of terrorists using biological and chemical agents could change patterns of notifiable diseases in the future. Some biological agents such as smallpox and anthrax represent serious threats to our society if utilized by terrorists. The public health system of our nation has assumed an increasingly important role in preparing for this type of threat. The various biological agents that may be utilized by terrorist organizations have different vectors of transmission and represent a wide range of potential health effects, both short term and long term. In addition, the use of biological and/or chemical agents as well as other threats such as the use of nuclear materials could have secondary health impacts in our lives. The full range of potential ramifications from all these possibilities presents a very complex array of challenges for the nation's health and public health systems.

Likely further declines in reportable infectious diseases will occur with the use of immunizations for such diseases as chicken pox. For other diseases, such as gonorrhea, the challenge continues, particularly with physiologic resistance to many current drug treatments. And, of course, the AIDS epidemic dramatically illustrates the potential threat from new infectious diseases. Other particularly gruesome infectious diseases, such as the Ebola virus and SARS, have come to the forefront in recent years, clearly demonstrating how we can be challenged by disease even with the advancing state of our knowledge. Some, such as TB, are resistant to current treatments.

LIFESTYLE PATTERNS AND DISEASE

Numerous behaviors and lifestyle patterns affect our health. Examples discussed previously in this chapter include exposure to violence, vehicular accidents, alcohol, drugs, and infectious agents.

An excellent example of the association between disease and behavior is the consumption of tobacco products. Cigarette consumption has been associated with numerous illnesses, including cardiovascular disease, lung cancer, and oral cancer. Reduction in cigarette and other tobacco product consumption has been a national goal for 40 years.

Government policy has been directed toward reducing morbidity and mortality by intervening in people's destructive behavior. Interventions include the use of taxation, public education, and restrictions on product production and distribution.

A reduction in cigarette consumption in the United States has occurred during the period of aggressive intervention, as reflected in Table 3.28.

Table 3.28. Current Cigarette Smoking by Persons 18 Years of Age and Over, According to Sex and Age: United States, Selected Years

Sex and Age	Percent of Persons 18 Years of Age and Over	
	1965	2003
Males		
18 years and over, age adjusted	51.6	23.7
18–24 years	54.1	26.3
25–34 years	60.7	28.7
35–44 years	58.2	28.1
45–64 years	51.9	23.9
65 years and over	28.5	10.1
Females		
18 years and over, age adjusted	34.0	19.4
18–24 years	38.1	21.5
25–34 years	43.7	21.3
35–44 years	43.7	24.2
45–64 years	32.0	20.2
65 years and over	9.6	8.3

Many current smokers may be consuming greater quantities of tobacco products than the typical smoker did in past years. Many of those giving up tobacco products were casual users.

The net effect on morbidity and mortality from tobacco product consumption is difficult to estimate. However, any reduction in use of these products is positive for the nation's health overall, probably substantially so.

HEALTH, LIFESTYLE, AND SOCIAL STRUCTURE

The relationship between lifestyle and health is well established with regard to practices such as tobacco products consumption, as discussed previously. Numerous other lifestyle issues also significantly impact health. Alcohol consumption and illicit drug use are examples of personal decision making and patterns of behavior that have tremendous adverse effects on health and on the nation's economy.

Alcohol consumption, beyond a moderate level, is associated with numerous physiological complications including cirrhosis of the liver, various cancers, intestinal disorders, and brain function deterioration. Equally severe psychological and social complications ranging from divorce to poor job performance are also common. Alcohol abuse results in illness and injury to others, including—but certainly not limited to—vehicular accidents, workplace injuries, poor fetal outcomes associated with fetal alcohol syndrome, and spousal and child abuse.

Like alcohol abuse, illicit drug use results in a spectrum of adverse consequences for our society. In addition to many of the adverse consequences already mentioned for alcohol abuse, illicit drug use leads to high levels of violent crime, general social dysfunction, and many other untoward consequences.

The implications of tobacco, alcohol, and drug abuse alone are wide-ranging and contribute to the destruction of the fabric of our society and of individuals' lives. And these three areas constitute only

a portion of dysfunctional behavior that impinges on health, with consequent increased morbidity and mortality.

The range of other behaviors that adversely affect health is tremendous. Enhanced morbidity and mortality have been associated with various complications of dietary behaviors such as elevated consumption of fat, sodium, and sugar, leading to an epidemic of obesity and associated problems. Sexual behaviors are associated with the spread of communicable diseases such as AIDS, gonorrhea, syphilis, and other sexually transmitted diseases, leading to increased levels of infertility, cancer, and other complications. Societal stress is associated with deterioration of the immune system and consequent morbidity and mortality, workplace violence, marital difficulties, spousal abuse, and other problems.

Thus, the etiology of much of our morbidity and mortality can be traced to behavior, social interaction, lifestyle, and other nonphysiological determinants. Solving the primary physiological causes of illness and disease may be easier than adequately addressing these social and behavioral ones. The challenges to modify behavior are great, and the complications introduced by our modern society make the task ever-more difficult. As we move through the new century, the failure of our society in the twentieth century to adequately address the social, behavioral, and economic causes of disease and illness will continue to haunt us.

MEASURING THE IMPACT OF ILLNESS ON SOCIETY

The impact of health, disease, and illness and the measurement of these effects have tremendous power in aiding the allocation of resources and in assessing the relative importance of various diseases, from both human and financial perspectives. Many quantitative approaches to measuring the impact of disease and illness on human populations have been developed, some of which are illustrated in this section of the chapter to provide a perspective on the relevance and methodologies for such efforts. Resource allocation and policy analysis exercises in particular can benefit from these approaches to quantifying the impact of disease. Such effort is not intended to draw attention away from the personal aspects of disease and illness, but rather to facilitate an analytic and objective assessment of the relative impact of different threats to our population. The analyses include such economic techniques as cost-benefit analysis and the illustrations presented in this section are in no way intended to comprehensively review all the techniques applicable to these kinds of analyses.

Measuring how people perceive their own health is one of the many approaches utilized in assessing the impact of illness and disease on a population. Although this approach can be utilized for specific disease conditions, it is also beneficial in looking at differential health status across various population groups as a means to measure the aggregate impact of illness in the population.

Table 3.29 presents self-assessed health status among selected population groups over a 10-year time period. Substantial differences in self-assessed health status, as measured by the percent of individuals reporting fair or poor health, is evident among different age, race, and income groups as measured by poverty status. Changes over time have not been as dramatic as these subgroup differentials. The impact of illness and disease clearly increases significantly with age and is greater for certain minority groups than for whites. The difference by sex is nominal.

Another indicator of the impact of illness and disease on populations is reflected in Table 3.30. For selected causes of death the number of years of life lost to the U.S. population by population subgroup is presented. In other words, the number of years of life lost from people dying from diseases of the heart in the white population subgroup is approximately 1,115 lost before age 75 for every 100,000 population under age 75. This is one of a number of indicators of the impact on longevity

Table 3.29. Self-Assessed Health Status According to Selected Characteristics: United States, Selected Years

Characteristic	1991	2001
	\multicolumn{2}{c}{Percent of persons with fair or poor health}	
Age		
Under 18 years	2.6	1.8
18–44 years	6.1	5.4
45–54 years	13.4	11.7
55–64 years	20.7	19.2
65 years and over	29.0	26.6
Sex		
Male	10.0	9.0
Female	10.8	9.5
Race		
White	9.6	8.2
Black	16.8	15.4
Asian only	7.8	8.1
Poverty status		
Poor	22.8	21.0
Near poor	14.7	15.5
Nonpoor	6.8	6.2

from each of the listed causes of death. If this cause of death did not exist, the number of years of life that the population would live before dying from other causes of death would be higher for every 100,000 people by the indicated number of years. Years of life lost by population group and disease category provide a relative measure of the impact, almost in practical human terms, of each disease category on our life spans in this country. The relative impact of each disease is also measurable for various population subgroups such as for race groups, as indicated in this table.

The impact of illness and disease can be measured in other ways as well. For example, the days of disability attributable to various ailments can be estimated. Disability days attributable to influenza, arthritis, or other diseases can reflect the relative

Table 3.30. Years of Potential Life Lost before Age 75 for Selected Causes of Death, According to Race: United States, Selected Years 1980, 2001

Race and Cause of Death	1980	2001	Race and Cause of Death	1980	2001
	Age-adjusted years lost before age 75 per 100,000 population under 75 years of age			Age-adjusted years lost before age 75 per 100,000 population under 75 years of age	
White Males			*Black Males*		
All causes	9,554.1	6,941.6	All causes	17,873.4	12,579.7
Diseases of heart	2,100.8	1,115.0	Diseases of heart	3,619.9	2,248.9
Ischemic heart disease	1,682.7	773.0	Ischemic heart disease	2,305.1	1,260.6
Cerebrovascular diseases	300.7	175.6	Cerebrovascular diseases	883.2	491.3
Malignant neoplasms	2,035.9	1,610.2	Malignant neoplasms	2,946.1	2,228.4
Trachea, bronchus, and lung	529.9	427.5	Trachea, bronchus, and lung	776.0	557.5
Colorectal	186.8	135.0	Colorectal	232.3	219.6
Prostate	74.8	53.1	Prostate	200.3	164.1
Chronic lower respiratory diseases	165.4	184.7	Chronic lower respiratory diseases	203.7	220.5
Influenza and pneumonia	130.8	72.7	Influenza and pneumonia	384.9	152.1
Chronic liver disease and cirrhosis	257.3	164.4	Chronic liver disease and cirrhosis	644.0	181.5
Diabetes mellitus	115.7	156.2	Diabetes mellitus	305.3	392.6
Human immunodeficiency virus (HIV) disease	—	88.4	Human immunodeficiency virus (HIV) disease	—	743.5
Unintentional injuries	1,520.4	1,049.0	Unintentional injuries	1,751.5	1,133.4
Motor vehicle-related injuries	939.9	585.1	Motor vehicle-related injuries	750.2	571.7
Suicide	414.5	373.5	Suicide	238.0	201.5
Homicide	271.7	204.0	Homicide	1,580.8	963.6

impact on disability as compared to mortality for each of these disease categories. Other measures of the impact of disease might include days of work lost attributable to each disease category. Thus, various measures of mortality and morbidity impact for each disease or disease category by population subgroup can provide significant insight into broader issues of the impact of health and disease. Economists may carry these analyses further by translating these measures into financial assessments such as, for example, measuring the cost of lower productivity or reduced revenue in a production setting from these days of work lost.

Measuring the impact of disease and illness is essential in establishing national priorities for research and for delivery of health care services.

Such analyses can facilitate the establishment of criteria for the allocation of dollars and can measure the relative importance of disease entities in financial and human terms.

ACCESS TO HEALTH CARE SERVICES

As mentioned previously, various aspects of the measurement and assessment of access to health care services are extremely important in assessing the health care system's response to disease and illness and to the development of national health policy. Assessing access to health care services can facilitate the determination of the degree to which the system responds to both consumer and professional assessments of need and demand for health care. Differentials in the measurement of access between population groups can reflect issues of equitable access to care and failures of the health care system to respond to perceived or actual needs on the part of consumers. Access trends over time, likewise, can reflect changes in the functioning of the health care system and its effectiveness in addressing the needs of the population.

The concluding section of this chapter addresses issues of access to care, a core theme of this book, particularly as reflected in utilization of care in response to perceived needs by individuals with various diseases and illnesses. Trends in access to care, like trends in disease and illness patterns, are key assessment variables in our monitoring and evaluation of the health care system over time.

Models of Access

Numerous quantitative models of health services access have been developed over the years. These models typically emanate from analytical assessments based on psychological, sociological, financial and economic, or psychological perspectives and assessments of individual's access to health care services. Some researchers have attempted to provide more comprehensive and integrated models of access by combining a variety of perspectives as well.

As might be expected, discipline-oriented models of access to care reflect the variables typically assessed by such a disciplinary researcher. For example, sociological models of access to health care typically examine sociological variables such as population characteristics and interpersonal relationships and influences. Psychological models of access would focus more typically on perceptions by patients of severity of illness, health beliefs, attitudes and values, and health knowledge. Economic models of utilization and access typically address such factors as insurance coverage and income, health systems organization, and financing arrangements. Table 3.31 lists illustrative variables

Table 3.31. Discipline Oriented Models of Access to Care

Discipline	Variables
Demographic	Age, sex, marital status, family size, residence
Social structural	Social class, ethnicity, education, occupation
Social psychological	Health beliefs, values, attitudes, norms, culture
Economic	Family income, insurance coverage, prices of services, provider/population ratios
Organizational	Organization of physicians' practices, referral patterns, use of ancillaries, regular source of care
Systems	All or most of the above

typically measured by each discipline's approach to assessing health system access.

In most instances, for the variables listed in Table 3.31, extensive and relatively expensive survey questionnaires are required to collect and process the information necessary for the conduct of the analysis. In reality, and from a practical perspective, demographic, financial, and patient variables are those that are most typically utilized in assessing access to health care on an ongoing basis. These utilization variables are usually obtained from enrolled client populations in health services plans or from large-scale national surveys conducted by the federal government or by other organizations.

The predictive power of many models of utilization and their ability to influence national health policy are somewhat limited. And the often high costs associated with collecting and analyzing the data limit their actual application. Newer practice information systems are facilitating data collection and analysis. These models are valuable in providing a mechanism or forum through which to analyze issues of access and national health policy. The conceptualization of access to care and, even in a limited analysis, the use of some discreet readily available measures of utilization do provide valuable insight into access concerns that our nation faces.

As noted earlier, many complex models of access to health care have been developed, primarily by academic researchers, over the years. These include behavioral and sociological models that focus on the health behaviors of various population groups modified by their environments. These environmental factors include such measures as economic well-being and perceptions of health status. Measuring many of these variables is difficult and potentially expensive on an ongoing basis. But, as noted previously, these models hold great value in helping us understand how the health care system responds to consumer needs.

Many models, particularly those using sociological and economic concepts, focus on the resources available in the health care system and their organizational and financial arrangements. Characteristics of the population under scrutiny are also included in many models of utilization and access. Personal characteristics include such factors as health practices and prior utilization as well as demographic variables. Social structure and an individual's response to his or her environment may also be measured in the context of his or her ability to cope with health problems. Interaction with other individuals, other social influences, and social and cultural backgrounds may be considered as well. Health beliefs, attitudes, and knowledge have a significant effect on how an individual responds to health care needs and to signs and symptoms.

Many access models include a careful examination of the availability of community and personal resources. These variables include supply measures such as the availability of physicians and hospitals. They also include individuals' financial access to care as measured by income, health insurance, the availability of regular sources of care, and other practical considerations. Managed-care arrangements and other characteristics of the health care system are also considered in the development of these models.

Analysis of access to care frequently addresses professional assessments by physicians, nurses, and other health care practitioners of a patient's signs and symptoms of illness. Some models seek to incorporate patients' own perceptions of their health care needs, separate from professional evaluations. Professional assessments include quantitative assessments as a result of a physical exam or the conduct of laboratory tests. Numerous other aspects of professional assessment may also be included in more sophisticated modeling. Of course,

Table 3.32. No Usual Source of Health Care Among Children, Selected Characteristics: United States, Average Annual 2002–2003

Characteristic	Under 18 Years of Age	Under 6 Years of Age
	Percent Without Usual Source	
All children	5.7	4.1
Race		
White	5.2	3.9
Black	6.7	3.3
American Indian or Alaska Native	*	*
Asian	10.3	*
Race and Hispanic origin		
White, non-Hispanic	3.4	2.7
Black, non-Hispanic	6.7	3.3
Hispanic	12.1	8.3
Poverty status		
Poor	10.6	7.1
Nonpoor	3.3	1.9
Health insurance status		
Insured	3.1	2.0
Private	2.4	1.3
Medicaid	5.0	3.3
Uninsured	29.2	25.5

*Too small sample.

professional assessment of individual needs may differ from the patient's own perceptions of what kind of care he or she needs.

Actual Measures of Access to Care

More common measures of access to health care services are used in this section to illustrate access and to examine trends over time. Selected measures of access are presented for the usual sources of care among children, use of mammography, and dental visits for selected United States populations.

Table 3.32 illustrates the increased availability, as measured by having a usual source of care, of health care services for white as compared to minority children. Lower income individuals also have less access to care as measured by this indicator.

Finally, Table 3.33 measures access to dental services. Again, poorer people have lower access as measured by visits in the prior year. While these data do not adjust for dental health need, it is likely that lower income individuals do have poorer dental health.

Extensive data are available from various surveys, especially those conducted by the federal government, for tracking changes in access to care for various population groups. This information is extremely valuable for national policy making and to contribute to the overall debate about the design of the health care system. Examples of current access-related issues reflected in these data would include lack of access to dental care for individuals without financial resources (a considerable percentage of the population, which is currently increasing); having no insurance coverage (or who are underinsured for

Table 3.33. Dental Visits in the Past Year According to Patient Characteristics: United States, 2003

Characteristic	2–17 Years of Age	18–64 Years of Age	65 Years of Age and Over
Total	75.0	64.8	58.0
Sex			
Male	74.1	60.9	58.4
Female	75.9	68.6	57.7
Race			
White	76.0	65.9	59.8
Black	70.5	58.1	38.7
American Indian or Alaska Native	69.9	58.0	49.2
Asian	72.9	63.6	57.4
Race and Hispanic origin			
White, non-Hispanic	79.4	69.3	60.9
Black, non-Hispanic	70.6	58.3	38.3
Hispanic	64.5	48.3	46.0
Poverty status			
Poor	65.8	44.5	37.1
Nonpoor	80.8	72.0	67.8

health care services); and lack of adequate access to health care in the areas of long-term care and mental health services.

Access is a key issue that has challenged our nation's health care system throughout history. As a nation, we have long struggled with issues of who has the right to access which health care services and under what conditions. Assuring adequate access to care is an issue that permeates all aspects of health care policy and delivery.

Managed-care organizations constantly struggle with the trade-offs involved in controlling access to care versus assuming increased costs. Social programs have long addressed issues of access. Medicare and Medicaid, as social programs, had their origins in the realization that access to health care for some population groups did not meet national social goals.

The formulation and measurement of indicators of access to care is a challenging area for health services researchers, but one that contributes substantially to improving the operation of the health care system. Addressing the challenges of access provides a key focal point for constant analysis of the nature of the health care system and our national goals for that system. Ultimately, it is the issues of access and cost that we must successfully address to ensure that all citizens receive a level of health care services adequate for their most fundamental needs. It is also important to recognize that issues of access are intimately connected to factors associated with the quality of care, with satisfaction on the part of providers and consumers, and with national, political, economic, and social goals.

SUMMARY

This chapter has traced many of the primary patterns of population dynamics and illness in our society during the twentieth century. A fundamental understanding of these trends is essential in interpreting the optimal structure of health services delivery systems as discussed in the remainder of this book. Understanding the relationships between these epidemiological trends and the physiological and psychological nature of the human body and of the determinants of health services utilization is important in defining the overall nature of a population's use of health care and, in turn, forms the basis for the organization and financing, and eventually evaluation, of that system.

REVIEW QUESTIONS

1. Describe the major trends in population demographics over the past 80 years.
2. How have fertility rates changed since the World War II?
3. What are the most important trends in mortality over the past century?
4. What disease patterns would you anticipate occurring over the next 30 years?
5. How do changes in disease incidence and prevalence translate into health care utilization patterns?

REFERENCES & ADDITIONAL READINGS

Bailey, P. G. (2005). Medicare and national coverage. *Health Affairs, 24,* 295–296.

Bloche, M. G. (2004). Healthcare disparities—science, politics and race. *New England Journal of Medicine, 350,* 1486–1488.

Cunningham, P., & Hadley, J. (2004). Expanding care versus expanding coverage: How to improve access to care. *Health Affairs, 23,* 234–244.

Zuckerman, S., & Shen, Y. C. (2004). Characteristics of occasional and frequent emergency department users: Do insurance coverage and access to care matter? *Medical Care., 42,* 176–182.

PART TWO

Financing and Structuring Health Care

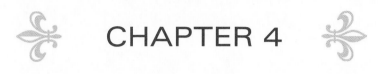

CHAPTER 4

Financing Health Systems

Alma Koch

CHAPTER TOPICS

- Health Expenditures
- Health Insurance
- Medicare
- Medicaid
- Physician Reimbursement
- Initiatives in Health Care Finance
- Strategies for Health Care Reform

LEARNING OBJECTIVES

Upon completing this chapter, the reader should be able to

1. Understand national health expenditures.
2. Understand governmental health plan programs.
3. Analyze provider reimbursement mechanisms.
4. Analyze health care reform.
5. Conceptualize avenues for improving health insurance plans.

The system for financing health services in the United States reflects the fragmentation of health care as a whole. It is a patchwork of financing mechanisms varying by sponsorship and provider type. It also reflects the age, health, and economic status of the specific patient groups that are being served. In view of the growing number of Americans who are uninsured for health care, one may say that it is a disappointing financing system. However, these observations do provide a touch point for studying the financing apparatus as it now exists. If one looks at the "system" in light of the role of tradition and the values of the American people, as well as the political philosophy of the times, the organization of health finance in the United States comes into better focus.

This chapter examines the size and scope of the health care financing system in the United States. Special attention will be paid to differences and similarities in the public and private financing components of the system, reimbursement of various provider categories, and trends that we may expect to see in the future.

HEALTH EXPENDITURES

Size of the U.S. Health Care Industry

The health care industry is the largest service employer in the country. In the number of people employed, the health care industry ranks second after total durable and nondurable goods manufacturing (U.S. Census Bureau, 2004–2005). In 2004, Americans spent $1.878 trillion on health care, comprising 16 percent of the gross domestic product (GDP) and amounting to $6,280 per capita (Smith et al., 2006). The United States spends far more on health care than other industrialized countries. For example, in 2000–2001, the United Kingdom and Japan fell at the lower end of the spectrum, spending 7.6 percent of their respective GDPs on health

care. Canada, France, Germany, and Switzerland, came closer to U.S. figures with 9.7, 9.5, 10.7, and 10.9 percent of their respective GDPs spent on health, with most other industrialized nations falling in the established range (U.S. Census Bureau, 2004–2005).

Growth in Health Expenditures

Since 1940, national health expenditures have grown at a rate substantially outpacing the gross domestic product (GDP). Table 4.1 shows that prior to World War II, only 4 percent of the GDP was devoted to health care, both public and private. By 2004, the proportion of the GDP expended for health care increased by 12 percentage points. Since the onset of Medicare and Medicaid in mid-1966, national health expenditures have grown particularly rapidly, from about 6.3 percent of the GDP to the present figure. Most of this growth is explained by increased intensity in the provision of health care services, excess medical inflation, and the aging of the U.S. population. Only a small fraction of growth in health care can be attributed to actual growth in the U.S. population. This brief stability in the 1990s was precipitated both by a slowdown in the rate of growth of health care spending and an upswing in overall economic growth. During the recession of the early 2000s, health care continued to grow as the economy slowed. Since 2000, health care spending has risen a whopping 2.2 percentage points, ending a six-year period of relative stability at around 13.5 to 13.8 percent of the GDP.

A variety of qualitative factors is believed to have contributed to the disproportionate growth in health care spending relative to the growth in GDP. These include (1) rapid development and dissemination of medical technology that expanded the treatment of disease, (2) rising expectations about the value of health care services, (3) government financing of health care services, (4) the nature of third-party reimbursement, (5) the growth in the proportion of elderly, (6) the lack of competitive forces in the health care system to increase efficiency and productivity in the delivery of services,

Table 4.1. Aggregate and Per Capita National Health Expenditures, United States, Selected Years

Year	Total (Billions)	Per Capita	GDP (Billions)	Percent of GDP
1940	$4.0	$30	$100	4.0
1950	$12.7	$82	$287	4.4
1960	$26.9	$141	$527	5.1
1970	$73.2	$341	$1,036	7.1
1980	$247.2	$1,052	$2,784	8.9
1990	$699.4	$2,689	$5,744	12.2
2000	$1,358.5	$4,729	$9,817	13.8
2004	$1,877.6	$6,280	$11,734	16.0

SOURCE: Adapted from "National Health Spending in 2004: Recent Slowdown Led by Prescription Drug Spending," by C. Smith et al., 2006, *Health Affairs, 25*(1), p. 187.

and (7) the maldistribution of physicians and other providers of health services.

Monetary Flow

Payment Sources

Figure 4.1 quantifies the monetary inflow (i.e., "Where it came from") and outflow (i.e., "Where it went") in the United States for total health spending in 2004. Private health insurance finances 37 percent of all health expenditures, with out-of-pocket payment financing another 13 percent. These private sources, together with other (mostly philanthropic) sources, account for the 54 percent of all health expenditures that are privately financed in the United States. The other 46 percent is financed publicly by federal, state, or local governments. The largest single public program is Medicare (the federal social security health insurance plan for the elderly, the disabled, and other groups), followed closely in size by Medicaid (the federal/state welfare program for health care), and other government programs.

Spending for Medicare and Medicaid has been increasing even more rapidly than total national health expenditures. In 2004, Medicare and Medicaid together comprised 35 percent of the total health care bill; in 1967 the two programs represented only 15 percent of the total health care bill. Out of approximately 288 million people in the

United States in 2002, over 31 percent (91 million people) were enrolled in either or both programs. Medicare's role was clearly most substantial for hospital care; Medicaid's role was most prominent for nursing home care, and the growth in these two services has indubitably been spurred on by the two public programs.

Outlays

In terms of outlays, 41 percent of the money spent for health in 2004 was used to purchase hospital and nursing home services, although hospital expenditures, which totaled $571 billion, have dropped substantially as a proportion of health care expenditures in the past 20 years. Another 40 percent was divided among physicians' services and other personal care items (i.e., dental services, other professional services, vision services, home health care, drugs, eyeglasses and appliances, and other miscellaneous health care services and products). While physician services have increased slightly over the years, "other" health care costs have burgeoned. Prescription drugs, with 11 percent, has been on the rise in recent years. The remaining 8 percent goes for administration and health insurance.

Personal Health Care

Figure 4.2 shows financing trends since 1950 for personal health care expenditures (PHCE), which

Where It Came From

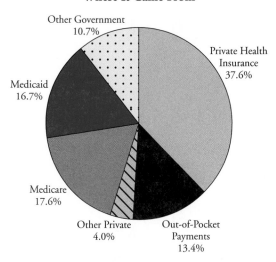

Where It Went

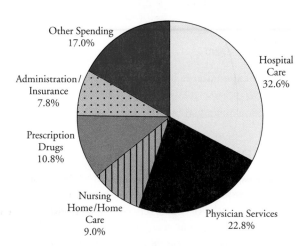

Figure 4.1. The Nation's Health Dollar, 2004

SOURCE: Adapted from "National Health Spending in 2004: Recent Slowdown Led by Prescription Drug Spending," by C. Smith et al., Jan./Feb. 2006, *Health Affairs, 25*(1), p. 187.

include total health expenditures minus program administration, public health activities, research, and construction. Government plus private insurance have grown enormously in the postwar era, funding about 80 percent of all PHCE. Direct payments by

patients have dropped commensurately to about 15 percent of PHCE (Smith et al., 2006).

For 2004, sources of funding for major providers of PHCE are depicted in Figure 4.3. Government funding dominates hospital reimbursement with 56 percent financed by Medicare, Medicaid, and other government programs, in that order. Another 36 percent of the national hospital bill is footed by private health insurance. Physician outlays are clearly dominated by the private sector. Private insurance, direct patient payments, and other private sources account for more than 66 percent of physician funding; Medicare, which in recent years has diminished as a financier of physicians' services, picks up another 20 percent. Nursing home funding reflects the "rich man, poor man" dichotomy of the long-term care industry, wherein patients must "spend down" their assets in order to qualify for government assistance. About 70 percent of nursing home revenues are funded by direct patient payment and Medicaid. Private long-term care insurance, which was practically nonexistent 10 years ago, has skyrocketed to 8 percent of nursing home funding. Medicare's share of nursing home funding is not for long-term care; Medicare pays for short-term nursing care in skilled nursing facilities for patients who can be rehabilitated.

HEALTH INSURANCE

Origins of Health Insurance

Health insurance originated in Europe in the early 1800s when mutual benefit societies arose to lighten the financial burden for those stricken with illness. The focus was on low-skilled, low-income workers who were industrially employed. (Providers in Europe wanted to keep high-skilled employees in the private medical market.) The first government health insurance program arose in Germany in 1840, mandating workers below a certain income level to belong to a "sickness fund." The concept of health insurance as linked to employment in the industrial sector persists internationally to this day.

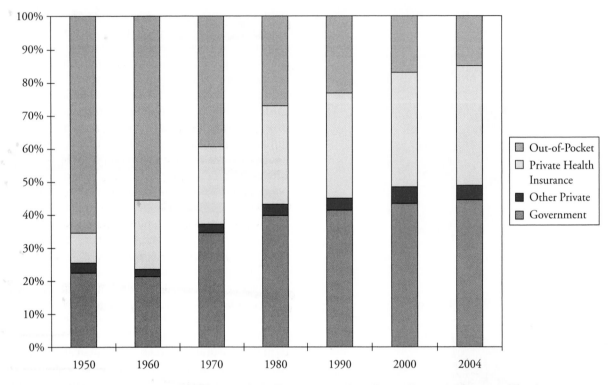

Figure 4.2. **Percentage Distribution of U.S. Personal Health Care Expenditures by Source of Funds, Selected Years**

SOURCE: Adapted from "National Health Spending in 2004: Recent Slowdown Led by Prescription Drug Spending," by C. Smith et al., Jan./Feb. 2006, *Health Affairs*, *25*(1), p. 191.

The health insurance networks of many nations grew out of this linkage and still reflect an emphasis on nonagricultural employment and coverage of the worker, irrespective of dependents (Roemer, 1977; Roemer, 1978).

Today in the United States, the framework of health insurance stems clearly from its European antecedents and breaks down into three categories which, in some sense, reflect employment status. Voluntary health insurance (VHI) is private health insurance usually denoting current industrial employment; social health insurance (SHI) reflects participation in a government entitlement program linked to previous (or current) employment; public welfare health care programs connote lack of employment, low-income employment, or the inability to gain employment stemming from a disabling condition.

Distributing Risk

Insurance is a way of pooling or distributing risk. Risk is the probability of incurring a loss. Risk stems from two kinds of occurrences: (1) unanticipated events such as fires, car accidents, or airplane crashes, and (2) anticipated events such as death, old age, and sickness. Health or, more correctly, illness is an anticipated event associated with old age and death. Thus, we know that illness is a likely event, but we don't know when it will strike, to whom it will happen, or how severe it will be. Therefore, health is uncertain for the individual, but not for a group. Groups are actuarially (i.e., statistically) predictable.

Moral Hazard

In the theory of insurance, it is assumed that risks are independent of each other: (1) What befalls one

Hospitals

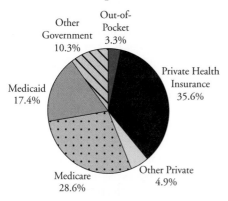

Physicians

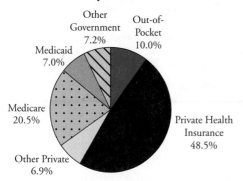

Nursing Homes

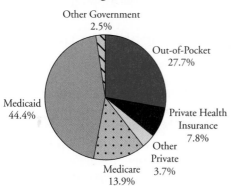

Figure 4.3. Personal Health Care Expenditures for Total U.S. Population by Type of Service and Source of Funds

SOURCE: Adapted from "National Health Spending in 2004: Recent Slowdown Led by Prescription Drug Spending," by C. Smith et al., Jan./Feb. 2006, *Health Affairs, 25*(1), p. 191.

person does not affect another, and (2) that for a single individual, risks are independent. Neither assumptions are true in health insurance because one person's sickness may spread contagiously and illness in one part of the body may weaken another part. These phenomena, together with the moral hazard inherent in medical care, make health insurance and health costs, in general, extremely volatile. Moral hazard means that, to the extent that the event insured against can be controlled, there exists a temptation to use the insurance. (The classic example of moral hazard is setting fire to a failing business in order to collect the insurance.) Health insurance usage is highly discretionary; doctors and patients can conspire (intentionally or not) to use the insurance. An example is where a private patient with a traditional type of policy is kept in the hospital an extra day because it would be difficult or inconvenient for the family to receive the patient back home on the earliest possible discharge day. In this example, the insured extra day in the hospital, at a cost of $900 or more to the carrier, saves a loss in earnings for the family, and the expense is borne by purchasers of the policy, as reflected in the price of the premium.

Benefit Structure

Because of moral hazard, health insurance usually pays less than the total loss incurred by levying out-of-pocket or direct costs on the patient. In fee-for-service provider reimbursement, these take the form of deductibles and copayments. A deductible is a sum of money that must be paid, typically every year, before the insurance policy becomes active. Deductibles have long been criticized in health insurance for posing an impediment to first-contact care, discouraging the patient from seeking care until the condition becomes severe. Since higher costs may be incurred for more severe illness, deductibles have been postulated to contribute to health cost inflation, rather then stimulating parsimonious consumer utilization. A copayment is paid as the beneficiary uses the insurance. For example, in a policy with a traditional indemnity benefit, a fixed cash amount is paid to the beneficiary per procedure or per day in the hospital (e.g., $800 for a one-night stay in the hospital following a hernia repair). If the hospital charges $1,100, then the patient must pay a copayment of $300. Thus the patient is liable for any amount in excess of the indemnity payment. An insurance plan with a service benefit reimburses on a percentage basis and the patient pays coinsurance. Using the preceding example, the insurance plan would pay 80% or $880 of the surgeon's charges, leaving only $220 in coinsurance to be paid by the patient. Thus, if the percentage rate is high, the reimbursement structure of service benefits usually works to the patient's advantage compared to indemnity benefits.

Pure types of indemnity or service benefits are becoming increasingly rare. Nowadays, to control health cost inflation, there is a growing trend toward hybrid benefit structures, combining both service and indemnity features. A plan may, for example, pay a percentage of charges up to a specified limit, beyond which point the patient becomes responsible for the balance. Preferred provider organizations (PPOs) utilize this technique, often in concert with low price ceilings, to reimburse nonparticipating providers. Using the example again, the PPO might pay 80% up to an $800 limit on charges for a nonparticipating hospital. The plan would pay $640 and the patient would thus incur a $460 copayment. However, if the patient utilizes a hospital participating in the PPO, the plan might pay 90 percent of the discounted fee of $1,000 (i.e., a contractually determined "allowed amount" of $900), resulting in a copayment of only $100 for the patient.

Premium Determination

Due to the financial implications of choosing one type of health insurance plan over another and because the possibility of moral hazard is a real one in health care utilization, health insurance plans are particularly vulnerable to the phenomenon of adverse selection. Adverse selection may be at work when an insurance policy experiences a higher number of claims due to sickness than would be probable on a random basis. If an employee is offered an alternate choice of plans, for example, a "sicker"

person or a potentially higher utilizer of health care services is likely to elect the plan with more generous provisions (i.e., lower deductible, copayments, and limitations or fewer exclusions), even if the employee's share of the premium is higher. Therefore, more liberal fee-for-service plans may experience an adverse selection of sicker enrollees compared to a more restrictive managed care plan, such as a PPO, or a health maintenance organization (HMO). This may result in ever-spiraling claims for the liberal plan as costlier people join and as healthier individuals defect to the lower-cost alternative plans.

Because of adverse selection, most health insurance plans today are experience rated: The premiums are based on the demographic characteristics, such as age and sexual composition, of the employer group or on the actual experience of the group in that plan in prior years. Community rating, originated by Blue Cross and Blue Shield (the Blues), bases premiums upon the wider utilization of the defined geographic area (e.g., census tracts, city, county, etc.). Today, most fee-for-service plans are experience rated, even the Blues, which must contend with stiff price competition from commercial carriers. HMOs use community ratings more widely for their enrolled groups than commercial carriers, but even this is fading as HMOs face stiff price competition in the for-profit arena.

Voluntary Health Insurance

Voluntary or private health insurance (VHI) in the United States can be subdivided into three distinct categories: (1) Blue Cross and Blue Shield, (2) private or commercial insurance companies, and (3) health maintenance organizations. The respective sponsorships of these types of VHI may be providers, third parties or middlemen, and patients or independent carriers. Nowadays, it is common for the Blues and commercials to own and operate HMOs and other managed care plans.

Growth and Development

The year 1929 was a landmark year for VHI. In spite of active opposition from the American Medical

Association (AMA) to any type of health insurance from 1920 onward, both Blue Cross and the HMO movement got their start in this last pre-Depression year. Blue Cross was initiated by Baylor teachers in Dallas, Texas, who organized to provide hospital care for three cents a day. Michigan and New Jersey were next in the movement for hospital insurance. In 1934, the depths of the revenue depression for hospitals, the American Hospital Association (AHA) united these plans into the Blue Cross network. Today Blue Cross has broken away from its original AHA sponsorship, but the hospital-sponsored underpinnings remain strong in many locales (Roemer, 1977; Roemer, 1978).

In Oklahoma also in 1929, the Farmer's Union started its Cooperative Health Association, the first HMO. Independently, in the same year in Los Angeles, two Canadian physicians founded the Ross-Loos group practice and sold the first doctor-sponsored health insurance plan with prepayment to the Department of Water and Power and Los Angeles City workers.

As these and other plans grew during the 1930s, the AMA reversed its opposition to VHI in response to dwindling physician and hospital incomes and, in 1939, the California Medical Society developed and sponsored a plan known as Blue Shield to pay doctor's bills in a hospitalized environment (Roemer, 1977; Roemer, 1978).

By 1946, private health insurance plans were experiencing astronomical growth as wage and price restrictions in the post–World War II period spurred the growth of fringe benefits, especially in unionized industries. Insurance companies, already having the inside track in sales and actuarial information in life insurance, went headlong into the health insurance business in competition with Blue Cross and Blue Shield.

Population Coverage

About 85 percent of the entire U.S. population in 2002 was covered by some type of health insurance, including private health insurance and public programs. In 2002, about 71 percent of the U.S. population under 65 had some form of VHI, more than 93 percent of whom had their health insurance linked to group health policies (usually linked to employment) (U.S. Census Bureau, 2004–2005). Firms that do not offer any health benefits at all tend to be small and nonunionized, hire seasonal workers, and employ relatively large numbers of low-wage employees with no college education. About 64 percent of the elderly, who with few exceptions are covered by Medicare, hold private insurance coverage (known as "Medigap" insurance) to supplement their Medicare benefits.

An unfortunate effect of employment-linked private health insurance is that people who are least able to pay for health care have the least insurance due to lack of employment (or full-time employment). The alternatives for these people are to purchase a nongroup or individual plan, usually a less generous and more expensive option in terms of out-of-pocket premiums, or to accept the risk of doing without any health insurance. Estimates vary, but according to the U.S. Census Bureau (2004–2005), about 15.2 percent of the total U.S. population in 2002 (44 million people) had no health insurance coverage at all, either public or private, for the entire year.

Benefits

Private health insurance coverage varies widely in terms of benefits provided, the extent of reimbursement for covered services, and exclusions or limitations. General health insurance plans are designed to provide limited protection for the most expensive services and usually cover inpatient hospital and physician services, and outpatient hospital services, including laboratory procedures. Limits may apply to a group of related services such as those provided during the course of a hospitalization. The most commonly covered services for the privately insured are linked to inpatient hospitalization: room and board, surgeons' and other physicians' fees, and outpatient diagnostic services.

Most comprehensive health insurance policies extend basic benefits to such services as physician office visits, outpatient mental health care, prescribed medicines, durable equipment and supplies, ambulance services, and the like. Thus, they are designed to protect against large medical bills as well as many expenses associated with routine types of medical care. For a typical claim, the insurer typically pays a specified share of total covered expenses (e.g., amounting to 75 percent or more of the bill). The patient pays the remainder or copayment. The beneficiary also pays a deductible amount—typically $300 for an individual or $600 for a family—at the beginning of each year. Deductibles and copayments comprise the share of the expenses not covered by the health insurance plan, subject to a maximum amount known as the "out-of-pocket limit" or "stop-loss provision." A limit of this kind may range from $1,500 to $3,000. The deductible and other provisions apply to expenses for all covered services. In contrast, Medigap plans, often purchased by Medicare enrollees, are designed to reimburse only the deductibles and copayments associated with Medicare covered services.

Hospital indemnity plans are another type of private insurance coverage that is noteworthy. Hospital indemnity plans offer specified cash payments (e.g., $200 per day) for each day of inpatient hospitalization, regardless of the expenses actually incurred. Thus, it is a type of disability insurance wherein the payment is not linked to the amount or type of medical services provided, but rather to length of the hospital stay, and the payment is not generous in relation to the actual hospital expenses.

Prepaid Plans

HMOs and similar prepaid plans provide fairly comprehensive coverage in return for a prepaid fee, usually without deductibles and coinsurance for most services. Therefore, HMOs offer coverage against the risk of large health care financial losses. Prepaid health plans peaked in enrollment in 2000 and have been losing membership ever since. In 2003, there were about 454 HMOs in the United States, covering about 72 million people, or about one-quarter of the population (U.S. Census Bureau, 2004–2005). This compares to about 50 HMOs in

1973, prior to the passage of the HMO Act, which required employers with over 25 employees to offer a dual choice of health plans including one HMO, if one was available locally.

It was anticipated that the concept would foster incentives toward prevention and cost consciousness on the part of physicians who are encouraged to be frugal in the use of secondary services, particularly hospitalization. However, because the prepayment of premium did not necessarily translate into capitated provider reimbursement and tight prospective budgeting, cost-containment experience is mixed due to legislative and economic incentives that are sometimes perverse (Hillman, Welch, & Pauly, 1992).

Social Health Insurance

The U.S. government sponsors two major mandatory social health insurance programs: (1) Workers' Compensation for the costs and pain of suffering job-related accidents, and (2) Medicare for the elderly, disabled, and other special groups. Several states sponsor social insurance programs in the areas of temporary disability (California) or health insurance (Hawaii and Vermont).

Workers' Compensation is offered to some extent in all 50 states. It is usually the first type of social insurance enacted in a nation and the vast majority of nations worldwide have some form of industrial accident insurance. The first workers' compensation law in the United States was passed by New York in 1914 in response to the tragic Triangle Shirt factory fire in which 146 women lost their lives. In 1950, Mississippi became the last state to enact worker's compensation. About 80 percent of the U.S. workforce is covered to some extent by worker's compensation, leaving the remaining workers, many of whom are agricultural, casual, and domestic workers, without coverage. Unfortunately, it is often these same people who are not covered by any type of health insurance (Roemer, 1978).

Workers' Compensation provides two basic benefits: (1) cash replacement of a portion of wages lost due to disability and (2) payment for all or part of the medical care necessary. Workers' compensation may be underwritten by a private insurance company, a state government insurance fund, or a corporate contingency fund. Premiums are usually determined by experience rating.

In 1935, national health insurance almost became a reality as part of the Social Security Act. Due to strong opposition from the AMA and conservative members of Congress, national health insurance was scrapped from the act by President Roosevelt, who did not want to risk passage by Congress. In 1939, and every two years for several Congresses thereafter, the Wagner, Murray, Dingell national health insurance bill was proposed in Congress. The timing of this bill coincided with the growth curve of private health insurance enrollment, which precluded a pressing interest in national health insurance. However, private health insurance was largely sponsored by employers and thus did not serve the nonworking population, particularly the aged. Nonetheless, about 50 percent of

the elderly enrolled in voluntary health insurance programs during the 1957–1964 pre-Medicare period (Roemer, 1978).

In 1957, Representative Forand of Rhode Island introduced the bill that was the precursor of Medicare (Title XVIII of the Social Security Act). On July 30, 1965, Medicare became the first entry of the federal government into the provision of social health insurance rather than medical assistance (public welfare medicine) such as offered by the Kerr-Mills Act of 1960—Medical Assistance for the Aged.

Strictly speaking, only Medicare Part A—Hospital Insurance (HI)—is social health insurance. (See Figure 4.4.) Part B—Supplementary Medical Insurance (SMI)—is neither compulsory nor funded by a trust fund. Over 82 percent of the funds for SMI comes from the U.S. general treasury and the other 18 percent comes from premiums collected from Medicare Part A recipients who elect to pay Part B premiums out of their monthly Social Security checks (Smith et al., 2006).

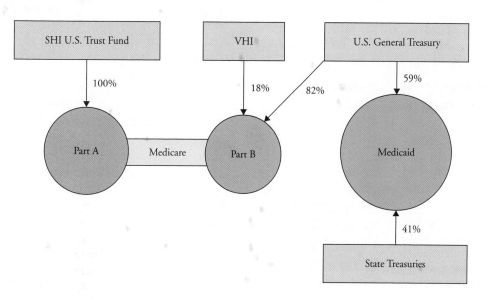

Each circle represents the relative size of the program in dollars.

Figure 4.4. Flow of Federal and State Financing for Medicare and Medicaid, 2004

Medicare utilizes an indirect pattern of finance and delivery, wherein the Centers for Medicare and Medicaid (CMS), a branch HCFA, contracts with independent providers. Medicare recipients also access providers independently. CMS sees to it that the provider is paid, but the providers are neither owned nor hired by the government, as in SHI systems utilizing the direct pattern of delivery. Generally speaking, if the private medical market is strong at the time when SHI is enacted, an indirect pattern of delivery emerges. If the market is weak, a direct financing route emerges.

Welfare Medicine

Public assistance or welfare medicine is sponsored by a plethora of federal, state, and local government programs, but the most far-reaching program is Medicaid (Title XIX of the Social Security Act). Administered at the federal level by CMS, Medicaid is financed by an average federal contribution from the general treasury of 59 percent and from state treasuries at an average contribution of 41 percent. (See Figure 4.4.) Federal matching varies from 50 to 77 percent, depending on the income of the individual state (USDHHS, 2005a). General treasury funds are generated from personal income tax, corporate income tax, and various excise taxes and, to the extent that these taxes are borne by higher income individuals and organizations, Medicaid represents a type of transfer payment to the poor.

The distinction between welfare medicine and social health insurance, both of which are public programs, is an important one and rests on the philosophical difference between a transfer payment and entitlement. Medicaid is a transfer payment "in kind," meaning that medical services are provided as a welfare benefit in lieu of cash. Welfare recipients also receive cash subsidies to pay for their living expenses, but medical benefits are paid directly to the provider so that the recipients will not be tempted to spend the money on expense items other than health care. (Food stamps are another "in kind" benefit, providing vouchers solely for the purpose of purchasing food and groceries.)

Thus the transfer payment is a type of "relief" that government bestows upon the poor; it is a form of charity.

Social health insurance is an entitlement program, not charity. It is a right earned by individuals in the course of their employment. The funds for SHI programs are contributed by a payroll tax (for 2004, 2.9 percent of total wages—a stable percentage for many years), which in the case of Social Security is divided equally between the worker and the employer. Worker's Compensation too is financed, at least in part, by worker contributions. When the worker retires or suffers a temporary or sustaining injury related to employment, SHI becomes active for the worker and dependents. The fundamental aim of a compulsory government-provided or supervised SHI program is social adequacy—to provide members of society with protection against hazards so widespread as to be considered risks that individuals cannot afford to deal with themselves. Eligibility in SHI is derived from contributions having been made in the program and benefits are a statutory right not based on need. Recipients are thus entitled to the benefits of SHI. Over half the countries in the world have a SHI system for financing health care, at least for some categories of employees (Roemer, 1978).

In reference to Figure 4.4, it is interesting to note that the federal share of funding (coming from the U.S. General Treasury) for Medicare Part B has increased substantially in recent years, despite premium increases.

MEDICARE

Medicare, the principal SHI program in the United States, provides a variety of hospital, physician, and other medical services for (1) persons 65 and over, (2) disabled individuals who are entitled to Social Security benefits, and (3) end-stage renal disease victims. In 2004, Medicare financed $309 billion in health services, comprising 39 percent of all publicly financed health expenditures and 19.2 percent of PHCE. Medicare reimbursed 28.6 percent of all hospital expenditures, and 20.5 percent of all physician expenditures in 2004 (Smith et al., 2006).

Part A: Hospital Insurance

Ninety-nine percent of the aged population of the United States is enrolled in Part A of Medicare, Hospital Insurance (HI). Part A finances five basic benefits for the covered population:

1. Ninety days of inpatient care in a "benefit period." (A benefit period is a spell of illness beginning with hospitalization and ending when a beneficiary has not been an inpatient in a hospital or skilled nursing facility for 60 continuous days. There is no limit to the number of benefit periods a beneficiary can use.)

2. A lifetime reserve of 60 days of inpatient care, once the 90 days are exhausted.

3. One hundred days of posthospitalization care in a skilled nursing facility.

4. Home health agency visits.

5. Three pints of blood, as part of an inpatient stay.

Since the inception of the Medicare program, hospital insurance has required the beneficiary to participate in cost sharing. The patient is required to pay an inpatient hospital deductible in each benefit period that approximates the cost of one day of hospital care ($952 in 2006). Coinsurance based on the inpatient hospital deductible is required for the 61st to 90th day of inpatient hospitalization and is always equal to one-fourth of the deductible ($238 in 2006). For the 21st to 100th day of skilled nursing facility (SNF) care, the coinsurance equals one-eighth of the deductible ($119), and for the 60 lifetime reserve days, the patient pays one-half of the deductible ($476) for each day of inpatient hospitalization. As previously mentioned, the majority of Medicare enrollees have private Medigap policies, which primarily cover some or all of the deductibles and coinsurance under

Medicare. In 2002, about 7.2 million of the aged and disabled have both Medicare and Medicaid coverage in combination (a group known as "crossovers" or "Medi-Medi"), and Medicaid usually assumes responsibility for the cost-sharing arrangements under Medicare (USDHHS, 2005b).

While hospital expenditures have grown enormously since the inception of Medicare in 1966, skilled nursing facility, home health agency, and outpatient benefits have all shifted significantly as a percent of total Medicare benefit payments. For example, in the early days of Medicare, SNF and home health care were just a sliver of total Medicare expenditures; now they comprise 10.5 percent of the total (Smith et al., 2006).

Part B: Supplementary Medical Insurance

Ninety-four percent of Part A beneficiaries are enrolled in Part B—Supplementary Medical Insurance (SMI). SMI was designed to complement the HI program. It provides payments for physicians, physician-ordered supplies and services, outpatient hospital services, rural health clinic visits, and home health visits for persons without Part A. SMI requires the beneficiary to meet a deductible (currently $124) each year, in addition to paying a monthly premium ($88.50 in 2006). Under "buy-in" agreements, most state Medicaid programs pay the premiums for Medicaid enrollees who qualify to participate in SMI (USDHHS, 2005b; USDHHS, 2006a).

In recent years, Medicare Part B has widened payment for preventive services including bone mass measurements, cardiovascular screenings, colorectal cancer screenings, diabetes screenings, glaucoma tests, Pap tests, prostate cancer screenings, screening mammograms, and flu, pneumococcal, and hepatitis B shots. Physical exams are offered on a one-time basis within the first six months that the enrollee has Medicare Part B.

Not covered by any part of Medicare Part B are dental care, routine eye examinations and eyeglasses, hearing aids or hearing exams, and long-term care services, such as custodial care in a nursing home. However, hospice benefits became available for persons who were terminally ill in 1983. Enrollees in Medicare can elect the hospice benefit for two 90-day periods and one 30-day period, with a subsequent extension period during the individual's lifetime.

Since the inception of Medicare, Part B has grown faster than Part A. In 2004, Part B represented 44 percent of Medicare expenditures, whereas Part A (focusing on hospitals) has shrunk commensurately (Smith et al., 2006).

Part C: Medicare Advantage Plans

In 1987, Medicare added Part C, offering Medicare Risk Contracts as an option to traditional Medicare Parts A and B. This allowed private HMOs to offer comprehensive services to Medicare enrollees in many parts of the country that had already established HMOs offering group coverage. Originally known as "Medicare+Choice," the name was changed to "Medicare Advantage" as part of the Medicare Prescription Drug, Improvement, and Modernization Act of 2003 (MMA). Under this legislation and beginning in 2006, PPOs and other managed fee-for-service plans were added to Part C.

Medicare HMOs enjoyed rapid growth in the 1990s, but in 2000, HMO contractors began dropping out the program due to lack of profitability. Since 1999, the program has shrunk by 1.6 million members. In 2005, 188 Medicare Advantage contracts were in operation, serving 5.7 million members or 13.6 percent of Medicare beneficiaries (as compared to about 66 percent of the Medicare population that has access to an Advantage plan). Indicating favorable selection, Medicare Advantage plans attract fewer beneficiaries with disabilities (7.2 percent in 2005) than traditional Medicare fee for service with 16.9 percent. The greatest penetration of beneficiaries enrolled occurs primarily in the West—California, Oregon, Nevada, and Hawaii—along with Pennsylvania and Rhode Island (USDHHS, 2005a; USDHHS, 2005b).

Part D: Medicare Prescription Drug Benefit

The centerpiece of MMA is, of course, the addition of Part D: Medicare Prescription Drug Coverage, initiated on January 1, 2006. The passage of the act in 2003 surprised health care interest groups that, despite a campaign promise from President George W. Bush, predicted that such an expansion of Medicare would never occur in a Republican-controlled Congress. While drug companies and health insurers have much to gain from this act, the real financial winners are Medicare beneficiaries, who have increasingly been burdened by the rising cost of prescription drugs.

The most interesting feature of the prescription drug benefit is the so-called "doughnut hole" or gap. After paying a $250 deductible, Medicare picks up 75 percent of next $2,000 in costs. Then comes the gap of $3,100, wherein Medicare pays nothing and the patient is liable for the whole amount out of pocket. Once the patient has reached the $5,100 threshold, Part D pays about 95 percent of drug costs. In this way, severely ill patients are protected against catastrophic expenses in procuring prescription drugs. As a response, Medigap plans have reorganized their benefit structures to fill the hole.

Enrollment in Part D is voluntary, and premiums are collected monthly by Medicare. However, enrollees have a wide variety of prescription drug plans from which to choose and the premiums vary widely by plan and by region. In 2006, the average national premium is estimated by CMS to be $37 per month or $444 per year—a sizable amount of money. Thus, the private health insurance industry participates in two ways—by offering the prescription drug plans and by sponsoring Medigap.

Now in its initial stages of implementation, the Medicare Prescription Drug Benefit has been subject to criticism for (1) glitches in enrollment and reimbursement procedures, (2) overload of information and confusion for beneficiaries in choosing a private prescription drug plan, (3) unpreparedness of pharmacies, and (4) problems in enrollment for

Medicaid buy-in (and other state-sponsored) low-income groups. However, the biggest criticism of MMA is not in the implementation, but in the actual law. MMA decrees that health insurers and governments cannot negotiate volume discounts with drug companies in purchasing drugs. This was considered by many to be anticompetitive and a financial give-away to the pharmacy industry.

Provider Reimbursement

Hospitals

Until 1983, Medicare operated primarily on a fee-for-service basis for physicians' and related services, and on a cost-based retrospective basis for hospital services. Hospitals were reimbursed for any reasonable costs incurred in the provision of covered care to Medicare patients. Commencing in 1983, payment rates were prospectively determined on a per-case basis. The Medicare hospital Prospective Payment System (PPS), discussed in detail later in this chapter, uses diagnosis-related groups (DRGs) to classify cases for payment. Except for four major classes of specialty hospitals (children's, psychiatric, rehabilitation, and long-term), all hospitals must participate in PPS to qualify for Medicare reimbursement, billing Medicare directly.

Physicians

To constrain SMI inflation, the Deficit Reduction Act of 1984 introduced the concept of "participating physicians," who are those who "accept assignments" for all services (i.e., claims) for all Medicare patients in that doctor's practice, with no exceptions. Several pecuniary and marketing incentives to participate were introduced and resulted in substantial increases in assignment. Nationally, the rate of participating physicians increased from 51 percent in 1983 to 92 percent in 2003, amounting to 99.4 percent of all Medicare Part B claims. A non-participating physician can continue to treat Medicare patients, accepting assignments or not on a claim-by-claim basis, but Medicare will reimburse only 95 percent of the amount given to participating physicians (USDHHS, 2003).

Under Medicare Part B, physicians may elect one of two reimbursement strategies. The first is to accept the Medicare Fee Schedule (MFS) as payment in full (i.e., participating physicians accepting the assignment); The second is to bill Medicare directly and receive 80 percent payment from the Medicare intermediary. The beneficiaries are liable for the remaining 20 percent coinsurance, also according to the MFS. On unassigned claims, the beneficiary is additionally liable for the difference between the physician's charge and the Medicare allowed charge.

Intermediaries or fiscal agents, such as Blue Cross or a commercial insurance company, that are contracted by the Medicare program to review and pay the bills, process claims. Enrollees can also join HMOs and similar forms of prepaid health care and special reimbursement provisions apply to these organizations. The Tax Equity and Fiscal Responsibility Act of 1982 (TEFRA) included major revisions to the Medicare law to encourage growth in the number of HMOs and other comprehensive medical plans enrolling Medicare beneficiaries. TEFRA also set limits on Medicare reimbursements for hospital costs at the per-case level—the harbinger of DRGs under PPS.

Utilization

The average Medicare enrollee spent about $6,805 in 2004. As in any other insurance program, however, utilization is uneven. A study of 1992 data showed that one-third of the enrolled population had small claims of $500 or less, and another 22 percent had no claims at all. The highest 9.8 percent of users had reimbursements of $10,000 or more and these enrollees consumed 68.4 percent of program payments (USDHHS, 1995). Other studies have demonstrated that high Medicare reimbursements are related to terminal illness. A seminal study by Lubitz and Prihoda (1984) found that reimbursements for persons in their last year of life averaged 620 percent higher costs than those who survived the period under study. Fuchs (1984) showed that the greatest proportion of medical care costs is incurred in the year prior to death, regardless of the age of natural death. For Medicare enrollees, the average reimbursement for those in their last year of life was 6.6 times as large as for those who survived at least two years. Thus, one may surmise that the principal reason why health expenditures rise with age is that the proportion of persons near death increases with age. Other studies have found a great deal of consistency over time in the utilization of health expenditures by the highest users, with the top 1 percent accounting for 20 or more percent of health care dollars (Gornick et al., 1985).

MEDICAID

Program Structure

Medicaid was enacted into law on July 30, 1965, as Title XIX of the Social Security Act, and became part of the existing federal-state welfare structure to assist the poor. Until Medicaid, there had been little federal participation in health care for the poor. This public obligation was delegated to the states as part of their police powers. Prior to Medicaid, many doctors donated their services or used a sliding scale of fees in treating the poor and, as a rule, hospitals admitted charity cases. However, under the purview of the states, health care for the poor varied widely from state to state and manifested all the forms of discrimination tolerated in each locale. The Kerr-Mills Act of 1960—Medical Assistance for the Aged—was the forerunner of the Medicaid model and was later subsumed under Title XIX.

Eligibility

In 2002, about 18 percent of the U.S. population (amounting to 51.5 billion people) was enrolled in Medicaid at some time during the year (Kaiser Family Foundation, 2006; U.S. Census Bureau, 2004–2005). Supported by federal grants and administered by the states, Medicaid is limited to specific groups of low-income individuals and families. Medicaid is welfare medicine and thus has no strict entitlement features. (In recent years, the word

"entitlement" has been used indiscriminately, particularly by politicians and the media, in reference to all social welfare programs, including Medicaid.) Recipients must prove their eligibility for Medicaid according to their income and, prior to 1976, states were even permitted to put a lien on a recipient's home or other personal property.

The program was designed to cover those groups who are eligible to receive cash payments under one of the two existing welfare programs established under Social Security: Aid to Families with Dependent Children (AFDC), now known as TANF, Temporary Aid to Needy Families, and Supplemental Security Income (SSI). In most instances, receipt of a welfare payment under one of these programs means automatic eligibility for Medicaid. The mandatory eligibility groups covered by Medicaid include (1) families with children which receive AFDC; (2) pregnant and postpartum women and children under 6 years of age, whose incomes do not exceed 133 percent of the Federal Poverty Level (FPL); (3) aged, blind, and disabled individuals who receive SSI; and (4) certain other specifically defined groups.

Figure 4.5 compares the distribution of Medicaid recipients to that of expenditures by eligibility category. Needy families—adults and children—were the largest group of Medicaid recipients (72.4 percent) in 2003 but accounted for a relatively small part of the Medicaid budget (28.1 percent), which is a reflection of the relatively good health of most Medicaid children. Due largely to high utilization of nursing home services, 24.3 percent of total Medicaid outlays was attributable to the aged, who comprise only 9.8 percent of the Medicaid population. Outlays for the blind and disabled totaled 42.1 percent of Medicaid expenditures, a disproportionately large amount as compared to the number of recipients (17.9 percent) (USDHHS, 2005a). These facts serve to dispel the conventional wisdom that families on welfare incur the lion's share of Medicaid expense. The impoverished aged and the disabled (which includes the mentally retarded) have no alternative but to expend large per capita amounts in the Medicaid program.

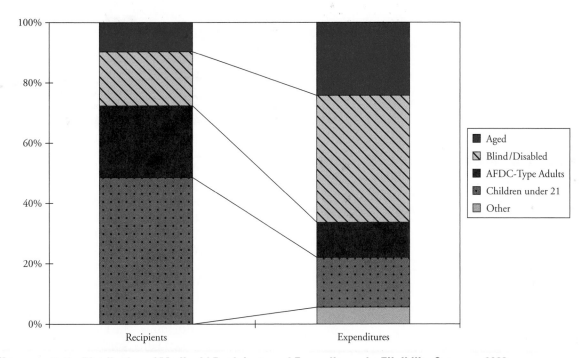

Figure 4.5. **Distribution of Medicaid Recipients and Expenditures by Eligibility Category, 2003**

SOURCE: *2005 CMS Statistics*, U.S. Department of Health and Human Services, Centers for Medicare & Medicaid Services, retrieved March 20, 2006 from http://www.cms.hhs.gov/MedicareMedicaidStatSupp/downloads/2005_CMS_Statistics.pdf

States may choose to provide Medicaid to certain "optional eligibility groups. Most of these optional groups share characteristics of the mandatory groups (parents and children, aged, blind, and disabled), but the income eligibility ceilings are higher (e.g., 1.33 to 1.85 times the federal poverty level of $16,090 for a family of three in 2005). "Medically needy" persons comprise another optional group—those who "spend down" their income and wealth, due to medical bills, to the medically needy standard. Under federal guidelines, states set income and asset levels for cash assistance and medical eligibility. Because there is considerable variation in the coverage of optional groups by the states and in income standards across Medicaid jurisdictions, the degree to which programs cover the poverty population varies considerably.

Benefits Provided

Services

Title XIX of the Social Security Act mandates that every state Medicaid program provide specific basic health services:

- Hospital inpatient care
- Hospital outpatient services
- Certified nurse practitioner services
- Laboratory and X-ray services
- Nursing facility services for those aged 21 and older
- Home health services for those eligible for nursing services
- Physicians' services
- Family planning services and supplies

- Rural health clinic services
- Early and periodic screening, diagnosis, and treatment for children under 21 years of age
- Nurse midwife services
- Certain federally qualified health center services
- Medical and surgical services furnished by a dentist

States may determine the scope of services offered (e.g., limit the days of hospital care or the number of physician visits covered) and provide a number of other elective services. The most commonly covered optional services include

- Clinic services
- Nursing services in a care facility for the aged and disabled
- Intermediate care facility services for the mentally retarded
- Inpatient psychiatric services
- Optometrist services and eyeglasses
- Prescribed drugs
- Prosthetic devices
- Dental care

Administration

Medicaid operates primarily as a vendor payment program. Payments are made directly to providers of service for care rendered to eligible individuals. With certain exceptions, a state must allow Medicaid recipients freedom of choice among participating providers of health care. Managed care plans, which are foremost among the exceptions, usually hold the ability to restrict freedom of choice to contracted providers.

Methods for reimbursing physicians and hospitals vary widely among the states, but providers must accept the Medicaid reimbursement level as payment in full. Payment rates must be sufficient to enlist enough providers so that comparable care and services are available to the Medicaid population as are available to the general population in the area. Notwithstanding, Medicaid physician reimbursement rates are usually less generous than those of Medicare.

In long-term care facilities, individuals are required to turn over income in excess of their personal needs and maintenance needs of their spouses (the monetary level being determined by the state) to help pay for their care. States may require cost sharing by Medicaid recipients, but they may not require the mandatory eligible to share costs for mandatory services. As noted previously, most state Medicaid programs have buy-in agreements with Medicare in which Medicaid assumes the responsibility for the Medicare cost sharing for persons covered under both programs (Gornick et al., 1985; Waldo, 1990).

States participate in the Medicaid program at their option. All states except Arizona (which has a demonstration project of capitated health delivery that excludes long-term care services) currently have Medicaid programs. The District of Columbia, Puerto Rico, Guam, the Northern Marianas, and the Virgin Islands also provide Medicaid coverage.

The states administer their Medicaid programs within broad federal requirements and guidelines. These requirements allow states considerable discretion in determining not only eligibility, also but covered benefits and provider payment mechanisms. Some states also include in the Medicaid program persons known as "state-only" enrollees, who do not meet federal requirements and hence do not qualify for federal matching funds. As a result of state options and policy decisions, the characteristics of Medicaid programs vary considerably from state to state. Medicaid expenditures also vary widely across the states and states' benefit mix offerings change frequently.

Growth of Medicaid

From 1980 to 2004, Medicaid expenditures grew almost twelvefold, exceeding growth in Medicare, which grew by ninefold over the same period. A disproportionately large share of this growth took place in the 1990 to 1995 period. During this time, Medicaid recipients as a percent of the total civilian population rose by 35 percent, which was principally attributable to an expansion of those covered in the mandatory eligible groups. In 2005, about 57 million people received Medicaid benefits at some point within the year, with an average monthly enrollment of 45 million (USDHHS, 2005a).

Providers

Hospital care (inpatient and outpatient) accounted for a much smaller proportion of 2004 Medicaid expenditures (33.9 percent) than Medicare hospital outlays (52.9 percent). Home health care and nursing home care—including skilled nursing facilities, intermediate care facilities, and intermediate care facilities for the mentally retarded (i.e., ICF/MR)—commanded 23.8 percent of Medicaid expenditures for 2004 (Smith et al., 2006).

Medicaid continues to be the largest payer of long-term care services, financing 46 percent of total U.S. nursing home care in 2004. Although growth in spending for nursing facility care has slowed considerably in recent years, since the early 1970s Medicaid has funded the lion's share of all public spending for nursing home care. Compared with other services that Medicaid provides, Medicaid payments for long-term care are also the most costly per user. In 2002–2003, 66 percent of all U.S. nursing home residents received Medicaid as their primary payer source, spending close to $28,000 per year for nursing home care. For ICF/MR beneficiaries, the payment averaged a whopping $92,789. In 2002, the highest growth rates in payments were for ICF/MR care and prescription drugs (Kaiser Family Foundation, 2006; USDHHS, 2005a).

State Spending

Since 1975, Medicaid has been fastest growing component of aggregate state spending. In 2002, Medicaid spent $213.5 billion (or $3,947 per enrollee) of combined federal and state funds for vendor payments for personal health care. New York paid the highest dollar amount per enrollee ($7,505) and California paid the lowest ($2,472). Across the board, Medicaid pays providers poorly—only about 71 percent of what Medicare pays—for all services, with three states paying less than half of what Medicare pays (Kaiser Family Foundation, 2006).

Cost Containment

To curtail Medicaid growth, cost-containment initiatives began in early 1980s. During this time important experiments were launched in prepaid managed health care; utilization review; case management; reimbursement via diagnosis-related group (DRGs); and new services for the elderly, disabled, and persons with AIDS. In 1990, Congress enacted careful and selective expansion of Medicaid coverage, particularly for low-income (and pregnant) women and children. Currently, the focus is on shifting Medicaid funding from the federal coffers to state budgets and encouraging states to model their systems using principles of managed care. Today, more than 60 percent of Medicaid enrollees are covered by some type managed care, although the range varies from 0 to 100 percent of enrollees among the states (Kaiser Family Foundation, 2006).

PHYSICIAN REIMBURSEMENT

Paying the doctor traditionally calls upon one of three reimbursement mechanisms: fee-for-service, prepayment, or salary. Health insurance plans, either public or private, may utilize any or all of the three reimbursement types. According to Reinhardt (1985), there is no optimal system for paying the doctor.

Fee for Service

Fee for service (FFS) is widely used throughout the world for paying the doctor and is typically the physician's preferred mode of payment. In FFS, the unit of remuneration is the medical act, either a service or a procedure. In the days before health insurance for physician reimbursement was widespread, most physicians had a sliding fee scale wherein the poor paid lower fees than wealthier patients. With the advent of health insurance in both the public and private sectors, physician payment became more regulated and physicians adopted one schedule of charges for all payers, whether they were individuals or third parties. By the 1980s, however, fees schedules began to vary widely by the type of health plan or insurance organization, public or private.

One the advantages of fee-for-service reimbursement is that the remuneration adjusts automatically for case complexity, linking the provider's reward closely to the output of services. The billing system, in turn, provides a great deal of "transparency" of the physician's profile of practice. The ease with which patients may change physicians in a traditional fee-for-service system enables them to directly exercise considerable economic clout over practitioners (Reinhardt, 1985).

Indemnity

Insurance policies that reimburse on a fee-for-service basis offer payment either by indemnity or service benefits or by fixed fees. Indemnity payment stipulates a certain dollar value per procedure, usually according to a "table of allowances." These allowances may vary widely among insurance plans. In traditional indemnity, the provider can charge anything above the stipulated allowed amount and collect the remainder directly from the patient. Often, the table of allowances is based on a "relative value scale," in which each procedure is rated according to a point system—relative value units (RVUs)—that reflects the relative technical difficulty and time cost of the procedure, with each point worth so many dollars. The dollars amount per RVU (known as the conversion factor) may also vary widely among insurance plans. This type of system is easy to administer and update for inflation and changing practice patterns, but no provision is made by the insurer to protect the patient from outlandish charges.

Service benefits pay a percentage per procedure, usually 80 percent of "usual, customary, and reasonable" (UCR) fees. In this scheme, the UCR fee schedule protects the carrier from unlimited liability in the wake of high charges and may also give the patient information about reasonable fee norms. UCR means that the fee is "usual" in that doctor's practice, "customary" in that community, and "reasonable" in terms of the distribution of all physician charges for that service in the community. The latter is commonly expressed as a percentile (e.g., the policy will pay up to the 75th percentile).

Hybrid fee-based systems came into vogue with the advent of PPOs, combining features of both indemnity and service reimbursement for cost containment. In a hybrid system, the intermediary contracts with the participating physician (or provider) to accept a discounted version of the UCR table of allowances. The plan considers these "allowed amounts" to be the maximum covered expenses. For a participating provider, the PPO will typically pay 90 percent of the allowed amount for most procedures, with the remaining 10 percent paid by the patient as coinsurance. This arrangement protects both the intermediary by effectively capping the reimbursement (as in an indemnity payment) and the patient by limiting the liability for the difference beyond 10 percent of the allowed amount.

Fixed Fees

In some reimbursement plans, physicians can only charge, and will only be paid, according to fixed fees, usually with little cost or no sharing on the part of the patient (e.g., $10.00 per physician office visit). If the provider accepts the plan, then the fee schedule must be accepted. This arrangement exists in Medicaid plans in a number of states, and many private plans also stipulate fixed fees in order to protect the patient and to contain costs. Many HMO plans also mandate fixed fees, especially for specialists contracted with the health plan.

Prepayment

In prepayment or capitation, the person served, rather than the medical act, is the unit of remuneration. The capitation payment takes care of reimbursement for a stipulated length of time, usually per month. Using capitation as a reimbursement methodology, HMOs have encouraged physicians to form networks linked to hospitals and have also spurred the popularity of independent practice associations (IPAs), in which the participating physicians actually sponsor and administer the HMO. Advantages to prepayment are that it is administratively simple, it facilitates advance global budgeting, and it gives physicians incentive to control the cost of medical treatments. If patients are allowed to switch primary care physicians from time to time, they still retain some economic clout over physicians (Reinhardt, 1985).

Salary

Salary is payment to the doctor for time consumption, irrespective of the units of service or the number of patients. On a large scale, salaried practice almost always takes place in a highly organized network like the National Health Service in Great Britain. On a smaller scale in the United States, urban public hospitals that serve indigent populations often have large attending staffs that are salaried. Countries in which salaried practices are common rarely include specialists in this payment mechanism. Instead, general practitioners or primary care providers have a "panel" of patients in the community. Advantages to salaried reimbursement for physicians are that it is administratively simple, the medical treatments selected are not influenced by relative profitability, and it encourages cooperation among physicians. Furthermore, salaries facilitate advance budgeting for health expenditures (Reinhardt, 1985).

Monitoring

All payment mechanisms have faults and each must be monitored for abuses. In FFS, the incentives are for overwork by the physician and overutilization by the patients. FFS fosters unnecessary or duplicative service to the point where the high volume of services may actually affect the quality of care adversely. Unfortunately, in the United States, malpractice suits have encouraged defensive medicine, wherein overutilization and extra fees are simply passed on to the consumer in higher insurance rates. Also, if fees for all procedures do not stand in constant proportion to costs incurred, the choice of treatment may favor more profitable procedures. For these and other reasons which foster inflation, fee-for-service reimbursement is very difficult to budget in advance.

In prepayment, on the other hand, underutilization must be monitored because the incentive is to decrease costs and services provided against revenues from capitation payments. In many prepayment schemes, any cost savings realized are distributed to the participating physicians, which may be an inducement to cut costs too far. In HMOs where only the primary care physicians are capitated, there also exists the incentive to excessively refer patients to specialists. Likewise, capitation gives physicians incentives for "dumping" patients with complex, costly conditions onto other providers. Finally, the administrative system for prepayment yields little insight as to the transparency of the physician's practice profile. As a result, HMOs may mandate that physicians submit monthly encounter data on patient visits and/or procedures delivered as a condition of participation in the health plan.

In salaried practice, incentives favor underwork or seeing too few patients. Doctors literally "get paid by the hour," resulting in no inducement toward higher volume. Unless the salary is linked to output and patient satisfaction, patients lose economic clout over the physician, who, in turn, may render care as an act of noblesse oblige. Like capitation, salaried practice gives little transparency as to the physician's practice profile (Reinhardt, 1985).

INITIATIVES IN HEALTH CARE FINANCE

Factors in Health Care Inflation

The implementation of Medicare and Medicaid in 1966 heralded a 50-year era of unprecedented health care cost inflation. In a seminal article, Aaron (1993/94) attributes the continually rising costs of health care to three main factors:

1. The technological transformation of medical care, including new diagnostic techniques and new methods of treatment.

2. The demand of consumers for low-benefit care.

3. The lack of budget limits on hospitals and fee controls on physicians.

He also notes that high administrative costs, compensation for medical malpractice, and bad health habits of the populace are not important factors in the rising costs of care.

Cost Containment Measures

In the 1970s, the federal government experimented with a number of programs and reimbursement methods to contain health care costs. Major programs included (1) the establishment of reasonable cost limits for hospitals; (2) the initiation of state and local networks of health planning agencies, along with the "certificate-of-need" procedure for augmenting capital plant and equipment; (3) the establishment of the Professional Standards Review Organization (PSRO) program to review care and to eliminate unnecessary hospital days for federally funded patients; and (4) the encouragement of the growth of HMOs to promote the use of preventive services and to decrease the utilization of hospital inpatient care. It can safely be said that the programs of the 1970s were unsuccessful in containing health care costs.

Early in the 1980s, during the Reagan administration, legislative efforts to change the monetary incentive system in health care began in earnest. While the 1980s witnessed considerable flux in health care financing, along with inducements to reduce overutilization, cost-containment efforts showed mixed results (Rice, 1992). Furthermore, they held painful consequences for many groups of people. To this day, the balance between reasonable costs and equitable access has not yet been struck. Managed care, particularly capitated prepaid care, holds better incentives for efficiency, productivity, and management coordination. Yet, even with more closely managed utilization, better quality management, and the continual expansion of government programs, universal access to health services remains illusive.

Procompetition

Early in the 1980s, Enthoven (1981) and other health economists exposited strategies of procompetition that were meant to restrain health care costs by creating competitive market conditions via direct incentives both for consumers and employers that purchase group health insurance policies. Among these strategies were the imposition of a "tax cap" on employer income tax deductions for health insurance expenses, raising the threshold for individual income tax deductions, and offering multiple choices by employers in health insurance plans. While the threshold for personal income tax deductions for medical out-of-pocket expense was raised to 7.5 percent of gross income, the other strategies, while not formally enacted, had a profound effect on the thinking of health policy makers. The programs of the 1980s reflect this conservative philosophy and, in most cases, the scorecards for their success are mixed, at best.

Beginnings of the Prospective Payment System

The Tax Equity and Fiscal Responsibility Act (TEFRA), signed into law in September 30, 1982 (and enacted the next day), set limits on Medicare reimbursements on a per-case basis for hospital costs and also placed a limit on the annual rate of increase for Medicare's reasonable costs per discharge. TEFRA was expected to reduce Medicare reimbursement by 4.5 percent in real dollars over the ensuing three years. Due to the fast enactment of the Prospective Payment System (PPS) one year later, it was difficult to evaluate the impact of the act. However, TEFRA was the harbinger of prospective payment and a number of features of the latter program were borrowed from it. These features were part of the Section 223 limits on hospital costs. They included (1) grouping hospitals by bed size and size of locale, (2) wage adjustments by locality, and (3) an adjustment for case-mix index. Today, most hospitals that are excluded from the Medicare Prospective Payment System are reimbursed according to TEFRA regulations.

The Section 223 limits were calculated according to a complicated formula whereby the labor-related component for the hospital region, adjusted by a geographic wage index, was added to a regional nonlabor component. The product was then multiplied by a case-mix index, specific to each hospital. These figures were all specified by the Health Care Financing Administration (HCFA) and the U.S. Department of Health and Human Services and published in the Federal Register. The formula used to calculate the Section 223 limits was substantially retained for figuring reimbursement rates for the Prospective Payment System.

HCFA developed institutional-specific case-mix indexes based on a diagnosis-related group (DRG) system designed at Yale University. The DRG classification system sorts patients into uniform, clinically compatible groups that have been categorized on the basis of traditional resource use by patients with similar diagnoses. The original Yale DRGs were modified to reflect variation solely in Medicare cases. For each hospital, HCFA used a 20 percent sample of the Medicare billing forms submitted for calendar year 1980. Using the 10,167 ICD-9-CM diagnosis codes from these claims and each hospital's Medicare cost report, HCFA developed the case-mix index. In essence, this case-mix index was intended to compare a particular

hospital's case-mix with that of all other hospitals in the nation. Table 4.2 shows how five hypothetical hospitals with five DRGs, each varying in volume by hospital, can calculate their case-mix indexes, which reflect the relative severity of each hospital's caseload. Hospital D, with 62.5 percent of its cases in the high-weighted DRG 3, claims the highest case-mix index of 1.6031. This contrasts with Hospital A that, with almost 70 percent of its cases in the low-paying DRGs 2 and 4, holds a case-mix index of 0.8900. Extending this calculation to all cases in all hospitals participating in PPS, the average case-mix index always equals 1.0000. The dollar amount ascribed to a DRG of 1.0000 is recalculated on a yearly basis.

The Prospective Payment System

The Prospective Payment System (PPS) was enacted on October 1, 1983, two years ahead of schedule. The Social Security Amendments of 1983 initiated the new system and contained provisions to base payment for hospital inpatient services on predetermined rates per DRG. In 2003, out of a total of 6,051 hospitals in the United States, 75 percent were participating in PPS. The remaining 1,514 hospitals in the United States still participate in Medicare under the TEFRA reimbursement arrangements (USDHHS, 2003). These "exempt or not yet transitioned to PPS" hospitals include psychiatric facilities, long-term facilities, children's hospitals, critical access facilities, short-term hospitals, and other special medical facilities that have an approved waiver.

PPS represents a major departure from the traditional reimbursement system—cost-based reimbursement—in that payment bears no direct relationship to length of stay, services rendered, or costs of care. For a given discharge, a hospital with actual costs below the designated PPS rate for a given DRG is permitted to keep the difference in payment. If discharge costs exceed the payment level, the hospital is required to absorb the loss. Payments for hospital-based physician services

Table 4.2. Calculation of Medicare Case-Mix Index[a]

Hospital	DRG 1	DRG 2	DRG 3	DRG 4	DRG 5	Total (Percent)	DRG Weighted Expected Cost per Case ($)[b]	Case-Mix Index[c]
A	2.5	27.3	10.5	41.5	18.2	100	1660.40	0.8900
B	21.0	0.9	30.1	2.0	46.0	100	2401.30	1.2872
C	40.6	5.0	2.3	47.2	4.9	100	1346.30	0.7227
D	5.1	18.4	62.5	10.0	4.0	100	2990.70	1.6031
E	30.4	65.0	1.0	1.6	2.0	100	929.00	0.4980
Average proportion for all hospitals	19.92	23.32	21.28	20.46	15.02	100	1865.54	—
DRG cost weight	$1000	$800	$4100	$1500	$2000	—		—

[a]Adjusted to make these five DRGs hypothetically represent all 356 Medicare DRGs.

[b]For hospital A, calculated as follows:

$$0.25(1000) + 0.273(800) + 0.105(4100) + 0.415(1500) + 0.182(2000) = \$1660.40$$

[c]For hospital A, calculated as $1660.40 divided by $1865.54 = 0.8900.

SOURCE: *Tax Equity and Fiscal Responsibility Act of 1982, Management Strategies for Health Care Providers*, 1982, New York: Deloitte Haskins & Sells.

(e.g., radiology, anesthesiology, pathology, etc.), which previously had been reimbursed according to a cost-based fee system, are included in the hospital's PPS rate. Nowadays, these physicians are reimbursed by Medicare via Part B, billing Medicare directly for their services. Other costs—capital depreciation expense, direct medical education costs, and costs associated with serving a "disproportionate share" of the poor—are exempt from PPS provisions and have their own payment formulas, which mimic the formulas used for DRGs.

Standardized Payment Amount

PPS pays a standardized amount for each DRG. Standardized amounts are updated each year by CMS. This amount is further divided into two components—a labor-related amount and a non-labor-related amount. To compute the payment amount for a DRG of 1.0000, the labor-related amount is multiplied by a wage index, specific to each locality, and the product is added to the non-

labor-related amount. For the 2006 fiscal year, for example, a hospital in Los Angeles is subject to a large urban labor-related amount of $3,297.84, times a wage index of 1.1660, plus a non-labor-related amount of $1,433.63. Thus, the DRG payment for a hospital in Los Angeles is $5,278.91. This "final" figure is adjusted by a number of factors including a capital depreciation factor and an adjustment factor for certain high-cost patient cases known as "outliers." Hospitals may also qualify for indirect medical education for serving a disproportionate share of low-income patients, and add-on payments for the acquisition of new technology.

DRG Weights

The DRG weight classifications originally used in TEFRA were updated for use in PPS using a stratified sample of 400,000 medical records drawn from patient discharges in 332 hospitals during the last half of 1979. To date, 550 DRGs have been developed, expanding on the original 467 principal diagnoses. A contracted fiscal intermediary, such as Blue Cross or a commercial insurer, assigns a DRG from a bill submitted by the hospital for each case. Using classifications and terminology consistent with the ICD-9-CM and the Uniform Hospital Discharge Data Set, the intermediary assigns the DRG using the Grouper Program (an automated classification algorithm), which compares information contained in the bill with appropriate DRG criteria. Criteria include the patient's age, sex, principal and secondary diagnoses, procedures performed, and discharge status. (Figure 4.6 presents a schematic diagram of the Grouper Program.) For all but a few DRGs that require clarification by the hospital before the payment amount is determined, the intermediary determines the payment amount and pays the hospital.

Outliers

Bills for "outliers," which result in extra payment for the hospital above the standard DRG rate, require special consideration. In the 2005 fiscal year (FY), 4.1 percent of the pool of total DRG payments is reserved for outliers. The hospital must identify cost outliers and request payment. (It is important to note that the classification of DRGs depends largely on the principal diagnosis, which may not

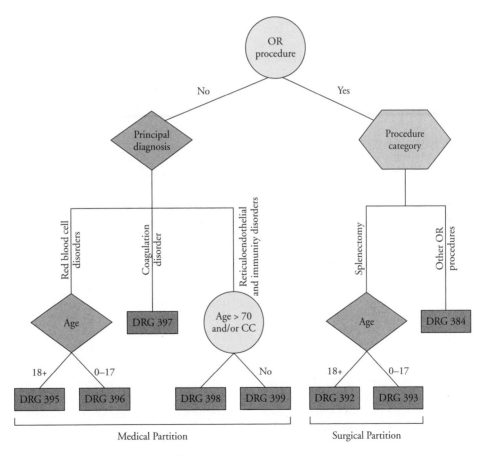

Figure 4.6. Flowchart of the Grouper Program

SOURCE: Reprinted with permission of American Medical Association. *Diagnosis-Related Groups (DRGs)*, 1984, Chicago: Author.

be the diagnosis consuming the most resources, thus making the discharge an outlier.)

For a discharge to be considered as an outlier, the rules are very stringent. For FY 2005, CMS set the outlier threshold to equal the prospective payment rate for the DRG (including adjustments) plus $25,800 in extra documented costs (Deloitte & Touche, 2005a).

Expansion of PPS

A clear incentive in the PPS system was for hospitals to expand services beyond inpatient care, thus increasing and unbundling reimbursement from Medicare. Outpatient care provided ample opportunities for marketing expansion, including disease-specific ambulatory programs, satellite clinics, family planning activities, chemical dependency treatment, and laboratory or other ancillary services. Post-acute hospital care provided more opportunities, including skilled nursing, rehabilitation, home health services, and other services which facilitate earlier discharge of patients. All these services grew enormously, providing additional sources of revenue for hospitals in the post-PPS period.

Gradually, CMS saw the wisdom of using PPS-style reimbursement methods for a wide array of providers. Today, Medicare uses standardized amounts, relative weights, geographic labor indexes, and case-mix grouping techniques for inpatient rehabilitation facilities, skilled nursing facilities, long-term care hospitals, home health agencies, hospices, and all types of outpatient hospital procedures and ambulatory surgery centers.

Long-Term Results of PPS

The implementation of PPS demonstrates the unpredictability of results stemming from changes in health finance. The major deleterious incentives anticipated in the early days of PPS included (1) multiple, unnecessary admissions of the same patient for a set of related procedures resulting in more discrete DRG payments—a practice known as churning; (2) skimming more profitable, less severely ill patients in each DRG, or dumping high-cost patients; and (3) reducing length of stay, tests, and procedures per admission to dangerously low levels, increasing mortality and morbidity.

Empirical findings as to the validity of these assertions have shown few ill effects of PPS or are inconclusive due to the rapidly changing nature of the health care sector. Prior to PPS, hospital admissions had been falling for all payers for a number of years and once PPS was enacted, Medicare admissions went down as well. In the year immediately following the enactment of PPS, hospital admissions declined by more than 11 percent, reversing the steady rise in Medicare admissions in the years prior to PPS. By 2002, hospital discharges per 1,000 enrollees fell to 315, down from 347 in 1985 While anecdotal evidence of skimming and dumping have surfaced, widespread usage of these practices by hospitals for Medicare patients has not been documented (DesHarnais et al., 1987; Guterman & Dobson, 1986; Guterman et al., 1988; USDHHS, 2003).

Length of stay has been falling for Medicare since the inception of the act. Under the PPS system, an even steeper decline in average length of stay (down 17 percent for the first three years of PPS), combined with reduced admissions, has resulted in declining inpatient volume nationwide. Reduced length of stay has been achieved through shorter stays across the board, rather than efforts aimed specifically at patients who have the longest stays (i.e., the most severely ill). From 1990 to 2002, length of stay continued to decline from 9.0 days per admission to 5.9 days. These phenomena indicate that PPS has been effective in encouraging hospitals to become more efficient in the provision of inpatient care (USDHHS, 2003).

The Medicare Case-Mix Index increased sharply and the percentage of hospital days spent in special care units increased after the implementation of PPS, possibly due to more judicious selections of candidates for inpatient hospitalization. Other studies of severity of illness at admission and discharge also show increases in the post-PPS period. The discharge of patients "quicker and sicker" has fostered rapid growth in the use of skilled nursing and subacute facilities. Home health agency services, which enjoyed rapid growth through 1997, have since been in retrenchment due to reduced Medicare reimbursement rates under PPS (USDHHS, 2005b).

A number of criticisms have been levied against the incentives inherent in the DRG system. To the extent that individual DRGs reflect procedures actually performed rather than diagnoses, the choice of treatment may vary according to the "profitability" of that DRG and treatment decisions may not be made on purely clinical grounds. In a similar vein, physicians, in their clinical notes, and medical records administrators, in abstracting data for the DRG grouper program, might call on coding strategies to ensure DRG creep to higher-level, revenue-enhancing diagnoses.

Financial Performance

Hospitals have generally fared well financially under PPS, but the distribution of results is uneven. The spate of hospital bankruptcies that were predicted at the inception of PPS has not taken place, but acquisitions and mergers have been rampant in the health care industry in recent years.

PPS appears to have decelerated the rate of increase in Medicare inpatient hospital expenditures. Although outpatient payments, which are excluded from PPS, have mushroomed, total Medicare benefit payments are increasing at a slower rate due to the sharp decline in growth of Part A payments. Hospital inpatient expenditures comprise about 40 percent of Medicare payments—only slightly more than total SMI payments in 2002 (USDHHS, 2003).

Medicare Physician Reimbursement

From 1975 to 1990, Medicare's total payments for physician services grew at a faster rate than payments for hospital services. By 1990, physician services reached a high of almost 23 percent of total Medicare spending. Over the same period, hospital care dropped as a drastically as a share of total Medicare expenditures. There was general agreement that physician payment under Medicare needed to

be revised. In 1990, Congress directed the administration to study physician payment reform when it established Medicare's DRG-based prospective payment system for hospital care.

Resource-Based Relative Values

On January 1, 1992, Medicare initiated a new system for reimbursing physicians using a resource-based relative-value (RBRV) scale. This payment method divides resources needed to produce physician services into three components: physician work, practice expenses, and malpractice insurance costs. For each procedure, each of the three components is characterized by a numerical value representing its relative contribution to the expenses incurred in delivering the service (Table 4.3). In addition, as shown in Table 4.4, the relative values of the three components are each adjusted for geographic cost/price variations. The total units drive the fee, which is derived by multiplying the total units by a conversion factor. The final fee is thus a geographically weighted summation of the three components of the RBRVs times the conversion factor or each unit of service. For 2006, the conversion factor is $36.18 per unit (Deloitte & Touche, 2005b; Hsiao et al., 1988a; Hsiao et al., 1988b).

For surgery, the RBRV payment schedule also establishes a uniform definition of "global surgery" to ensure that identical payments are made for the same amount of work and resources expended in furnishing specific surgical services on a nationwide basis. The initial evaluation or consultation by a surgeon is paid separately from the global surgery package. The global fee includes all preoperative visits and all medical and surgical services related to a procedure, covering a 90-day postoperative period for all visits by the primary surgeon.

Simulations done by the Harvard University developers of the new reimbursement system (Hsiao et al., 1988a) showed that certain types of physicians would be financial winners and losers under RBRVs. Pathologists, radiologists, thoracic surgeons, cardiovascular surgeons, and ophthalmologists stood to lose, whereas physicians specializing in evaluation and management, such as internists,

Table 4.3. Relative Value Units Used in the Medicare Fee Schedule: Selected Procedures, 2006

Description	Physician Work	Practice Expense	Malpractice Insurance	Total Units*
Appendectomy	9.99	4.32	1.31	15.62
CABG, arterial, four or more	37.44	18.34	5.42	61.20
Cesarean delivery	17.34	7.85	4.12	29.31
Colonoscopy	2.82	5.09	0.26	8.17
Hysterectomy and vagina repair	15.74	7.79	1.91	25.44
Knee arthroscopy/surgery	8.18	5.05	1.25	14.48
Magnetic Resonance Image, jaw joint	1.48	11.72	0.66	13.86
Psychiatric treatment, 45–50 min	1.86	0.60	0.04	2.50
Repair detached retina	14.82	11.33	0.73	26.98
Repair inguinal hernia	8.56	4.08	1.13	13.77

*Total units reflect the hypothetical number of RVUs existing in an area where all three GPCIs are 1.000.

SOURCE: *Medicare Physician Fee Schedule, 2006*, U.S. Department of Health and Human Services (USDHHS), Centers for Medicare & Medicaid Services. Retrieved on March 20, 2006, from http://new.cms.hhs.gov/ PhysicianFeeSched/PFSRVF/itemdetail.asp?filterType=none&filterByDID=-99&sortOrder=ascending&itemID= CMS057575

family practitioners, and immunologists would gain considerable amounts over their previous Medicare earnings.

Hsiao (1992) later published an article criticizing HCFA for setting the monetary conversion factors at unreasonably low levels and that Medicare continued to reimburse invasive services with more units than research justified, according to the RBRVs actually assigned in the Medicare Fee Schedule. This practice by CMS continues to this day, and now most types of physicians are feeling the pinch of restricted Medicare fees, which are down more than $2.00 per unit since 2001.

STRATEGIES FOR HEALTH CARE REFORM

National Health Insurance

National health insurance (NHI) is a concept that has been espoused by many for more than 70 years for containing health care costs and for providing universal access for the U.S. population. NHI came close to becoming part of the Social Security Act of 1935, and numerous bills, representing a spectrum of schemes, have been introduced and seriously debated by most congressional sessions ever since. In the mid-1970s the issue of NHI became so heated that both political parties introduced some bills that were strikingly similar. NHI bills ran the gamut from expanding Medicare to new population groups (e.g., children under 5 years of age) to a national health service (NHS) concept like that of Sweden or Great Britain where the government owns the hospitals and pays the doctors directly.

When President Carter was elected in 1976, many in the health arena assumed that NHI would be an eventuality in a Democratic administration, but early on, it was evident that Carter took little interest in health issues. In the 1980s and early 1990s, the Reagan and Bush administrations were active in introducing cost-containment measures, such as PPS and RBRVs for Medicare, but until the Clinton administration, no serious consideration was given to sweeping reform of the entire system.

Table 4.4. **Geographic Practice Cost Indexes (GPCIs) Used to Weight the Components of RBRVs: Selected Cities and Areas, 2006**

Locality	Physician Work	Practice Expense	Malpractice Insurance
Arizona	1.000	0.992	1.069
Atlanta, GA	1.010	1.089	0.966
Birmingham, AL	1.000	0.846	0.752
Boston, MA	1.030	1.329	0.823
Chicago, IL	1.025	1.126	1.867
Colorado	1.000	1.014	0.803
Dallas, TX	1.009	1.062	1.061
Detroit, MI	1.037	1.054	2.744
Houston, TX	1.016	1.014	1.298
Iowa	1.000	0.868	0.589
Los Angeles, CA	1.041	1.156	0.954
Miami, FL	1.000	1.046	2.269
Minneapolis-St. Paul, MN	1.000	1.005	0.410
New Orleans, LA	1.000	0.946	1.197
New York, NY (Manhattan)	1.065	1.298	1.504
Puerto Rico	1.000	0.698	0.261
San Francisco, CA	1.060	1.543	0.651
Seattle, WA	1.014	1.131	0.819
Vermont	1.000	0.968	0.514
Washington DC, Area	1.048	1.250	0.926

SOURCE: *Medicare Physician Fee Schedule, 2006,* U.S. Department of Health and Human Services (USDHHS), Centers for Medicare & Medicaid Services. Retrieved on March 20, 2006, from http://new.cms.hhs.gov/apps/pfslookup/step0.asp

American Medical Association

An unprecedented issue of the *Journal of the American Medical Association* (*JAMA*) appeared in May 1991. The entire issue was devoted to health system reform proposals, a subject traditionally anathema to organized medicine. Most proposals called for a revised system administered by private insurers with employer/employee premium sharing, supplemented by some form of government financing for nonworking individuals and families. With few exceptions, the proposals called for universal access to health care and for the provision of health insurance to all employees. Looking to the political left, it was interesting that no plan advocated a national health service model. On the right, only one of the plans called for increased privatization and freedom of choice.

In what can only be called a courageous editorial, Lundberg (1991, p. 2566), then the editor of the *JAMA*, summed up the findings:

Although there may be consensus that our society must provide basic medical/health care for all of our people, we seem not to be close to a consensus on how to do it. Virtually all comprehensive health care proposals involve major legislation of some sort. Since consensus means "general agreement or unanimity; group solidarity in sentiment or belief," it is unlikely that, either as a society or as a profession, we will ever reach a true consensus on how to proceed, so we must not wait for one. To pass federal legislation requires only a simple majority in both houses of Congress plus presidential approval.

The Clinton Health Security Plan

Health care reform became one of the hottest domestic political issues of the early 1990s. Pressures for reform came from a wide variety of groups including providers, the elderly and disabled, labor unions, state and local governments, and insiders within the Washington establishment. Even the health insurers and managed care organizations called for change. The two main targets of discontent were (1) the growing numbers and financial burden of uninsured and underinsured Americans, and (2) the high cost of health care that eroded American competitiveness in the international marketplace.

In response to these pressures, President Clinton introduced the President's Health Security Plan (White House Domestic Policy Council, 1993), which was largely the work of a task force headed by Hillary Rodham Clinton. The plan was subject to a great deal of criticism (and negative television advertising) from a large number of wealthy special interest groups, with the result that the plan died in Congress within a few months.

The essence of the plan was to create regional health alliances (i.e., health insurance purchasing cooperatives), wherein various competing insurance plans would be offered, at various premium supplements, to all participating employers and thus their employees. The model was based, in part, on the California Public Employees Retirement Program (CalPERS) health insurance, which had been quite successful for more than a decade in containing costs, maintaining quality, and offering a wide range of comprehensive traditional and managed care plans to its members. The Clinton plan would also have created a separate risk pool for the uninsured.

Perhaps the ultimate reason that the Health Security Plan failed was that its implementation depended on global prospective budgeting for health care at a national level, the moneys from which would be dispersed to state budgeting agencies and then on to the regional alliances. Many influential opinion makers maintained that the United States had no viable administrative apparatus whereby such complex prospective budgeting could take place. They predicted that a large and costly new government bureaucracy would emerge.

The irony of the failed outcome of the Clinton plan is that, in many regions of the country, such health alliances have emerged within the private sector, spurred by consolidation of health plans and providers into large health systems and managed care plans.

President Clinton, in the face of his defeated plan, was active in pushing health reform legislation incrementally, based on the research conducted for the Health Security Act. Among areas of federal legislative reform enacted late in the Clinton administration were (1) increasing the portability of health benefits from one employer to another, (2) encouraging growth for Medicare managed care plans, (3) expansion of mental health benefits in health plans so that they are comparable to physical health benefits, and (4) incentives to form Health Savings Accounts (HSAs).

HSAs, drawing the greatest amount of conservative political approval, are similar in concept to Individual Retirement Accounts, offering income-tax-exempt trusts to pay for qualified medical expenses. Individuals and families have to purchase high-deductible health plans that meet federal specifications. Yearly deductibles (e.g., $2,000 per family per year) are subject to annual out-of-pocket expenses of $10,200 per family (not including the price of the health insurance premium). In return, families get to deduct $5,250 in income taxes. In 2005, more than 1 million Americans were covered by HSAs. In 2006, HSAs—touted as a method for reducing the numbers of the uninsured—are proposed for growth by the George W. Bush Administration (AHIP, 2005a, AHIP, 2005b).

Medicaid Reform

The Welfare Reform Act of 1996 placed new restrictions on eligibility for AFDC, SSI, and other federally funded welfare programs, including Medicaid. Furthermore, greater discretion was given to the states as to how to organize and enact welfare programs. Chief among the provisions was that Medicaid be delinked from cash assistance programs and that states be required to redetermine Medicaid eligibility for all welfare recipients. Another new federal provision was that states may deny Medicaid and cash assistance to current legal immigrants. Legal immigrants who arrive after the bill is enacted are subject to a five-year waiting period before they become eligible for means-tested programs. (This provision held cost-cutting opportunities for states with high rates of immigration, like California and Texas.)

SCHIP

In 1997, President Clinton was successful in passing one expansion of publicly funded health care as part of welfare reform—the State Children's Health Insurance Program (SCHIP), which provided states with $40 billion in federal funding over 10 years to expand coverage for low-income children. SCHIP provides a capped amount of funds to states on a matching basis. Implementation of SCHIP is meant to reduce the number of low-income children lacking insurance coverage, even if they earn too much to qualify for Medicaid. Unlike previous expansions, which built upon existing Medicaid programs, states can set up separate programs to serve SCHIP enrollees. States that choose to participate have greater flexibility in designing benefit packages and may impose some cost sharing, resembling private insurance plans more than Medicaid. The majority of states take advantage of SCHIP. In 2004, SCHIP funded $6.6 billion in separate state programs and Medicaid expansions, covering 6.2 enrollees. (USDHHS 2005b.)

The Uninsured

Health reform cannot be discussed without addressing the growing plight of the uninsured. For the entire year of 2002, approximately 15.2 percent of the U.S. population, comprising about 44 million people, was not covered by health insurance, either public or private. This percentage is up from 1987, when about 12.9 percent of the population was uninsured for health care. Groups that predominate among the uninsured are Hispanics and, to a lesser extent, African Americans; those 18 to 24 years old; and those with low household incomes. The South and the West are also disproportionately represented, with the highest concentrations of uninsured (accounting for more than one-third of the total) in California, Texas, and Florida. Although uninsurance cuts across all income levels, the majority of the uninsured were poor or in the lower-middle income bracket. (U.S. Census Bureau, 2004–2005) (A detailed account of the uninsurance issue will be presented in the following chapter.)

International Comparisons

A great deal of interest in recent years has been focused on the reasons U.S. health spending is so much higher than that of other industrialized nations, even those with much older populations and universal access to care (Reinhardt, Hussey, & Anderson, 2004). When compared with the 29 countries in the Organization for Economic Cooperation and Development (OECD) from 1990–2002, U.S. per capita health spending exceeded other countries by huge margins. At the high end of per capita outlays, Switzerland spent only 68 percent of the U.S. amount, and Canada and Germany each spent 57 percent. In the lower half of the OECD spectrum, Japan and the United Kingdom spent only 44 and 41 percent, respectively, on per capita health care.

Reinhardt and colleagues (2004) give five major factors that are driving U.S. health spending: (1) the high level of GDP per capita in the United States; (2) the comparatively high price of health services; (3) the lower supplies of health professionals, facilities, and equipment in the United States; (4) administrative complexities and costs;

and (5) the unwillingness of Americans to ration care. Furthermore, in an update of the article, Anderson and colleagues (2005) debunked the popular misconception that the costs associated with malpractice litigation are responsible for high U.S. health care costs, as compared to the OECD countries.

SUMMARY

Financing health services in the United States includes a plethora of institutions and activities. The growth of employer-based private health insurance has stimulated unprecedented growth in health expenditures and biomedical advancement for the nation in the postwar era. The advent of Medicare and Medicaid in 1966, heralded a period of even more rapid growth, along with unbridled inflation, that persists to this day.

Inequities in access to health care (once thought to be alleviated by Medicare and Medicaid along with the extensive provision of voluntary health insurance for employed groups) have not been resolved. Universal health coverage has not been realized, and a substantial and growing percent of the U.S. population go uninsured. State revenues have grown at rates slower than state-funded health care costs, inducing across-the-board reductions and more restrictive eligibility requirements for state Medicaid programs. The Prospective Payment System, the new Medicare Fee Schedule for physicians, selective contracting, and managed care plans have demonstrated short-lived successes in stalling the continued growth in health care spending. However, health care expenditures as a percent of GDP continue to grow with no end in sight. Furthermore, effective means for identifying and monitoring the adequacy and appropriateness of health care have not been developed.

The cry for health care reform resounds in all sectors of the U.S. economy. While most policy makers agree on universal access, they are far from an agreement on how to finance the system, reimburse the providers, and impose cost controls. Whatever transpires in the future is likely to revolve around the fundamental politic of health finance: private versus public, entitlement versus social welfare, and fee for service versus prepayment.

This chapter has provided a historical and methodological framework for understanding and analyzing health care finance in the United States today. Many of the principles that have been presented apply to financing health systems worldwide, no matter how turbulent the future of health care proves to be.

REVIEW QUESTIONS

1. Describe the size of the U.S. health care industry in financial terms, and discuss the growth in health care expenditures.
2. Describe the flow of finance in health care in the United States, referring specifically to payment sources and outlays for health care services.
3. Describe the three main types of health insurance in the United States, referring specifically to voluntary health insurance, social health insurance, and welfare medicine.
4. Briefly describe Medicare Parts A, B, C, D.
5. Briefly describe the Medicaid program.
6. Discuss the methods of physician reimbursement in the United States.
7. Provide an overview of the prospective payment system.
8. Describe the resource-based relative-value scale payment method.

REFERENCES & ADDITIONAL READINGS

Aaron, H. J. (1993/1994, Winter). Paying for health care. *Domestic Affairs*, 23–78.
AHIP Center for Policy and Research. (2005a). Summary: Number of HSA plans exceeded one million in March 2005. Retrieved May 4, 2005, from http:/www.ahipResearch.org.
AHIP Center for Policy and Research. (2005b). Comparison of tax-advantaged health care spending

accounts. Retrieved January 11, 2005, from http:/www.ahipResearch.org.

American Medical Association. (1984) *Diagnosis-related groups (DRGs) and the prospective payment system.* Chicago: American Medical Association.

Anderson, G. F., Hussey, P. S., Frogner, B. K., & Waters, H. R. (2005). Health spending in the United States and the rest of the industrialized world. *Health Affairs, 24*(4), 903–914.

Deloitte Haskins & Sells. (1982). *Tax Equity and Fiscal Responsibility Act of 1982: Management strategies for health care providers.* New York: Deloitte Haskins & Sells.

Deloitte & Touche. (2005a, August 4). CMS Final FY 2006 inpatient PPS update includes 3.7-percent increase, DRG revisions, post-acute-care transfer policy expansion, and other significant changes. *Washington Commentary,* pp. 1–23.

Deloitte & Touche. (2005b, November 7). CMS issues final FY 2006 physician fee schedule update containing 4.4-percent payment reduction. *Washington Commentary.*

DesHarnais, S., Kobrinski, E., Chesney, J., et al. (1987). The early effects of the Prospective Payment System on inpatient utilization and the quality of care. *Inquiry, 24,* 7–16.

Enthoven, A. (1981). The competition strategy; status and prospects. *New England Journal of Medicine, 304,* 109–112.

Fuchs, V. R. (1984). "Though much is taken": Reflections on aging, health, and medical care. *Milbank Memorial Fund Quarterly, 62,* 143–166.

Gornick, M., Greenberg, N. J., Eggers, P. W., et al. (1985). Twenty years of Medicare and Medicaid: Covered populations, use of benefits, and program expenditures. *Health Care Financing Review* (Ann. Suppl.), 13–59.

Guterman, S., Dobson, A. (1986). Impact of the Medicare Prospective payment system for hospitals. *Health Care Financing Review, 7,* 97–114.

Guterman, S., Eggers, P. W., Riley, G., Greene, T. F., & Terrell, S. A. (1988). The first 3 years of Medicare prospective payment: An overview. *Health Care Financing Review, 9*(3), 67–77.

Hillman, A. L., Welch, W. P., & Pauly, M. V. (1992). Contractual arrangements between HMOs and primary care physicians: Three-tiered HMOs and risk pools. *Medical Care, 30*(2), 136–148.

Hsiao, W. C., Braun, P., Becker, E. R., et al. (1992). Results and impacts of the resource-based relative value scale. *Medical Care, 30*(11), NS61–NS79.

Hsiao, W. C., Braun, P., Dunn, D., Becker, E. R., DeNicola, M., & Ketcham, T. R. (1988a). Results and policy impications of the resource-based relative-value study. *New England Journal of Medicine, 319*(13), 881–888.

Hsiao, W. C., Braun, P., Yntema, D., & Becker, E. R. (1988b). Estimating physicians' work for a resource-based relative-value scale. *New England Journal of Medicine, 319*(13), 835–841.

Journal of the American Medical Association. (1991, May 15), *265*(19), May 15.

Kaiser Family Foundation. (2006). *State health facts.* Retrieved February 26, 2006, from http://www. statehealthfacts.org/cgi-bin/healthfacts.cgi.

Lubitz, J., & Prihoda, R. (1984). Use and costs of Medicare services in the last two years of life. *Health Care Financing Review, 5,* 117–131.

Lundberg, G. D. (1991). National health care reform: An aura of inevitability is upon us. *Journal of the American Medical Association, 265*(19), 2566–2567.

Neuschler, E. (1990). *Canadian health care: The implications of public health insurance.* Washington, DC: Health Insurance Association of America.

Reinhardt, U. E. (1985). The compensation of physicians: Approaches used in foreign countries. *Quality Review Bulletin, 11,* 366–377.

Reinhardt, U. E., Hussey, P. S., & Anderson, G.F. (2004). U.S. health care spending in an international context. *Health Affairs, 23*(3), 10–25.

Rice, T. (1992). Containing health care costs in the United States. *Medical Care Review, 49*(1), 19–65.

Roemer, M. I. (1977). *Comparative national policies on health care.* New York, Marcel Dekker.

Roemer, M. I. (1978). *Social medicine: The advance of organized health services in America.* New York, Springer.

Smith, C., Cowan, C., Heffler, S., Catlin, A., & National Accounts Team. (2006). National health spending in 2004: Recent slowdown led by prescription drug spending. *Health Affairs, 25*(1), 186–196.

U.S. Census Bureau. *Statistical abstracts, 2004–2005.* Retrieved February 6, 2006, from http://www.census.gov/prod/www/abs/statab.html.

U.S. Department of Health and Human Services. (USDHHS), Centers for Medicare & Medicaid Services. (2003). *Data Compendium.* Retrieved February 27, 2006, from http://www.cms.hhs.gov/DataCompendium/02_2003_Data Compendium.asp#TopOfPage.

U.S. Department of Health & Human Services (USDHHS), Centers for Medicare & Medicaid Services. (2005a). *2004 Medicare & Medicaid statistical supplement.* Retrieved February 26, 2006, from http://www.cms.hhs.gov/MedicareMedicaidStatSupp/05_2004%20Edition.asp#TopOfPage.

U.S. Department of Health & Human Services (USDHHS), Centers for Medicare & Medicaid Services. (2005b). 2005 CMS statistics. Retrieved February 6, 2006, from http://www.cms.hhs.gov/MedicareMedicaidStatSupp/downloads/2005_CMS_Statistics.pdf.

U.S. Department of Health and Human Services (USDHHS), Centers for Medicare & Medicaid Services. (2006a). *Medicare & you.* Retrieved February 1, 2006, from http://www.medicare.gov/publications/pubs/pdf/10050.pdf.

U.S. Department of Health & Human Services. (USDHHS), Centers for Medicare & Medicaid Services. (2006b). *Medicare physician fee schedule.* http://new.cms.hhs.gov/apps/pfslookup/step0.asp.

U.S. Department of Health and Human Services (USDHHS), Health Care Financing Administration, Office of Research and Demonstrations. (1995, February). *Medicare and Medicaid statistical supplement. Health care financing review.* (HCFA Pub. No. 03348), Vol. 17.

Waldo, M. O. (1990). Addendum: A brief summary of the Medicaid program. *Health care financing review* (Ann. Suppl.), *12,* 171–172.

The White House Domestic Policy Council: The president's health security plan. (1993). New York: Times Books.

CHAPTER 5

Private Health Insurance and Managed Care

Alma Koch

CHAPTER TOPICS

- Principles of Insurance
- Health Insurance in the United States
- Health-Related Insurance Programs
- Health Plan Benefits Design
- Managed Care
- The Future of Health Insurance
- The Uninsured
- The Prospect of National Health Insurance

LEARNING OBJECTIVES

Upon completing this chapter, the reader should be able to

1. Understand the history, structure, and role of health insurance.
2. Appreciate the commercial health insurance industry.
3. Differentiate various health insurance provisions, terms, conditions, and product types.
4. Understand related insurance products.
5. Analyze the appropriate role of managed care in the nation's health care system.
6. Understand the variety of arrangements included under the term *managed care*.
7. Appreciate the roles of all key players, especially the consumer, in managed care.
8. Understand the underlying mechanisms of managed care.
9. Appreciate the challenges facing this industry in the future.

The United States is clearly the world leader in financing health services using the private health insurance (PHI) vehicle. In 2004, PHI financed 35 percent of the nation's health care dollar, covering, to some extent, almost 85 percent of the population. PHI is by far the most comprehensive source of medical care financing for working Americans and it plays a pivotal role in influencing the direction and structure of the United States medical care system.

Since 1980, managed care has insinuated itself on all health insurance products in the private sector. Today, even the most generous indemnity-type plans require prior review of elective hospital admissions (this being the minimum intervention in the managed-care process). Employee health benefits and managed care are inextricably linked for a large (but shrinking) majority of working American families. The possibility of uninsurance is a real threat to many workers who may experience either periods of unemployment or jobs that do not offer health insurance benefits at all. Thus, a clear understanding of private health insurance and managed care is becoming essential, not just for health policy makers and health executives, but also for everyday people as they look at careers and families, evaluate the health insurance options available to them (if any), and prepare for their retirement.

PRINCIPLES OF INSURANCE

Risk is the possibility of a loss. Thus it is the risk that one insures against. Insurance is a mechanism for managing the financial exposure to risk via two basic principles: (1) transferring risk from an individual to a group, and (2) sharing losses on some equitable basis by all members of the group. Depending on the purchaser's tolerance for risk and on one's ability to withstand the economic consequences of an actual loss, the amount and type of insurance required can vary widely.

When health insurance began in the United States, it was purchased to protect an individual from an expensive loss requiring hospital care. As PHI evolved to cover more people and a wider variety of medical expenses, it began to hold certain violations of the principles of insurance.

- The loss is supposed to be something out of the ordinary, as well as something to be avoided. Ill health, however, is a commonplace event for most people, and in many cases the loss being insured against is not necessarily an event to be dreaded (e.g., a routine visit to the doctor).

- Losses are supposed to be independent events: from person to person and from one event to another within the same person. In contrast, the very nature of infectious illness (or, in the extreme, an epidemic) implies a great degree of dependency among insured losses.

- The loss should be of such financial magnitude that it is unrealistic to budget for it. First dollar medical plans violate this tenet. Vision care insurance, for example, skates the edge of this insurance principle.

Because of these principles, health insurance has evolved into a fundamentally different product than most other forms of insurance. And many health care observers have noted that these unique characteristics of health insurance, when added to the economic structures of the medical care marketplace, have made health insurance a chief contributor to the continuing growth of health expenditures in the United States. Ironically, the presence and growth of health insurance in the 1950s and 1960s provided a financial foundation for much of the medical industry that now fuels escalating costs. The presence of health insurance, in itself, creates a situation that stimulates demand and increases medical care prices, thereby raising the cost of health care and encouraging even greater insistence on more comprehensive coverage (Whitted, 2001).

HEALTH INSURANCE IN THE UNITED STATES

Modern private group health insurance started in 1929, when Dallas teachers contracted with Baylor Hospital to cover certain hospital expenses, thereby starting the first Blue Cross plan. During the 1930s and 1940s, health insurance coverage grew slowly, in terms of both the insured population and the types of coverage offered. In 1940, private insurers provided some form of health protection to 12 million people, less than 10 percent of the population. After World War II, a series of legal and tax incentives for both employers and employees provided inducements to purchase comprehensive health insurance benefits. In 1942, only 37 insurers wrote group health insurance coverage; by 1951, this number had climbed to 212. By 1950, the number of people covered by the nation's health insurers had climbed to nearly 77 million, or 53 percent of the U.S. population. Fueled by the strong union gains of the 1950s and 1960s, collectively bargained employee benefits packages quickly became the norm throughout American industry (Congressional Budget Office, 1991; Feldstein & Friedman, 1977; Greenspan & Vogel, 1980).

In 1960, 123 million Americans held some type of health insurance, generating about $5 billion in payments and accounting for nearly 21 percent of total personal health care expenditures. (See Table 5.1.) The 1960s were a boom time for the health insurance industry with coverage expanded to an additional 36 million Americans and payments tripled to $15 billion—more than 23 percent of total United States personal health care expenditures. This expansion was coincidental with the inception of Medicare and Medicaid in 1965, giving substantial impetus to the notion that affordable access to the health care system was a right for Americans.

The 1970s witnessed another 29 million Americans added to the roster of the health insured

Table 5.1. Private Health Insurance (PHI) as a Health Financing Mechanism for Personal Health Care Expenditures (PHCE), Selected Years

Year	PHI Expenditures ($ Billions)	PHI Expenditures (Percent of PHCE)
1960	5.0	21.0
1970	14.8	23.0
1980	62.0	29.0
1990	201.8	33.4
2000	398.7	35.1
2004	658.5	37.6

SOURCE: Adapted from *Statistical Abstracts, 2004–2005;* U.S. Census Bureau, retrieved February 24, 2006, from http://www.census.gov/prod/www/abs/statab.html and "National Health Spending in 2004: Recent Slowdown Led by Prescription Drug Spending;" by C. Smith et al., 2006, *Health Affairs, 25*(1), 186–196.

population along with new forms of health insurance products (principally dental and prescription drug insurance). By 1980, health insurance paid 29 percent of the nation's personal health care bill. Although the 1980s saw proportionately slower growth in the proportion of people with PHI, by 1990, PHI expenditures more than tripled to $202 billion. By 2004, PHI and employee benefit programs were responsible for financing nearly almost 38 percent of all personal medical care expenditures (PHCE).

Table 5.2 describes health insurance coverage from 1984 to 2003 among those under 65 years of age. The privately insured are contrasted with Medicaid beneficiaries and the uninsured. (Few Medicare enrollees are under age 65 and thus are excluded from the table.) PHI, including health benefits obtained through work, has been in steady decline in terms of the percentage of the population obtaining it. While Medicaid has expanded, particularly for those under 18 years, so has the percent of the population over 18 that is uninsured. Whites are more likely to be privately insured than any

Table 5.2. Private Health Insurance Coverage among Persons under 65 Years of Age, According to Selected Characteristics: United States, Selected Years 1984–2003

Characteristic	Private Insurance Total		Private Insurance Obtained through Workplace		Medicaid		No Health Insurance Coverage	
	1984	2003	1984	2003	1984	2003	1984	2003
	Number in millions							
Total	157.5	173.6	141.8	159.3	14.0	30.9	29.8	41.6
	Percent of population							
Total	76.8	68.9	69.1	63.3	6.8	12.3	14.5	16.5
Age								
Under 18 years	72.6	63.0	66.5	58.6	11.9	26.0	13.9	9.8
18–44 years	76.5	67.7	69.6	62.2	5.1	7.4	17.1	23.5
45–64 years	83.3	77.3	71.8	70.0	3.4	5.3	9.6	12.5
Race								
White only	79.9	71.5	72.0	65.6	4.6	10.4	13.6	16.0
Black or African American	58.1	54.9	52.4	51.5	20.5	23.7	19.9	18.4
American Indian/ Alaska Native	49.1	45.0	45.8	40.5	28.2	18.5	22.5	35.0
Asian	69.9	71.4	59.0	62.1	8.7	8.0	18.5	18.2
Hispanic or Latino	55.7	41.9	52.0	38.9	13.3	21.8	29.5	34.7

SOURCE: *Control and Health United States, 2005,* U.S. Department of Health and Human Services, Centers for Disease Prevention, National Center for Health Statistics, 2005, Hyattsville, MD: U.S. Department of Health and Human Services, pp. 379–385.

other racial or ethnic group, and they are more likely to receive group coverage through work. Blacks are more disproportionately represented in Medicaid than any other group, whereas Hispanics are far more likely to be uninsured. Although their numbers are relatively small, Native Americans are overrepresented in Medicaid and among the uninsured.

Methods for Categorizing Health Insurance

Most health insurance today is a combination of true insurance against illness and other employee benefit products, such as disability income. One

method characterizes health insurance according to the typical combination of products. The principal insurance vehicles that provide benefits associated with ill health are (1) basic employee benefits, including medical, dental, vision, and prescription drug benefits; (2) disability insurance—short- and long-term insurance offered as part of many employee benefit programs, as well as compulsory temporary disability insurance mandated by five states; and (3) workers' compensation. Employers pay partially or wholly for each category of insurance, with basic employee benefits reimbursing most of the expenditures attributed to health insurance.

The second major method for categorizing health insurance is by the type of organization sponsoring the coverage. First among such sponsors are the approximately 500 to 800 for-profit insurance carriers that comprise the commercial health insurance industry. Second, Blue Cross and Blue Shield plans also sponsor basic employee health benefits but traditionally enjoy a nonprofit tax status from that of the commercials. (However, the Tax Reform Act of 1986 removed the federal tax exemption for some Blue Cross and Blue Shield organizations engaged in providing commercial-type insurance.) Third, health maintenance organizations (HMOs) also offer health insurance, although not according to the same legal strictures as either the Blues or the commercials. HMOs are not guaranteeing to reimburse the insured for medical expenses. Rather, their obligation to the insured is more direct: to actually provide medical services to them. A fourth major entity in furnishing health insurance is employers (primarily large corporations) that self-fund or partially self-fund employee benefits for workers and their families. Although declining in importance, unions are a fifth type of health insurance sponsor. Finally, corporations and unions sometimes jointly sponsor and administer Taft-Hartley health and welfare funds.

The final method for categorizing health insurance is by funding mechanism: (1) fully insured, (2) partially insured, and (3) self-funded or self-insured. All three funding alternatives are used by private medical and dental plans (Park, 2000). Which type of funding is most attractive to an employer is primarily a function of the size of its employee population and the employer's degree of risk aversion.

Full Insurance

The standard, fully insured program remains the principal funding mechanism for the millions of small and medium-size businesses that form the foundation of employment for most Americans. For employers with more than 5,000 employees, pure self-funding is actuarially viable because medical expenses are relatively predictable. With 100 percent self-funding, employers basically choose some organization (an insurer or third-party administrator) to administer their medical benefits program and perform claim adjudication. Thus, the employer pays two types of employee benefits expenses: (1) medical service claim expenses submitted to the administrator for reimbursement and (2) an administrative fee (or "retention"). This fee can be computed as a per capita charge, a percent of claim payments, or a transaction-related fee.

Partial Insurance

Many employers, particularly those with 500 to 5,000 employees, are reluctant to assume the financial risk of a full self-funding. For them, partial self-funding is usually the funding mechanism of choice. The most common type of partial funding is the "minimum premium plan" that allows the employer to self-fund claim expenses up to a certain predetermined maximum amount, after which an insured policy assumes financial liability. Another variant of self-funding involves the purchase of stop-loss insurance for individual enrollees who exceed their maximum allowable out-of-pocket payments. The point is that the employer pays directly for all medical claims, except for those that exceed a predetermined threshold.

Self-Insurance

Self-insurance has been one of the principal trends in health insurance since the late 1970s. One inducement for self-funding is that the employer avoids the risk charges, various administrative fees, and profits paid to the insurer and rolled into the premium. Also, because self-funding is technically not insurance, employers can avoid the taxes assessed by states on premium revenue (usually amounting to several percentage points).

Perhaps the biggest enhancement of self-funding, the Supreme Court ruled in June 1985 that the 1974 federal Employee Retirement Income Security Act of 1974 (ERISA) exempted states from regulating self-funded group medical programs (Blumenthal, 2006; Rublee, 1985). The most important advantage of this preemption is the ability of employers to avoid state mandates to cover particular services (e.g., fertility treatment, mental health coverage, etc.) and make it easier for them to design new benefit packages. Thus, self-funding not only provides financial savings for large employers, but also permits the employers significantly greater flexibility in designing benefit plans and establishing employee cost-sharing responsibilities. By 2005, 54 percent of all covered workers (and 82 percent of workers in firms of 5,000 or more employees) were either partially or completely self-funded by their employers.

The Commercial Health Insurance Industry

There are several ways to describe the commercial health insurance industry. Perhaps the most fundamental distinction is between mutual and stock insurers. Mutual insurance companies, such as Prudential and Liberty Mutual, are essentially owned by their policyholders, in contrast to stock insurance companies, such as Aetna and United Health-Care, which are owned in the more traditional corporate fashion by stockholders.

Commercial health insurance companies are either "multiline" carriers or "single-line" insurers. Multiline insurers offer life insurance as well as other property/casualty products (e.g., auto, homeowners, worker's compensation, business liability, etc.). Many multiline insurers also operate a range of financial services, particularly in the pension and investment areas. In contrast, single-line health insurers offer health insurance and related employee benefits (e.g., disability insurance).

With the hundreds of companies that participate in writing health insurance policies, the commercial health insurance industry is lightly concentrated, with the top 10 largest health insurers accounting for about 18 percent of all private health insurance revenues in 2003.

Blue Cross and Blue Shield Plans

As noted earlier, Blue Cross initiated the modern era of private health insurance in 1929. Throughout the early portion of their history, Blue Cross plans focused attention on insurance for hospital costs, and Blue Cross itself was closely affiliated with the American Hospital Association. In 1939, Blue Shield began offering medical insurance protection for physicians' services. Blue Shield was affiliated with the American Medical Association because of its focus on insuring physician expenditures.

Since the 1960s, many Blue Cross and Blue Shield plans (known as "the Blues") have merged their activities, becoming essentially a single insurance entity in a state. By the 1980s, however, a number of Blues Cross and Blue Shield plans divorced themselves from each other, and in a few cases became bitter rivals within some states. Today, 64 Blue Cross and Blue Shield organizations operate in all 50 states and U.S. territories.

In recent years, the national Blue Cross and Blue Shield Association has become more aggressive about coordinating resources of individual plans (e.g., in the area of centralized claims processing). This cooperation has been necessary in order to compete effectively with large national commercial insurance companies, especially in procuring the business of employers that operate in more than one state. The Blue Cross and Blue Shield Association also developed a national HMO network for the same reason.

Unlike commercial insurance companies, which are regulated in most states by a state insurance department, most Blue Cross and Blue Shield plans are subject to special enabling state legislation. In addition to the close affiliations of the Blues with hospital and physician providers, the Blues have differentiated themselves historically from commercial insurers by establishing premium levels using a community rating methodology (in contrast to the experience rating most often used by commercial insurers) (Hall, 2001).

Another area of differentiation historically between the Blues and commercial insurers is the Blues' adoption of service benefits (i.e., percentage reimbursement for the total expense of covered benefits) rather than the indemnity benefits used by commercial insurers (i.e., payment of a fixed monetary amount for a covered claim). Today, however, many commercial insurers offer service or hybrid benefits, especially in their managed-care products.

One final point of distinction for the Blues is their traditional reluctance to underwrite quite as rigidly as commercial carriers, particularly with respect to refusing coverage for entire industry groups or for individuals. In some states, the Blues are the only health insurer of any significant size. All these historical differences between the Blues and commercial insurers, however, are rapidly disappearing.

The 1990s witnessed profound changes in the structure and organization of Blue Cross and Blue Shield plans. The number of Blues plans decreased steadily due to mergers between Blue Cross and Blue Shield on the state level, and Blues plans throughout the country are cooperating to market and administer their services (such as claims processing) jointly on a regional level. In addition, many Blues plans have already converted, or are seriously planning to convert, to for-profit status. In some cases, Blues plans are only spinning off for-profit subsidiaries, but the rationale is primarily to gain access to capital markets by selling stock to finance the investments in managed-care initiatives. It is likely that the Blues will continue to emphasize managed care with greater zeal than has historically been the case.

Health Maintenance Organizations

HMOs have been in existence for more than 75 years, since 1929, when the Ross-Loos Clinic in Los Angeles was founded. However, one can argue that the true roots of prepaid group practice began at the Mayo Clinic in the late 1800s.

Beginning with Kaiser's coverage of the health needs associated with workers building the Grand Coulee Dam in the 1930s, HMOs grew relatively slowly until the Nixon administration sparked new interest in capitated prepaid plans with the passage of the HMO Act of 1973. This act required employers with more than 25 employees to offer an HMO option if a local, federally qualified HMO was available. The legislation also required employers to contribute toward the HMO premium of its employees an amount equal to that contributed toward indemnity plan premiums—the so-called "equal contribution" rule.

In the 1990s, HMO growth slowed somewhat, due to several factors. The emergence of competing managed-care delivery systems, such as preferred provider organizations (PPOs) and point-of-service (POS) plans, provided employers with cost-effective, middle-of-the-road medical benefit plan options. Principal among the attractions to employers of these managed-care options is the enhanced employee freedom of choice regarding providers, particularly physicians. In addition, the wave of enthusiasm for HMOs regarding their success for cost containment was tempered when many HMOs' premiums reached levels as high as those of commercial insurers and the Blues. Finally, due to the financial and liability consequences of dealing with potentially insolvent HMOs, some employers substantially trimmed the number of HMOs offered to employees, particularly beginning in 1995 when the dual-choice mandating provision of the HMO Act of 1973 no longer applied to employers due to legislative amendments enacted in 1988. This same legislation also permitted greater employer flexibility in determining their required contributions to HMO premiums (Whitted, 2001).

Unlike the commercial carriers and the Blues that offer reimbursement for health care outlays, HMOs actually guarantee the provision of covered health services. Historically, like the Blues, HMOs have generally relied on community rating, rather than experience rating, to set premiums. (Indeed, the HMO Act of 1973 required federally qualified HMOs to price insurance by community rating.) Due to competitive pressures, HMOs are being pressured to engage in experience rating, which has been permitted since 1989 via amendments to the HMO Act of 1973. Another distinction between HMOs and their pure insurance colleagues is that HMOs are often regulated by an entirely different set of statutes and organizations than either commercial insurers or the Blues.

Not only can HMOs be freestanding organizations, but the Blues and commercial insurers also own and operate HMOs. Although the earliest large HMOs (such as Kaiser, the Health Insurance Plan of New York, and Group Health Cooperative of Puget Sound), as well as some of the newer, well-respected HMOs (such as the Harvard Community Health Plan in Boston), were organized as not-for-profit entities, many of the newer, rapidly expanding HMOs (such as United HealthCare) and most of the commercial insurance company-sponsored HMOs are for-profit organizations.

Private Health Insurance as a Financing Mechanism

Private health insurance is made up of the three principal entities just described (commercial carriers, the Blues, and HMOs plus self-funded plans). The importance of PHI as a source of financing for personal health care expenditures has increased slowly, but steadily.

As noted earlier, PHI began with coverage principally for hospital and physicians' services. In 1960, virtually all the total net PHI payments were devoted to these two types of health care. PHI has grown in importance as a source of financing for physicians' services. The largest percentage impacts of health insurance financing have occurred in the areas of dental services, nonphysician professional services, and pharmaceuticals. PHI for these expenses was negligible until about 1970, and even at that time, reimbursements from PHI were less than 7 percent of total payments in each of the three categories.

As political debates in the United States continue regarding health insurance, there has been considerable argument and criticism about the overhead generated by the PHI mechanism (Woolhandler & Himmelstein, 1991). From 1960 to 2000, the total overhead costs of PHI averaged about 12 percent of premiums, ranging from about 9 to 16 percent. This total includes administrative costs, taxes, profits, and other nonbenefit expenses (Lemieux, 2005). The full cost of PHI administration to Americans—including insurers' administrative costs, net additions to reserves, rate credits and policyholder dividends, premium taxes, and carriers' profits or losses—is estimated to be about 15 percent of total national health expenditures. None of this includes the formidable "hidden" costs to providers for filing claims, collecting data on quality of care, and submitting various financial reports to insurers.

Although there is no denying that some government health insurance programs such as Medicare deliver benefits at far less administrative cost per dollar of reimbursement than the PHI industry, health insurance by itself is not always a profitable business for insurers. This is particularly true at the high end of the market, where self-funded administrative-services-only customers generate relatively narrow profit margins for most group insurers. Indeed, the health insurance industry suffered a net underwriting loss (the difference between premiums and claims paid) in many years since 1976. Health insurance is beneficial for many insurers because it serves as a vehicle for selling other, more profitable products (such as life insurance) and because health insurance premiums generate revenues via investment income (Whitted, 2001).

HEALTH-RELATED INSURANCE PROGRAMS

Individual Coverage

A number of health insurance entities (including commercial carriers and the Blues) offer insurance coverage for individuals and their families (Pauly & Percy, 2000). Some of the nation's largest commercial accident and health insurers sell few or no individual policies.

Ordinary individual policies for basic medical (hospital and physician) coverage are extraordinarily expensive. This is because of adverse selection: Insurers assume that the individual knows something that the insurance plan doesn't about future health needs. Therefore, the insurer adds on premium for underwriting the additional risk. Policy premiums can easily reach $5,000 per year, even for HMO plans with extensive cost-sharing provisions. In addition, underwriting guidelines for individual policies have become increasingly stringent; so many people who might wish to purchase coverage are not able to do so (Saver & Doescher, 2000). In some states, the only recourse for such individuals is through high-risk state insurance pools. Many states have enacted broad-based pools for uninsurable individuals to provide some protection (Rogal & Gauthier, 2000).

A large dollar amount of individual insurance sold is supplementary in nature. Medigap insurance, usually sold as individual policies, are supplementary to basic Medicare Parts A, B, and D. Supplementary insurance policies pick up reimbursement for the many expenses and amenities that the primary plan does not cover (or covers only with significant cost sharing).

Demand for individual medical policies diminished with the enactment of COBRA (the Consolidated Omnibus Budget Reconciliation Act of 1985). Under this statute, employers with 20 or more employees must extend group health care coverage to former employees after they leave their jobs (voluntarily or not) and for dependents of employees following events such as death or divorce. Employers can charge a premium equal to the average cost of group health insurance for that employer.

Group Coverage

Table 5.2 on page 112 shows that in the United States employment is the principal source of insurance protection against medical and income losses associated with both on- and off-the-job illness and injury. The United States is the only major industrialized country in which voluntary, employment-based health plans are the primary source of health insurance for its citizens. Through sponsorship by a large number of different groups including employers, unions, employer/union Taft-Hartley plans, and multiple-employer trusts and other arrangements, about 63 percent of all Americans receive their health insurance protection via employer-based group coverage (down from 69 percent in 1984).

The rapidly accelerating costs associated with medical care and the tax-exempt nature of employee medical benefits have stimulated the expansion of group health coverage. For workers of medium-size employers, medical insurance protection is a commonplace benefit, and for large employers, health insurance is an almost universal benefit for full-time workers. But small employers tend to provide meager health insurance benefits, if they provide them at all.

HEALTH PLAN BENEFITS DESIGN

Today's core PHI health benefits consist primarily of medical and dental coverage. Larger employers may offer separate plans for coverage of prescription drugs, vision services, and (increasingly) long-term care. In addition, all health benefits can be bundled under one general medical plan. In 2004, more than 70 percent of PHI expenditures went toward hospital care and physician services.

The Indemnity Design

The indemnity plan, reimbursed by fee for service, is the oldest form of health insurance design. For most major types of providers (e.g., hospitals, physicians, nonphysician providers, laboratory and radiology services, etc.), traditional indemnity group policies hold benefits for enrollees that are somewhat uniform, but with different cost-sharing provisions for employees. The most generous plans (but also the type of plan rapidly losing favor with employers) are called "major medical" or base plans.

Under these arrangements, there is first-dollar coverage for hospitals and sometimes physicians, then more limited payments for other services (e.g., requiring 20 percent employee coinsurance). Perhaps the biggest disadvantage of base/ major medical plans is that many do not place any upper limit on the expenses borne by the patient in a calendar year.

Comprehensive Design

Today, the most prominent type of medical benefit plan—the comprehensive design—retains little, if any, first-dollar coverage. A comprehensive design usually has a relatively small annual deductible (e.g., $200) that pertains to all medical expenses; then it reimburses the patient a fixed percentage (usually 80 percent) of all medical claims that exceed the deductible, up to a maximum out-of-pocket patient expense (e.g., $2,000 per insured person). When the patient reaches this out-of-pocket maximum, 100 percent of all subsequent expenses are borne by the medical plan. Both base/major medical and comprehensive plans sometimes place lifetime maximums of $1 million or more on the total amount of benefits that will be paid to any individual.

Capitation Design

The benefit structure of medical plans offered by HMOs that receive their revenues by capitation is more comprehensive than in fee-for-service indemnity programs (although there are notable exceptions, particularly regarding the coverage of psychiatric and substance abuse illnesses). Second, the more generous HMO plans usually have no deductibles. Third, instead of coinsurance, HMOs feature fixed-dollar copayments for selected services such as physician office visits ($5 to $15 per visit) and medications ($5 to $10 per prescription). Finally, HMOs have traditionally displayed greater attentiveness to fostering health promotion and preventive services than indemnity insurers. Such covered expenses in HMO benefit plans include immunizations, well-child care, and annual physical examinations.

High-Deductible Health Plans

Although there are several types of high-deductible health plans (HDHPs) enabled by federal legislation, Health Savings Accounts (HSAs)—created as part of the Medicare Modernization Act of 2003—is the one of greatest interest to employers. HSAs give consumers financial incentives to choose their health care providers and manage their own health expenses. HSAs must be coupled with a high-deductible health plan (HDHP) to cover current and future health care costs. Under this arrangement, employers may create a tax-exempt trust created exclusively to pay for qualified medical expenses for employees who choose this option. Any unspent funds can be carried over by to subsequent years (Claxton et al., 2005).

Up to 100 percent of employee contributions are tax deductible, which holds significant financial advantages for people who can afford the direct costs. For 2005, employee deductibles must be at least $1,000 for self-only and $2,000 for family coverage, up to a maximum of $2,650 for a self-only account and $5,250 for a family. The maximum out-of pocket expense (i.e., deductible and copayments, not premiums) that can be incurred by an enrollee is $5,100 for self-only and $10,200 for a family. For the employer, contributions are excludable from gross income and not subject to payroll taxes, also holding financial advantages (AHIP, 2005b).

In 2005—less than 1 year into the program—the number of HSA plan enrollees topped 1 million. Although the group market is growing at a faster pace than the individual market, 54 percent of those covered by HSAs in 2005 are enrolled as individuals. About 37 percent of these individuals report that they were previously uninsured. In the small group market, 27 percent of policies were associated with small companies that did not previously offer coverage.

More than half of people covered by HSAs were age 40 or older. HSAs were meant for this group of affluent, employed middle-aged people who can take the risk of incurring high expenses for freedom of choice among providers under an indemnity plan. The tax benefits for this group are also substantial, yielding added incentives for growth in HSAs.

Dental Plans

Private insurance for dental expenses was not generally available until the 1970s. In 2004, dental insurance reimbursed nearly 50 percent of all dental services. Plan designs for dental insurance generally follow a comprehensive design. Usually there are three tiers of benefits. For preventive services (e.g., semiannual prophylaxis and routine dental X-rays), coverage is often 100 percent, without an annual deductible. For the two remaining benefit tiers, there is a small annual deductible ($50 to $100) per insured person) the patient must satisfy before any benefits are paid. Restorative services (such as amalgams), removable prosthetics, oral surgery, endodontics (such as root canals), and periodontics are then paid with relatively standard coinsurance (usually 80 percent). Expensive elective services such as crowns, inlays, and fixed prosthetics are reimbursed at only 50 percent by the dental plan. Cosmetic dentistry may be excluded from coverage entirely. Orthodontic services usually receive a limited lifetime benefit (e.g., $1,000), unless special orthodontic coverage is elected. Unlike medical benefits, dental plans are more restrictive in terms of annual limits on reimbursement. Dental HMOs (DMOs) and Delta Dental Plans offer broader services with fewer cost-sharing requirements than indemnity dental plans (Whitted, 2001).

Vision Plans

Insurance for vision care was first introduced by private insurers in 1957. Many health care observers believe that vision care is a prime example of what should not be covered by an insurance program, as vision care is relatively inexpensive for most Americans. For those covered for vision services, benefits generally include periodic examinations, eyeglasses, and contact lenses. With the advent of managed care, vision care may be available as a "carve-out" benefit, sometimes with a separate deductible. These vision care programs are usually offered in conjunction with large, national chains of vision care products, offering enrollees substantial discounts on these products if they are purchased through the preferred providers (Whitted, 2001).

Prescription Drug Plans

In 2004, PHI financed almost 48 percent of total prescription drug expenditures in the United States. In order to take advantage of managed-care cost savings, prescription drug benefits are often a carve-out of the regular medical benefit program. Coverage assumes one of two forms. In the traditional fashion, prescription drugs are simply a covered expense under the medical benefit plan. There may be individual copayments per prescription ranging from an average of $10 for a generic to $35 for a nonpreferred branded drug. Nearly all types of prescription drugs are eligible for reimbursement, with common exceptions being certain injectibles (except insulin), contraceptives, and experimental drugs. Prescription drugs for acute conditions (e.g., antibiotics) may be covered in part by the regular medical plan, with maintenance drugs available through mail order. Mail-order plans permit employers and employees to take advantage of steep discounts and some drug use review, while offering the convenience of home delivery. Mail-order programs have been particularly well received by older employees and retirees. The latest trend in pharmacy programs, however, is a full carve-out program for all prescription drugs, a feature that may or may not include a mail order companion product.

Long-Term Care Coverage

Long-term care (LTC) insurance has grown dramatically in recent years. In 2002, 104 companies sold more than 900,000 policies out of a cumulative 9.2 million policies sold since its inception in 1987. Approximately 80 percent of all LTC policies have been sold through the individual market, and about 70 percent of all individual policies remain in force (AHIP, 2004).

In 2002, the employer-sponsored group market surged to almost one-third of all policies sold. A large portion of this growth can be attributed to the launching of the LTC insurance program for federal employees. About 5,600 employers offer group LTC insurance to their employees, retirees, or both. For most of these plans, the employer contributes nothing to the premium (AHIP, 2004). However, for employers that do contribute to the premium, there are significant tax deductions and, for their beneficiaries, benefits are tax free up to specified limits (Pincus, 2000).

Unlike the service benefits of most group medical and dental plans, long-term care insurance is largely an indemnity product, offering a fixed daily reimbursement payment for LTC services. Invariably, all plans cover nursing homes, assisted living facilities, home health care, hospice care, respite care, and alternate care services. Other common benefits include case management and homemaker or chore services, certain medical equipment, survivor benefits, and caregiver training (AHIP, 2004).

Retiree Medical Coverage

For active employees between the ages of 65 and 70, the Tax Equity and Fiscal Responsibility Act of 1982 (TEFRA) required employers' group health insurance plans to remain the primary payers, with Medicare retaining only secondary coverage. In 1984, legislation further stipulated Medicare as the secondary payer for aged spouses of workers under age 65. These statutes are just two examples of how the federal government has shifted fiscal responsibility for the financing of medical care from government to the private sector.

Since the early 1990s, employers have been reevaluating the financial wisdom of providing continuing health insurance to retirees, particularly

for those under 65 who have taken early retirement (and therefore are ineligible for Medicare). This rethinking of retiree medical coverage has occurred because the unrelenting growth in health insurance benefits, which is two or three times as rapid as the increase in other costs of doing business, has forced employers to cut funding for retiree medical expenses.

Furthermore, for employers with significant numbers of retirees (such as automakers and insurance companies themselves), early retiree medical costs can significantly raise an employer's overall average financial liability for medical benefits. These pressures will strengthen with the flood of baby boomers now entering their sixties.

Regulations by the Financial Accounting Standards Board in 1993 (referred to as FASB 106) mandated that employers must accrue retiree health care liabilities as an expense against earnings from the date an employee is hired until that employee becomes eligible for benefits. With this accounting change, employers had to acknowledge the mounting burden of all medical benefits (not just retiree obligations) on employers' overhead expenses. For retirees under age 65, benefit protection is often the same as that for active employees. For retirees over age 65, employers' liability is diminished significantly because the group health insurance plan becomes secondary to Medicare coverage. For both groups, however, employers are reconsidering their funding options.

As a result of these combined forces, most employers are reexamining the wisdom of providing medical coverage for retirees. Among all firms with 200 or more workers that offer health insurance to active workers, only 33 percent offered retiree health benefits in 2005, as compared to 1988, when 60 percent offered such benefits (KFF & HRET, 2005). Several large U.S. employers have attempted, in high court and with considerable success, to rescind long-standing retiree health insurance programs entirely. Less draconian approaches to cut costs in this area include (1) not to offer retiree medical coverage for new hires, (2) to link coverage with length-of-service requirements, and (3) to require retirees to contribute a larger share of the costs of medical expense benefits.

The most fundamental choice facing most employers is whether to switch to a defined-contribution program, like pensions. This limits employers' future liabilities by making them more predictable (like pension benefits) and clearly places most of the concern over the ultimate magnitude of medical care cost escalation squarely on retirees. If defined-contribution programs for retiree medical benefits become the norm, retirees will need to be much more concerned about issues of plan design and cost containment than they have in the past. Active employees will also be required to assume more responsibility for funding their retiree medical benefits far ahead of when they will be incurred, just as workers must plan to ensure that they will retain enough retirement income via pension benefits and individual investment plans (Whitted, 2001).

Disability Insurance

Serious illness or injury for the employee creates financial hardship due to both the high costs of medical care and the loss of income. Thus, disability insurance is one of the oldest forms of health-related insurance. In contrast to the disability programs available through Social Security for long-term or permanent loss of income via disability, private insurance has focused on the short to medium term. Unlike most health insurance, disability insurance pays indemnity benefits, not service benefits. Neither short- nor long-term private disability programs reimburse for expenses associated with medical services. For decades, temporary disability insurance programs (including medical expense reimbursement) have been mandated by states such as Rhode Island, California, Hawaii, New Jersey, New York, and Rhode Island. These state-sponsored social health insurance programs, in turn, may contract with commercial carriers for health insurance services or managed care.

Short-Term Programs

Coverage for loss of income due to illness can be available to workers through two avenues: (1) sick leave or salary continuation benefits or (2) short-term disability insurance. While sick leave benefits usually replace all or most of an ill employee's wages, reimbursement is often limited to no more than a few weeks, at best. Eligibility for sick leave and accrued sick leave days are usually related to an employee's length of service.

Short-term disability programs protect workers for only relatively brief periods. Many short-term disability insurance plans have an employer length-of-service requirement, or waiting period, for employees before they are eligible for coverage (usually three months or less). Also, there is usually a short elimination period (1 to 7 days) between the onset of disability or illness and the date when benefits begin to be paid. In the most generous short-term income protection employee benefits, short-term disability benefits commence as soon as sick leave is used up, so that the ailing worker has no front-end gaps in income.

Long-Term Programs

Long-term disability insurance is often entirely employer-financed. Like short-term coverage, long-term disability insurance maintains a waiting period before employees are eligible for coverage. Plan participants may have an elimination period of six months.

In order to induce workers to return to the job and because long-term disability payments can be exempt from both state and federal taxation, benefits are paid at rates usually in the range of 50 to 67 percent of a worker's wages, subject to maximums. Due to the existence of Social Security disability programs, most long-term disability policies include provisions that permit benefits to be reduced commensurate with the amount of Social Security disability benefits paid. This provision is analogous to the coordination-of-benefits feature common in most medical and dental insurance policies.

Workers' Compensation Insurance

Like Medicare, workers' compensation insurance is a social insurance program. Workers' compensation was the first type of broad-coverage, health-related insurance plans in the United States. Worker's compensation programs were enacted by nine states in 1911, and by 1920, all but six states had inaugurated such a program (Workers' Compensation, 1991). Today, there are 55 workers' compensation programs in operation, one in each of the 50 states as well as in Puerto Rico, the District of Columbia, and the Virgin Islands. There are also two special federal workers' compensation programs covering government employees, longshoremen, and harbor workers. In addition, there are unique occupational illness and injury programs for coal miners suffering from pneumoconiosis (black lung disease) and railroad workers.

Workers' compensation insurance is compulsory for most private employment, except in a very few states. This protection provides workers and their families with three types of benefits: (1) indemnity cash benefits to help replace lost wages, (2) medical expense reimbursement, and (3) survivors' death benefits. Despite generally broad-based coverage, many state workers' compensation programs do not cover domestics, agricultural workers, and casual laborers. Initially focusing on workplace injuries, workers' compensation programs are increasingly being pressured financially by the long-term effects of occupational illness.

In most states, employers purchase workers' compensation insurance through private commercial insurers. In some states, however, commercial insurance is not permitted and the state assumes responsibility for the program. Each state establishes its own regulatory mechanisms, eligibility rules, benefit schedule, and funding alternatives.

Since 1980, the percentage of total medical expenditures that are reimbursed by workers' compensation has been increasing slowly, but steadily. This trend is due both to states' restrictions on cash compensation benefit levels and to the higher growth rate of medical care when compared to wages. Nearly all employee medical plans contain provisions that exclude coverage for medical care for work-related accidents, in order to avoid duplicate payments by both the medical plan and workers' compensation.

Workers' compensation expenses are accelerating like the costs of medical care in general. Thus, it is no surprise that many managed care techniques are now being modified for workers' compensation programs. However, some states mandate a higher degree of freedom for employees in their choice of providers than would be tolerated in managed care plans. Thus, some of the most aggressive transference of managed-care techniques from the employee benefits arena to workers' compensation is occurring in those states that provide employers with unilateral physician selection powers (Whitted, 2001).

MANAGED CARE

Although the term "managed care" has become increasingly familiar to anyone involved with health care in the United States, there are two major misunderstandings with regard to the term and its use. First, the term is sometimes used as though all forms of managed care are the same, or that managed care were a single organizational structure that functions like a tightly unified entity Unfortunately, nothing could be further from the truth. Managed care covers a wide variety of organizational forms, and in any one of the organizational forms, there are three or four separate subunits that make up the whole.

The second misunderstanding with regard to managed care often involves the impact of the arrival of managed care on the American health care system. Sometimes, managed care is discussed as if it were merely one more change in the way health insurance is organized and in the way that providers of health services are paid. Frequently, managed care is described as yet one more technical innovation in what has become an increasingly specialized field of insurance.

Unfortunately, viewing managed care as merely a new set of technical changes misses the point that managed care has brought about a major change in the way health care in the United States is delivered by providers and utilized by patients. It should be understood that although the technical changes included in managed care are very interesting, it is much more important to realize that the structural and policy changes in American health care are being promulgated by managed care.

What Is Managed Care?

It is virtually impossible to provide a definition of managed care that satisfies all participants in all circumstances because the applications of the term are so wide and varied (Fox, 1997; Miller & Luft, 1994). One definition might be, "Managed care is an organized effort by health insurance plans and providers to use financial incentives and organizational arrangements to alter provider and patient behavior so that health care services are delivered and utilized in a more efficient and lower-cost manner." This definition includes the central principles of managed care: It is an organized effort that involves both insurers and providers of health care; it uses financial incentives and an organizational structure in reaching its goal; and its purpose is to increase efficiency and reduce health care costs (Drake, 1997). Table 5.3 outlines the major objectives in managed care.

Table 5.3. Objectives of Managed Care

- Enhance cost containment
- Implement some forms of rationing
- Promote administrative and clinical efficiency
- Reduce duplication of services
- Enhance appropriateness of care
- Promote comprehensive contracting mechanisms
- Manage care processes by managing provider and consumer behavior

The Structure of Managed Care

The structure of managed care includes at least four tiers of players: (1) the purchaser or ultimate payer for health care; (2) the health insurance plans, including HMOs; (3) the providers of care (i.e., hospitals, physicians, and others involved in the direct delivery of personal health care); and (4) the patients receiving health care.

The purchaser of managed care is generally one of three groups: employers who purchase private health insurance for their employees, the federal Medicare program, or state Medicaid programs. Health insurance plans are licensed by individual states to offer medical benefits coverage that is bought by the purchasers. Health insurance plans design the benefit packages, market the plans, enroll the beneficiaries, arrange for the provision of health care services, and monitor the results. The providers of care are licensed health care professionals, organizations, and institutions that actually deliver the needed health care services to the individual beneficiaries under the terms of insurers' benefit packages. The patients are the individuals who are covered by health insurance plans and receive health services from providers. It has been suggested that a fifth important component part of the managed-care structure might be the health insurance brokers, as an increasingly high percentage of health insurance (particularly that provided by employers) is arranged through the technical and organizational assistance of brokers.

In many instances of managed care, these four (or five) components are separate organizational units, linked together by negotiated contracts. In HMOs, such as the Kaiser-Permanente Health Plan, the insurance and provision of care functions are seemingly joined together in a single organization that appears to be both the insurer and the entity providing services. In most other managed-care arrangements, this is not the case, and it is more useful to consider the insurance and the provision of services functions as organizational subunits that can be either more loosely or more tightly linked together.

How Managed Care Works

The process of making managed care work begins with certain important decisions made by the purchaser or employer (Enthoven & Singer, 1996). With these decisions, the purchaser must decide how many and what type of health insurance plans are to be offered to employees and how much the organization will pay in employee premiums. Today, purchasers are offering fewer health insurance plans and are paying a defined dollar contribution to each employee's premium, irrespective of which plan the beneficiary chooses, with the employee paying any difference.

Specifically, purchasers must decide whether they wish to give their beneficiaries a wide-open range of choices of providers or whether they wish to limit, in some fashion, the choices available to the beneficiaries. Figure 5.1 shows the continuum of managed care. The more restrictive plans may yield lower costs, but with a limited choice of providers and with greater controls on consumer behavior. Purchasers must also decide whether they want to have their beneficiaries in a plan that pays providers on a fee-for-service basis or by capitation, that is, a fixed amount per person per month (PMPM). Given these choices, the purchasers usually find themselves choosing between a preferred provider organization (PPO) or a health

maintenance organization (HMO). The PPO allows the recipient of health insurance a wider choice of providers and pays those providers on a modified fee-for-service basis; the HMO offers a more constrained range of providers and usually pays the provider organization on a PMPM basis.

Types of Managed-Care Plans

The two main types of managed-care plans offered to purchasers are preferred provider organizations (PPOs), and health maintenance organizations (HMOs) and point-of-service (POS) plans. These plans differ significantly in their major characteristics.

Preferred Provider Organizations

The PPO is essentially a fee-for-service type of health plan that allows a beneficiary to use a wide range of providers (or select from a narrower list of providers) that have agreed to give the purchaser a discount on regular fees. If the beneficiary chooses to use a provider on the preferred list, the plan, the provider, and the beneficiary all benefit. The health plan has generally contracted a discounted rate from participating provider's for their services. (A 20 percent discount is not uncommon.) In other words, the health plan uses its purchasing power to extract a lower price. In return, the providers hope

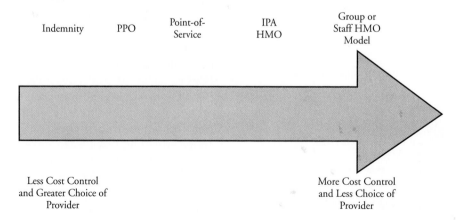

Figure 5.1. Continuum of Cost Control in the U.S. Health Care System

that the health insurance plan's members will choose them more frequently because they are now put on a special list of "preferred providers" available to the health plan's members.

Members benefit by choosing a preferred provider because their share of the cost (i.e., deductibles and coinsurance) is substantially reduced. A common coinsurance rate for members using a preferred provider is 10 percent of the also reduced contracted fee or "allowed amount" by the health plan. In other words, financial incentives are used to create a network that potentially benefits payers, providers, and enrollees.

For purchasers, the PPO is an attractive option because they are not forcing their beneficiaries to limit their provider choices or change their behaviors if they do not want to. However, if members do go outside of the preferred group, they will pay higher coinsurance rates on discounted maximum allowances per service.

Health Maintenance Organizations

Table 5.4, which outlines HMO plans by type and over time, shows that the number of HMO plans and their enrollment peaked around the year 2000 (with more than 30 percent of the population in HMOs). Enrollment has been in retrograde ever since, shifting since 1980 from the group practice model to the IPA and mixed models. Medicaid HMOs (often contracted to the private sector) have seen strong growth since 1990. Today, HMO plans are prominent in the Northeast and the West.

The HMO type of managed-care plan holds many significant differences from PPOs plans. Indeed, the differences are so major that it is confusing to describe them under the same general heading of managed care, as though both are closely related and are only minor variants of each other.

The HMO type of managed-care plan has a number of important premises built into its framework. The HMO depends on the fact that the health plan has developed a contract with a group of physicians to take total responsibility for a list of enrolled patients. The HMO form of managed care depends on an individual choosing to sign up with

Table 5.4. **Health Maintenance Organizations (HMOs) and Enrollment, According to Selected Characteristics, 1980–2004**

HMO Plans and Enrollment	1980	1990	2000	2004
Plans	*Number*			
All plans	235	572	568	412
Enrollment	*Number of persons in millions*			
Total	9.1	33.0	80.9	68.8
	Percent of population enrolled in HMOs			
Total	4.0	13.4	30.0	23.4
	Percent of HMO enrollees			
Model type				
Individual practice association	18.7	41.6	41.3	35.8
Group	81.3	58.4	18.9	22.2
Mixed	—	—	39.9	42.0
Federal program				
Medicaid	2.9	3.5	13.3	20.8
Medicare	4.3	5.4	8.1	7.1
Geographic region				
Northeast	3.1	14.6	36.5	30.1
Midwest	2.8	12.6	23.2	18.7
South	0.8	7.1	22.6	16.0
West	12.2	23.2	41.7	34.4

SOURCE: *Health United States, 2005,* U.S. Department of Health and Human Services, Centers for Disease Control and Prevention, National Center for Health Statistics, 2005, Hyattsville, MD: U.S. Department of Health and Human Services, p. 391.

one particular group of physicians and then to receive virtually all medical care—both primary and specialty—through that group of physicians, either directly or by referral. That particular group of physicians, in return, is paid a fixed fee per patient (capitation rate) that the group agrees to take on for total responsibility for health care. In the PPO, medical providers are paid fee for service and take no coordinating control for the total health of the enrollee.

In HMOs, the linkages between the health plan, the providers, and members are tighter and more formal. Just as in the PPO form, the three participants (health plan, providers, and patients) form a network of mutual benefit, but it is based on different principles. The health plan benefits because it is able to limit its financial exposure by prepaying the provider group a fixed amount per member per month (PMPM) for taking care of the enrolled population. The plan knows that no matter how much care the provider is required to give enrollees, the health plan will not be required to make any additional financial payments. From the provider's point of view, these prepaid contractual arrangements provide a steady stream of revenue, whether individual patients seek care or not. The provider organizations are able to plan on a more financially stable and long-term basis than they could if they were in a PPO plan (that depends on individual choices). The patient benefits as well, as there are usually small deductibles, if any, and low or no co-payments for each class of service (e.g., physician visit, laboratory tests, etc.). The patient knows, therefore, that once the premium is paid each month, there will be little or no additional fees required.

Providers have a wide variety of contractual arrangements that they may make with managed-care plans. Hospitals, for example, may agree to contract with PPOs and offer substantial discounts when PPO members are actually admitted or treated at contracting hospitals. On the other hand, hospitals may also contract with HMOs to provide hospital care for an enrolled population on a PMPM basis. Hospitals may, in turn, agree to take part in joint contracting efforts involving physician groups, independent practice associations (IPAs), or other medical care organizations that agree to take on an enrolled population via capitation, with the revenues being divided by mutual agreement between the physician organization and the hospital.

For their part, physicians have a variety of ways to take part in managed-care health plans, either singly or in larger groups. With PPOs, individual physicians or groups can simply contract with the health plan to take PPO members on a discounted fee-for-service basis. This type of arrangement is organized around individual patients making individual visits to a doctor and implies no long-term commitment between the physician and the health plan, or between the physician and an individual patient. By contrast, when physicians are faced with HMOs, their decisions are more critical because they have much broader and much longer-term implications.

In 2001, 88 percent of all physicians participated in at least one managed-care contract, accounting for 41 percent of average practice revenue. This was up sharply from 1998, when only 61 percent of physicians contracted for 23 percent of practice revenue (Kaiser Family Foundation, 2004). Physician relationships with HMOs vary widely according to state licensure laws and market conditions. But three HMO models—the IPA, the group model, and the staff model—are the most common forms of collaboration.

Table 5.5 shows the shifting that has taken place in since 1996 in the type of managed-care plans selected by covered workers. Traditional indemnity plans have continued to wane in availability by employers and selection by workers. This trend, coupled with the movement out of HMOs, has

Table 5.5. Health Plan Enrollment for Covered Workers by Plan Type, Selected Years

	1996	2000	2005
Traditional	27%	8%	3%
PPO	28	42	61
POS	14	21	15
HMO	31	29	21

SOURCE: *Employer Health Benefits 2005 Annual Survey,* Chart #6, Kaiser Family Foundation and Health Research Educational Trust, 2005, retrieved on January 16, 2006, from http://www.kff.org/insurance/7315/index.cfm

spurred the enormous growth of PPOs, which now cover more than 60 percent of workers. POS plans, which offer some freedom from the strictures of HMOs (and resemble PPOs if the member goes out of network), have maintained about 15 percent of the market.

The IPA Model. In the IPA, the physician in practice voluntarily joins a collaborative group of physicians, all of whom are in independent practice and all of whom join the IPA in order to be able to take part in large contracts with HMOs. In the IPA, the physician remains in independent practice and agrees to care for those patients whom the IPA attracts and assigns to that physician. The physician in practice usually has many other patients who come from other sources, some of whom may be paid for on a fee-for-service basis and others for whom payment may be from other managed-care arrangements, including HMOs. The IPA allows individual physicians the benefits of independence, multiple sources of patients, and involvement in other contracting arrangements. The individual physician may also be an owner of the IPA, but that is not usually a necessary condition of the physician's involvement with the IPA as a provider of care.

When IPAs first began to appear, it was believed that they might merely be a transitional form of medical organization that might gradually give way to tighter forms of group practice and staff model HMOs, but that has not been the case, as the IPA model holds great flexibility for physicians who may structure their financial revenues as they see fit. The longer IPAs are in existence, the more tightly they are organized and managed. However, the fundamental model of physicians in independent private practice who voluntarily join a collaborative contracting group remains the same.

The Group Model. Physicians also participate in HMOs by organized medical groups and having the groups contract with HMOs to provide care to an enrolled population. In this form of involvement in managed care, a physician chooses to become a formal member of an organized medical group that

practices together, shares premises, and may share patients and revenues. The formal contract with the HMO is between the medical group and the HMO, not with individual physicians. In other words, by joining a specific medical group, the physician is accepting the HMO contract. HMOs may prefer this type of arrangement, as the internal discipline of an organized medical group is usually much tighter than that of an IPA, with large numbers of doctors who work in separate locations. On the other hand, in the group model, medical groups may contract with multiple HMOs, so no one HMO holds undue influence.

The Staff Model. Although less popular than other organizational arrangements, the physician may decide to join a staff model HMO that actually employs its own physicians. In this model, the doctor decides to become directly associated with the HMO itself. In effect, the physician is becoming a salaried member of a larger corporation that, in turn, directly owns and operates hospitals, clinics, and other institutional providers in its market. In some instances, due to state medical practice laws, physicians may actually form a partnership that, in turn, contracts exclusively with the HMO (e.g., the Permanente Medical Group contracts exclusively with the Kaiser HMO corporation).

In summary, it can be seen from this brief review that managed care is not a unified monolithic organization, but rather a series of separate subunits, linked together by a series of decisions, contracts, and administrative structures. The result is a wide variety of managed-care activities and operations, subject to lower prices for enrollees and providers as freedom of choice in health care decision making diminishes. Therefore, in discussing issues related to managed care, it is important to specify which type and level of the managed care is actually being addressed, as the details and outcomes of such discussions may vary greatly.

Point of Service Plans

In general, point of service plans combine elements of both HMOs and PPOs. Usually the HMO is the platform plan in which the POS member obtains most health care. However, if the member chooses to receive care outside of the HMO provider group, then the beneficiary is exposed to higher cost sharing in the form of deductibles and copayments/coinsurance. If the member goes out of the HMO to a PPO provider contracted with the plan, fees will be subject to PPO allowed amounts. But if the member receives care from a provider that has no contract with the health plan, there is no limit to the fees that the provider can charge. Average premiums for POS plans lie, not surprisingly, between HMO and PPO premiums, but employee premium contributions for POS plans exceed those of PPOs (KKF & HRET, 2005).

Areas of Management in Managed Care

Managed care implies at least some management of the health care process. There are some functional areas of health care management, as well as certain concepts, and principles that are generally common to all types of managed-care programs. Areas of management in managed care include (1) provider contracting and network management, (2) utilization management, (3) quality management, (4) general administration (i.e., financial management and operations management), (5) health information systems, and (6) sales and marketing management.

Contracting in Managed Care

With the exception of staff model HMOs that employ their own physicians, managed care consists of a series of separate organizational entities that are linked only by legally negotiated systems of contracts. Contracts are a series of legally binding documents that set the terms and boundaries for everything that happens within the managed-care structure. Therefore, the negotiation of proper contracts and the clear understanding of all the details in the contracts by all parties is essential for the long-term success of managed-care plans. At the present time, the negotiation and creation of contracts between the various parties in managed care

are challenging and uncertain. Unfortunately, many clinical professionals in health care are not used to the negotiating and contracting process and, as a result, pay less attention to it than they should.

Probably the least informed and prepared party in the managed-care contract structure is the person covered by the health insurance policy. If the health insurance policy is considered a contract between the health plan and the enrollee, it is very important that the beneficiary understand what is in that contract. There is growing concern for methods of better education and preparation of patients in the interpretation of their managed-care plan, as well as an increased interest in discovering ways in which enrollees or the public can take a more active part in the actual negotiation with purchasers or providers of better contracts for themselves. One of the most interesting and potentially important areas of future activity in managed care is the possible increase in the power of groups of patients as members of the managed-care structure.

Utilization Management

Because the main objective of managed care is to reduce the unnecessary use of services and to provide health care in a more efficient fashion, utilization management of health services is central to the successful implementation of managed care. Control of costs, utilization, and, to an extent, consumer behavior depend heavily on influencing provider behavior, especially physician behavior. Table 5.6 lists common managed-care practices designed to control physicians. There are numerous considerations involved in influencing physicians, ranging from careful selection of efficient participating providers (known as "economic credentialing") to strict utilization review processes and controls on both providers and beneficiaries.

The control of the utilization begins with decisions that are made by the purchaser in regard to what services should be included in the benefits package. Increasingly, the range of services included as benefits is being narrowed by purchasers who are ever-more anxious to limit their financial exposure. Many times, health plans find themselves

Table 5.6. Influencing Physician Behavior in Managed-Care Practices

- Feedback and comparisons to the norm using quantitative data
- Physician recruitment and selective contracting policies
- Socialization to group goals and philosophy
- Positive rewards such as money, benefits, on-call preference, and leave time
- Promotion of teamwork and quality management
- Financing and reimbursement incentives
- Efficiency and productivity enhancements

blamed for not paying for certain health care services when the actual decision to limit such services has been made by the purchaser in designing the benefit package.

Health plans frequently require the provider to report on the use of expensive services such as inpatient care and high-technology diagnostic and treatment services. The basic contract between the insurance organization and the providers frequently stipulates the nature and extent to which providers must review their own utilization of services and provide summary data. Because medical groups are increasingly being paid on a capitation basis and are at risk for the financial consequences of high utilization, it is logical that the most active and aggressive control of utilization occurs within the medical group or IPA itself (Kerr, 1996). Thus, the utilization control processes used within the medical group or IPA can become increasingly stringent.

At the heart of any utilization control system is the concept of the primary care physician (PCP) or "gatekeeper." The gatekeeper concept rests on the idea that one physician—usually a PCP in family practice, general internal medicine, general pediatrics, or, for some women, obstetrics/gynecology—is responsible for providing all of the primary care for the patient. The PCP also determines when referrals to specialists are needed and then provides oversight and coordination for the use of the specialists on an ongoing basis. The gatekeeper

concept is designed to control the patient's use of expensive resources, to reduce the patient-initiated use of specialty physicians, and to ensure overall coordination of care.

Placing the PCP in the position of gatekeeper is increasingly being seen as a potential source of conflict of interest for physicians playing this role. If the primary care physician aggressively seeks to ensure that the patient has all possible diagnostic procedures and specialists' opinions, that PCP may also be draining the IPA or medical group's total financial pool under capitation. The PCP realizes very quickly that the more aggressively the patient's interests are pursued, the less advantageous it may be to the physician financially. The subject is one of serious concern to physicians and medical organizations.

Education of Enrollees

If managed care is to succeed in its goals, it is important that the insured be told very specifically what managed care is and what it is not. Because the use of health services under a managed-care arrangement may be quite different from fee-for-service health plans (and from other managed-care plans), it is important that patients be instructed about what services are covered and how care can be obtained. Often the purchasers leave it to the health plans to inform the enrolled members about the details of their health benefits, as well as the administrative procedures to which members must adhere in order to access benefits. Unfortunately, many managed-care plans fall woefully short in instructing their members about how their plans function. It is clear that if managed care is to succeed, a better job of information exchange and education must be done by both purchasers and managed-care plans alike.

Information Systems and Outcome Measures

One of the central characteristics of all forms of managed care is the absolute necessity of advanced information systems that will provide more accurate and timely data on the utilization of services and on the quality/outcomes of those services. Under fee-for-service health plans, including PPOs, the key information that is collected comes from claims data (i.e., actual transaction data listing providers' requests for reimbursement for specific items of service for each enrollee). Claims data allow great transparency of what goes on at the provider-patient interface. (Claims data usually reveal very little about the technical quality of the services provided or the outcome of those services on the health status of the patient.) Under HMO capitation reimbursement, on the other hand, the type of detail contained in claims data for enrollees, their services, and procedures are no longer collected, yielding no transparency of the provider's practice profile and clinical choices. Because of this, many capitated plans require providers to submit periodic encounter data that resemble claims. Unless audited, these encounter data may be of lesser accuracy than claims data.

Whatever data are collected, they must be combined and statistically analyzed to produce meaningful information on quality of care and actual health outcomes. The necessity of sophisticated health information systems is further heightened by the purchasers' requirements for detailed reports—often using standardized formats such as the HEDIS (Health Plan Employer Data and Information Set) collected from health plans on the appropriateness and quality of services provided. Likewise, managed-care plans are requiring provider groups and health systems to gather and report more sophisticated information on utilization, quality, and outcomes. These reports are used by health plans to evaluate providers better and to report back to the purchasers on the quality of services for which they are paying.

Only a small portion of the data being gathered at the present time is being utilized to its maximum potential. However, it is clear that health information systems will advance very quickly, given available and developing information technology and the increasing demands for more and better health data.

Capitation

Central to the HMO type of managed-care program is the concept of capitation, the payment of a PMPM fee to physicians or hospitals in exchange for their assumption of responsibility to provide a comprehensive of services as needed. In contrast to the fee-for-service form of reimbursement, capitation provides entirely different incentives to those providing care. Under fee-for-service, the more services that are provided, the more the provider is paid. Under capitation, the fewer services that are provided, the more funds there are left over for the provider. The incentive embedded in capitation is, therefore, for the provider to be more efficient and frugal in the use of health services in order to retain more revenue.

Within IPAs or medical groups, capitation can also be used to reimburse individual physicians in different ways. For example, it is quite common for an IPA to reimburse primary care physicians on a per capita basis but then reimburse specialists on a modified fee-for-service basis.

Risk Sharing

Of increasing importance and interest in managed care is the use of risk-sharing pools. These vary widely, but in general, they involve the establishment of a pool of money from which certain services are paid for throughout the year. Funds remaining at the end of the year are then divided, either between the providers and the health plan or between the physicians and hospitals with which they have joined in a collaborative effort.

Risk pools provide an incentive to reduce utilization, particularly with regard to hospitalization, specialty referrals, and high-technology diagnostic and treatment services. The extent to which risk pools are effective in reducing use and saving money is not clear. It is also unclear whether risk pools (together with capitation payments) result in under use of needed services. The greatest fear in managed care, both on the part of patients and of providers, is that the incentives to control overuse of health services will now lead to underutilization and denial of needed services, with the resulting decline in the health status of the covered population. Indeed, of all of the questions involved in managed care, this is the most critical to monitor.

THE FUTURE OF HEALTH INSURANCE

Several important issues must be considered with regard to the future development of private health insurance and managed-care programs. Among the important issues are consolidation among health plans, the impact of managed care on the provider system, Medicare and Medicaid managed care, managed behavioral health care, conflicts of interest, and protection of the public.

Consolidation among Health Insurance Plans

As managed care matures, one phenomenon that is developing rapidly is consolidation among health insurance plans. Consolidation measures how much of the industry is controlled by how many companies. For example, if the top five companies account for a high percentage of the total business (e.g., 70 or 80 percent), then the industry is highly consolidated. Every year sees more and more of the nation's health insurers merging with or acquiring other health insurers in what can only be described as a major change in the health care financing landscape.

This consolidation of health insurance providers and plans is a concern for several reasons. Foremost is the possibility that health plans will become so large that they have an unfair advantage in dealing with both purchasers and providers. The larger a health insurance plan becomes, the higher its financial assets and the more enrolled lives it controls. This means that the financial leverage among the plans may become unduly strong, making it difficult for an even balance among

purchasers, health plans, and providers to exist. In their defense, health plans very frequently say that they must consolidate because purchasers and providers are themselves consolidating into larger bargaining units; the plans must consolidate if they are not to be overwhelmed by the larger size and strength of their negotiating partners.

Consolidation that reduces the number of health plans controlling the market also reduces the competitive nature of the marketplace, which in itself may be a bad outcome for purchasers and the public. Healthy competition among providers of any service is critically important to the success of any market-oriented industry. This is no less true when considering the health insurance industry. A purchaser who goes into the marketplace seeking health insurance and confronting a limited choice of health insurance plans is less able to engage these plans in a dialogue on price and quality of services. If a purchaser is confronted with a wide variety of plans, health insurers would have to work harder to compete for the business.

Consolidation may also result in the reduction of variation among health plans, their product lines, utilization of services, and rules of procedure in bidding for contracts. In other words, uniformity in products and procedures may translate into higher profits. At a time when everyone is trying to learn about managed care and when there still seems to be considerable experimentation in insurance products, consolidation may preclude the opportunity to learn exactly what are the best forms of managed care for our various subpopulations. Experimentation may prematurely be ended before we have had a chance to learn the lessons that should be learned.

Obviously, there are major antitrust and monopoly issues to be considered in regard to consolidation. The formal legal and regulatory mechanisms in this area move so slowly that significant reshaping of the health insurance industry (particularly in the managed-care sector) is likely to occur before any formal governmental protections are able to come into effect (Kuttner, 1997). Also, because there are very few legal or regulatory precedents in the health insurance/managed-care sector, those formal governmental protections may be even slower to come into effect than in a well-established industry.

Impact of Managed Care on the Provider System

Because managed care is really a series of subunits that are linked together by a series of legal, contractual, and organizational mechanisms, a change in any one subunit tends to bring about changes in other subunits. This means that any change in the methods for financing health care through health insurance (such as the growth of capitated reimbursement mechanisms) will cause changes in the provider system as well.

In practice, what has happened among providers has been a growth of new organizational forms and new operating principles with regard to the provision of care in response to change on the financing side (Table 5.7). This has led to the growth in the size of physician groups, an increase in joint ventures of physician groups and hospitals, and a drive for increased efficiency of operation. Consequently, an

Table 5.7. Provider Concerns in Managed Care

- Enter into contracts carefully
- Know practice strengths and weaknesses
- Use clinical protocols and other control guidelines
- Establish performance goals and measures of success or failure
- Ensure that management information systems are adequate
- Continually monitor results and respond to information
- Reduce inpatient utilization
- Be cost conscientious
- Emphasize primary care
- Monitor and manage risk
- Maintain provider relationships
- Enhance consumer controls and satisfaction

overall rethinking about the most appropriate organizational structure for the delivery of personal health care services is now taking place.

This rethinking may have both positive and negative effects. On the positive side, the reorganization of the provider system may lead to greater efficiency and better effectiveness of that system and, therefore, to better patient care with improved outcomes. This scenario suggests that the previous organizational structure of health care under a fee-for-service stimulus may not have been the most efficient or effective and that managed-care-driven changes in the delivery system are a distinct improvement.

On the negative side, the drive for increased efficiency of operation, the emphasis on providing fewer services, and the overwhelming concern about economic issues may all serve to dampen or reduce the humane and compassionate aspects of health care as it was previously delivered in the United States. Under this scenario, the provider system for health services in the United States may become more coldly efficient and effective in an organizational sense, but less satisfactory in a personal and psychological sense to the people receiving services.

A point to remember here is that changes in the way in which health care providers are paid are not merely financial or economic in nature. They also drive organizational changes, and those organizational changes may be either for the better or the worse, depending upon how they develop.

Medicare and Medicaid Managed Care

Although much has been said about the impact of managed care in reducing health care for employers and private health insurance, the major impact of managed care may actually be felt in the two major public sector programs: Medicare and Medicaid. The impact on each of these programs may be quite different, given the different nature of the constituencies they serve and the specifics of their financing.

With Medicare expenditures increasing at a rapid rate and anticipating the baby boomers, the Health Care Financing Administration (HCFA) had wanted to have approximately half of all Medicare beneficiaries enrolled in managed-care programs (HMOs and PPOs) by the year 2007. HCFA felt that managed care should play a major part in the long-term solution of Medicare's financial woes.

The implications for patients served under Medicare are potentially good and bad (Wagner, 1996). On the positive side, Medicare beneficiaries may actually receive more benefits and services and may also have their patterns of care and the outcomes of that care more closely monitored and controlled. In other words, Medicare beneficiaries may actually get more appropriate care in managed-care plans and have more confidence in that care than in traditional Medicare.

On the negative side for Medicare beneficiaries is the effect of consolidation among provider organizations and medical groups. Medicare beneficiaries in managed care may find that solo-practice physicians are becoming a thing of the past, replaced by comparative supermarkets of physicians whose hallmarks include efficiency of a less personal kind. Moving into a Medicare managed-care program may mean that elderly Medicare patients have less time with their physicians as well as less personal connection to them.

Private companies that contract to Medicare do so to make a profit. In 2001, several corporate providers determined that federal capitation rates were inadequate to provide Medicare managed-care services in certain of their markets. Subsequently, these companies let their contracts with HCFA expire, leaving more than 500,000 HMO patients in these localities with no other option but traditional Medicare (with less comprehensive benefits and higher out-of-pocket costs). Whether this represents a realignment of the marketplace is unclear. Less-concentrated population centers and particularly rural areas have been hardest hit. The availability of adequate numbers of contracting providers and the capability to achieve a critical mass in enrollments, coupled with relatively low federal capitation rates, will continue to be factors determining the geographic reach of the Medicare managed-care program.

In the same fashion, Medicaid programs around the country are moving very rapidly to use managed care for their recipients' care, and it seems clear that the impact on Medicaid recipients will also be quite marked, if different from the impact on Medicare beneficiaries. In the case of Medicaid, changes from the increased use of managed care are more likely to be positive than negative.

In the past, Medicaid recipients generally received their care in a somewhat random and scattered fashion from local governmental hospitals, clinics, and emergency rooms; interested physicians; and a wide variety of free clinics and other community organizations. There was usually very little cohesion among the providers and very little coordination in the patterns of care being given.

Under managed care, Medicaid recipients have a firm and formal connection with a medical group or medical provider and are required to have a designated PCP as the coordinator of all their services. Required services are provided on a regular basis and will be monitored for outcomes. For the first time, Medicaid recipients have the ability to access continuous care from a single provider network. In a very real sense, managed care presents a great opportunity to improve the quality of care received by Medicaid recipients across the country.

Mental Health and Managed Care

One of the most interesting areas of managed care, and also one of the most rapidly expanding, is the implementation of managed care for mental and behavioral health services. Over the years, the general criticism of traditional mental health services has been that they are unstandardized, poorly supervised, and without any meaningful measures of outcomes. There was also an excessive use of expensive inpatient mental health services, stemming from the availability of health insurance payments for such services.

The shift to managed care in mental health services is causing significant concern among both patients and providers of mental health services and is also forcing patients and providers to learn a new set of procedures and policies for delivery of care. Rather than offer a wide-open patient-initiated selection of mental health practitioners, the managed behavioral health plans require beneficiaries to first use a triage process that attempts to determine the severity of the problem, the most appropriate form of treatment, and a connection to the most appropriate type of practitioner (e.g., psychiatrist, social worker, etc.). This means that the patient is no longer free to pick the practitioner of his or her choice and begin therapy at will. Now all those previous forms of behavior are organized, controlled, and monitored for treatment outcomes by the managed mental health organization itself.

From the patient's point of view, this means that there are more formal and supervised systems of determining the severity of the initial problem and a much more standardized process for initializing and continuing care. Also, there is a deliberate attempt on the part of the managed-care organization to determine the credentials of the mental health practitioners before they are accepted as providers by the plan. For their part, providers of mental health services may now find themselves dependent upon the managed-care plan for a flow of initial patients and then limited in their ability to provide care by the number of encounters that are authorized. Mental health practitioners see this as an imposition on their independence and their clinical judgment, and, for the most part, mental health professionals are not very positive or supportive in their views about managed mental health programs.

Conflict of Interest in Managed Care

One of the most important issues facing managed care in the future is the question of conflict of interest among the various participants in any type of managed care system (Gray, 1997). The conflict is centered around the need to reduce the use of various health services, products, and procedures. The economic survival and prosperity of all the major players in managed care depend upon the imposition of tight controls on the use of health services, with the implication that services have been overused in the past and that this overusage must be eliminated.

Although there is general agreement that many types of health services have been overused in the past, it is not always specifically clear which of those services qualify as "unnecessary" and, therefore, need reduction. The application of across-the-board methods to reduce the use of health services will affect both those services that may have been overused and overprovided in the past as well as those services that may not have been overused and overprovided. The net result may be that all health services utilization may be reduced, both those services that needed reduction and those that did not. The end result may be that patients who need some services may not get them in the future.

For the most part, purchasers/payers and health insurance plans have been unwilling to concede or even discuss the possibility of a conflict of interest affecting their participation in managed care, but increasingly physicians have been more vocal about the difficult situation in which they find themselves. Indeed, because physicians are directly involved with their patients on a face-to-face basis, it is very likely that the issues of conflict of interest will be most apparent in this part of any managed-care system. It is also very obvious that the discussion of conflict of interest in managed care will most likely be led by physicians, as it is there that the stresses and strains are felt most acutely (Kerr, 1996). For physicians, medical ethics versus economic pressures will be the focus of this discussion, but it certainly will not end there. Conflict of interest is rampant throughout the entire managed health care structure.

Protection of the Public

A final issue of importance to the future of managed care is the development of better mechanisms for the protection of patients and in the public interest. In recent years, it appears that individual patients and the public in general are somewhat at the mercy of a managed-care structure that is consolidating very rapidly at the purchaser, the health plan, and the provider systems levels (Bodenheimer, 1996). The only part of the managed-care structure that is not consolidating (and, therefore, not gaining clout in the marketplace) is that of individual enrollees and the public in general.

For most individuals who must make their way through the managed-care system in a relatively unaided fashion, the complexities of managed care leave them vulnerable and relatively unprotected. From the time when purchasers/payers select a health insurance plan under which the employees will be covered (sometimes without choice or options and other times with options that are not clearly explained), the individual is at a significant disadvantage because of the relative lack of information, experience, and sophistication in consuming medical services. Later, in dealing with individual health insurance plans and their consumer service departments, the individual is also at a disadvantage, as one is dealing with a health plan staff member who is more experienced and knowledgeable about the details of the health plan's operation. The plan employee may also have been given the specific direction to constrain or reduce the utilization of services and may have the best interest of the health plan uppermost in mind. The utilization review process, for example, may not be clearly described to the enrollee and may be implemented in widely varying forms with different medical outcomes.

All these circumstances tend to make members of managed-care health plans suspicious and distrustful even when the plans and the physicians are actually doing as much as they can to provide appropriate service. The sense of vulnerability among individuals, when they are confronted with the detailed machinations of managed care, may make them feel that they have fewer options and less influence over their care than they really hold.

One response to this sense of isolation and vulnerability among members of managed-care plans has been the passage of a series of legislative and regulatory efforts by Congress, state legislatures, and state regulatory departments to protect the interests of the public. Statutes mandating the minimum number of days that a woman may remain in the hospital after a normal delivery, for example, raise serious raise serious questions about their wisdom of legislating the details of personal care. Nevertheless, until people organize to protect themselves from this apparent imbalance of power, and until purchasers and managed-care plans do much more in the way of direct communication and assistance to patients and the public, the only channel of recourse available to the public will be through the rule of law.

THE UNINSURED

According to the U.S. Census Bureau, 45.8 million people in 2004 were without health insurance of any kind, up from 45.0 million in 2003. From 1987 to 1998, the uninsurance rate (12.9 percent in 1987) either increased or was unchanged from one year to the next. After peaking at 16.3 percent in 1998, the rate fell for 2 years, then increased for 3, hopefully stabilizing at 15.7 percent of the U.S. population in 2004.

"Forty-five million Americans are uninsured, and each one of these uninsured people is a tragedy waiting to happen" (Kennedy, 2005). It is unfortunate that after decades of relentless debate and discussion, the United States continues to battle the issues surrounding uninsurance. The nature of the problem, in addition to the characteristics of the uninsured, has been examined in countless pieces of literature. However, the problem has remained the same: There are far too many Americans living without health insurance coverage.

Minorities account for 50 percent of the 45 million uninsured Americans. Kennedy (2005) reports that, at any given point in time, approximately 32 percent are Hispanics, 20 percent are African

Americans, and 18 percent are Asians/Pacific Islanders.

The uninsured population is generally characterized by three main groups: the working uninsured, the nonworking uninsured, and the medically uninsurable. Many assume that the uninsured are poor and unemployed. However, statistics continuously disprove this assumption. In 2004, roughly 63 percent of the total uninsured population had an income above the federal poverty level (Porter, 2005). More importantly, 8 out of 10 uninsured individuals are in fact members of families participating in the workforce. As a result, this group constitutes more than 50 percent of the total uninsured population. These individuals are generally low-wage earners employed by organizations that do not offer health insurance. While the incomes earned by this group are typically above the poverty level, private health insurance continues to be a financially unattainable alternative (Wilensky, 1989).

The nonworking uninsured comprise the second largest group of the uninsured. Incomes for these individuals typically fall below the federal poverty level, and many are ineligible for state Medicaid

programs. Additionally, this group tends to experience longer periods without any form of employment (Wilensky, 1989).

The medically uninsurable constitute the smallest percentage of the uninsured population. These individuals have preexisting health conditions that prevent them from obtaining insurance through the private market. Health plans often confront them with exorbitant premiums, copayments, and deductibles. Consequently, their families endure unrelenting financial distress that may ultimately result in bankruptcy. This group also has a considerable impact on health care providers since much of the care they receive is mostly uncompensated. Thus, it is clear these individuals will be less likely to procure health insurance, placing an economic burden on our health care system (Wilensky, 1989).

The offering of health insurance by the employer is closely related to the size of the organization. Figure 5.2 shows that less than 50 percent of firms with fewer than 10 workers offer group health insurance. As firm size grows, so do the number that offer PHI, but even among the largest firms, not all offer this benefit. A federal survey on employer-sponsored

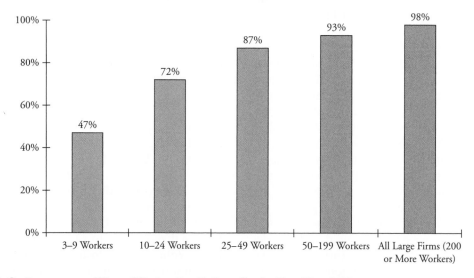

Figure 5.2. Percentage of Firms Offering Health Benefits, by Firm Size, 2005

SOURCE: *Employer Health Benefits 2005 Summary of Findings*, Chart #8, Kaiser Family Foundation and Health Research Educational Trust, Retrieved January 16, 2006, from http://www.kff.org/insurance/7315/sections/upload/7375.pdf

health insurance estimates that only 43.2 percent of establishments with fewer than 50 workers offer health insurance. Furthermore, the trend is downward. In 2000, 69 percent of all firms offered health benefits, and by 2005, that figure had diminished to 60 percent. Reasons cited by firms for not offering health insurance are that (1) premiums are too high, (2) the firm is too small, and (3) employees are covered elsewhere (KFF & HRET, 2005; USDHHS, 2003).

In 1999, the Institute of Medicine (IOM) issued a six-volume report on the uninsured U.S. population. The IOM found the presence of health insurance coverage to be one of the most significant factors in generating access to health care services. Despite the existence of free community clinics and other institutions offering discounted services, it is clear that the uninsured continuously experience reduced access to medical care (Wolman and Miller, 2004). Not surprisingly, the committee concluded that adults who lack coverage have worse health outcomes stemming from inadequate treatment for chronic diseases and higher age-specific mortality rates, as compared to their insured counterparts. The study found that urban areas serving large uninsured populations offer relatively fewer services (such as mental health and trauma care) when compared to urban areas with larger insured populations.

The figure 45 million uninsured represents only a snapshot in time and does not reflect the number of people who constantly move in and out of insurance coverage. Extensive survey research examined the stability of health insurance coverage in the United States from 1996 to 1999. Despite the tremendous number of uninsured Americans, relatively few were found to be continuously uninsured during this time period. Almost 85 million Americans under the age of 65 were uninsured for a minimum of one month throughout the 4-year period. This figure greatly surpasses the current estimate of 45 million. However, only 10 million individuals were continuously uninsured. Therefore, most of the participants who were uninsured in 1996 had one or more changes in coverage during this time period (Short and Graefe, 2003).

Table 5.8 provides a summary of coverage patterns among the uninsured. The "repeatedly uninsured" proved to be the most common among the seven patterns observed. This group accounted for 33 percent of the study population. The second largest group, comprising about 19 percent, followed the "single gap in coverage" pattern and were usually uninsured for 12 months or less. This gap

Table 5.8. Percentage Distribution of the Uninsured by Total Months Uninsured over 4 Years, According to Coverage Patterns, U.S. Population Under Age 65, 1996–1999

| | | Number of Months Uninsured | | | |
| | | Percent of Persons in Coverage Pattern | | | |
	Millions	1–4	5–12	13–24	25–48
Total persons uninsured	84.8	24	22	19	35
Coverage pattern					
Always uninsured	10.1	0	0	0	100
Transition into coverage	9.9	24	22	23	31
Transition out of coverage	7.3	24	20	19	37
One gap in coverage	15.9	64	22	10	5
Temporary coverage	4.8	0	4	8	87
Frequent changes	8.5	64	22	10	4
Repeatedly uninsured	28.2	4	33	34	30

NOTE: Row percentages might not sum to 100 because of rounding.

SOURCE: P. F. Short and D. R. Graefe, 2003. "Battery-Powered Health Insurance? Stability In Coverage of the Uninsured," by *Health Affairs, 22*, pp. 244–255.

was largely attributed to changes in Medicaid/SCHIP and employer insurance. Interestingly, the individuals who remained uninsured for the longest period of time manifested the "temporary coverage" pattern. These people, who were initially uninsured, experienced only one movement into coverage and subsequently remained uninsured for the duration of the study. Roughly, 87 percent were uninsured for more than 24 months.

The results of this study highlight the complexity of uninsurance in the United States. The variety in the different coverage patterns among the uninsured suggest that simply expanding coverage may not be an appropriate solution to the problem. The results do indicate, however, that efforts to target pockets of the uninsured with incremental coverage reforms must target the right people at the right time in order to even begin to reduce the uninsured population. Moreover, policymakers may also want to explore options that increase stability in coverage (Short and Graefe, 2003).

While relatively small incremental changes have been made, the number of uninsured individuals continues to rise. A lack of consensus among policy makers proves to be a major obstacle in establishing health care reform. Current policy initiatives typically support expansions of the current financing system. More specifically, strategies revolve around the establishment of refundable tax credits, the expansion of federal and state programs, and the expansion of employer-based insurance coverage (Cubanski, 2004).

THE PROSPECT OF NATIONAL HEALTH INSURANCE

According to Reinhardt (2003), neither moral sentiments among U.S. political leaders, economic self-interest among those who would ultimately pay for universal health insurance, nor political pressure from the uninsured will provide a sufficiently strong imperative to move the country toward universal coverage anytime soon. Despite the decades of persistent debate over how to solve the problem of uninsurance, the United States is still the only Western industrialized nation without national health insurance (Quadagno, 2004). Many would contend that universal coverage, under some form of national health insurance, is the best approach to insuring the uninsured. However, the twentieth century revealed at least 10 failed attempts to achieve a national health insurance program (Davis, 2001).

The IOM Committee report on uninsurance concludes with the committee's vision for achieving universal coverage and provides specific strategies to accomplish this goal. These include expanding Medicaid and SCHIP through the distribution of tax subsidies, instituting individual and employer mandates, and establishing a national single-payer health insurance system. Inherent in all these strategies are major shortcomings that threaten major stakeholders in the current health insurance system including private health plans, providers, states, and—considering the continuing pressure of health inflation—the entire U.S. economy. The general public may stand to lose as well, in terms of access to health services and satisfaction with care. It is clear these and other barriers (i.e., surrounding the benefit package and the wide geographic variations in practice patterns) will continue to preclude the adoption of a U.S. national health insurance policy in the near future (Chollet, 2005; Newhouse & Reischauer, 2004).

It is clear the United States has failed to reduce the rising number of uninsured Americans. Despite the wide variety of proposals, a lack of consensus among policy makers has proven to be the driving force behind this relatively unchanged crisis. It will take strong political leadership and a clear commitment from the federal government to resolve the issue of uninsurance. The sheer complexity of American health insurance dynamics has intensified the issue with the growth of the working uninsured population. As a result, the uninsured will continue to burden families, communities, and society. The prospect of universal coverage will essentially remain a vision of the future.

SUMMARY

Health insurance in the United States defines most individuals' health care systems. The complexity of insurance programs and arrangements is huge. The mechanisms that are included under these plans are undergoing constant revision and modification as the nation's health systems evolve. Most change in recent years, since the introduction of today's popular managed-care plans, has been evolutionary. Revolutionary change is possible, but unlikely although the political and cost pressures are continuing to mount, potentially eventually forcing a radical redesign of health care plans in this nation.

REVIEW QUESTIONS

1. What is insurance, and why is it used?
2. How does private health insurance violate the standard principles of insurance?
3. Describe the three methods for categorizing health insurance in the United States.
4. Briefly describe the differences among the commercial insurance industry, the Blues, and HMOs.
5. What is managed care? List the main objectives of managed care.
6. Briefly describe PPO and HMO plans.
7. List the common managed-care practices designed to influence physician behavior.
8. Describe the role of the gatekeeper.
9. Describe the impact of managed care on both the Medicare and Medicaid programs.
10. Discuss the conflict of interest inherent in managed care.
11. Briefly describe the characteristics of the uninsured population in the United States.

REFERENCES & ADDITIONAL READINGS

America's Health Insurance Plans (AHIP). (2004). *Long-term care insurance in 2002.* Washington, DC. Retrieved May 4, 2006, from http://www.ahipresearch/org.

America's Health Insurance Plans (AHIP). (2005a). *Comparison of tax-advantaged health care spending accounts.* Retrieved January 11, 2006, from http://www.ahipresearch/org.

America's Health Insurance Plans (AHIP). (2005b). *Number of HSA plans exceeded one million in March 2005.* Washington, DC. Retrieved May 4, 2006, from http://www.ahipresearch/org.

Blumenthal, D. (2006). Employer-sponsored health insurance in the United States—origins and Implications. *New England Journal of Medicine, 355*(1), 82–88.

Bodenheimer, T. (1996). The HMO backlash . . . righteous or reactionary? *New England Journal of Medicine, 335,* 1601–1604.

Chollet, D. (2005). Insuring the uninsured: Finding the road to success. *Frontiers of Health Services Management, 21,* 17–27.

Claxton, G., Gabel, J., Gil, I., Pickreign, J., Whitmore, H., Finder, B., Rouhani, S., Hawkins, S., & Rowland, D. (2005). What high-deductible plans look like: Findings from a national survey of employers, 2005. *Health Affairs,* Web Exclusive (W5), 434–441.

Congressional Budget Office, Congress of the United States. (1991). *Rising health care costs: Causes, implications, and strategies.* Washington, DC: U.S. Government Printing Office.

Cubanski, J. (2004). Is incremental change working? Or is it time to reconsider universal coverage? *Issue Brief* (Commonwealth Fund), *711,* 1–8.

Davis, K. (2001). Universal coverage in the United States: Lessons from experience of the 20th century. *Journal of Urban Health, Bulletin of the New York Academy of Medicine, 78,* 46–58.

Drake, D. (1997). Managed care: A product of market dynamics. *Journal of the American Medical Association, 277,* 311–314.

Enthoven, A., & Singer, S. (1996). Managed competition and California's health care economy. *Health Affairs, 15,* 40–57.

Feldstein, M., & Friedman, B. (1997). Tax subsidies, the rational demand for insurance, and the health care crisis. *Journal of Public Economics, 7*(2), 155–178.

Fox, P. (1997). An overview of managed care. In P. Kongstvedt (Ed.), *Essentials of managed health care.* Gaithersburg, MD: Aspen Publishers.

Gray, B. (1997). Trust and trustworthy care in the managed care era. *Health Affairs, 16,* 34–49.

Greenspan, N. T., & Vogel, R. J. (1980). Taxation and its effects upon public and private health insurance and medical demand. *Health Care Financing Review,* *1*(4), 39–46.

Hall, M. A. (2001). The structure and enforcement of health insurance rating reforms. *Inquiry, 37,* 376–388.

Kaiser Family Foundation. *Trends and indicators in the changing health care marketplace.* Retrieved January 16, 2006, from http://www.kff.org/insurance/7031/print-sec6.cfm.

Kaiser Family Foundation and Health Research Educational Trust (KFF & HRET). (2005). *Employer health benefits: 2005 annual survey.* Retrieved March 12, 2006, from http://www.kff.org/insurance/7315/index.cfm.

Kennedy, E. M. (2005). The role of the federal government in eliminating health disparities. *Health Affairs, 24,* 452–458.

Kerr, E. (1996). Quality assurance in capitated physician groups. *Journal of the American Medical Association, 276,* 1236–1239.

Kuttner, R. (1997). Physician-operated networks and the new anti-trust guidelines. *New England Journal of Medicine, 336,* 386–391.

Lemieux, J. (2005). *Perspective: Administrative costs of private health insurance plans.* Washington, DC: America's Health Insurance Plans. Retrieved March 12, 2006, from http://www.ahipresearch.org.

Miller, R., & Luft, H. (1994). Managed care plans: Characteristics, growth, and premium performance. *Annual Review of Public Health, 15,* 437–459.

Newhouse, J. P., & Reischauer, R. D. (2004). The Institute of Medicine Committee's clarion call for universal coverage. *Health Affairs,* Suppl. Web Exclusives (W4-179-83).

Park, C. H. (2000). Prevalence of employer self-insured health benefits: National and state variation. *Medical Care Research Review, 57,* 340–360.

Pauly, M. V., & Percy, A. M. (2000). Cost and performance: A comparison of the individual and group health insurance markets. *Journal of Health Politics Policy and Law, 25,* 9–26.

Pincus, J. (2000). Employer-sponsored long-term care insurance: Best practices for increasing sponsorship. *EBRI Issue Brief, 220,* 1–22.

Porter, E. (2005, December 18). Health care for all, just a (big) step away. *The New York Times,* Business/Your Money Sec., p. 4.

Quadagno, J. (2004). Why the United States has no national health insurance: Stakeholder mobilization against the welfare state, 1945–1996. *Journal of Health & Social Behavior, 45,* 25–44.

Reinhardt, U. E. (2003). Is there hope for the uninsured? *Health Affairs,* Suppl. Web Exclusives (W376-90).

Rogal, D. L., & Gauthier, A. K. (2000). Introduction: The evolution of the individual insurance market. *Journal of Health Politics Policy and Law, 25,* 3–8.

Rublee, D. A. (1985). Self-funded health benefit plans. *Journal of the American Medical Association, 255*(6), 787–789.

Saver, B. G., & Doescher, M. P. (2000). To buy, or not to buy: Factors associated with the purchase of non-group, private health insurance. *Medical Care, 38,* 141–151.

Short, P. F., & Graefe, D. R. (2003). Battery-powered health insurance? Stability in coverage of the uninsured. *Health Affairs, 22,* 244–255.

Smith, C., Cowan, C., Heffler, S., Catlin, A., & the National Accounts Team. (2006). National health spending in 2004: Recent slowdown led by prescription drug spending. *Health Affairs, 25*(1), 186–196.

U.S. Census Bureau. *Health insurance data. Health insurance coverage: 2004.* http://www/census.gov/hhes/www/hlthins.

U.S. Census Bureau. *Statistical Abstracts, 2004–2005.* Retrieved February 24, 2006, from http://www.census.gov/prod/www/abs/statab.html.

U.S. Department of Health and Human Services (USDHHS), Agency for Health Research and Quality from MEPS Survey. (2003). *Medical expenditure panel survey: 2003 employer-sponsored health insurance data.* (2003). Retrieved January 16, 2006, from http://www.meps.ahrq.gov.

Wagner, E. (1996). The promise and performance of HMOs in improving outcomes in older adults. *Journal of the American Geriatrics Society, 44,* 1251–1257.

Whitted, G. (2001). In S. J. Williams & P. J. Torrens (Eds.), *Introduction to health services* (6th ed.). Albany, NY, Delmar.

Wilensky, G. R. (1989). Underinsured and uninsured patients. Who are they, and how can they be covered? *Consultant, 29,* 59–62, 67, 70.

Wolman, D. M., & Miller, W. (2004). The consequences of uninsurance for individuals, families, communities, and the nation. *Journal of Law, Medicine, & Ethics, 32,* 397–403.

Woolhandler, S., & Himmelstein, D. (1991). The deteriorating administrative efficiency of the U.S. health care system. *New England Journal of Medicine, 324*(18), 1253–1258.

Workers' compensation. (1991). *Social Security Bulletin, 54*(9), 28–36.

THREE

Providers of Health Services

CHAPTER 6

Public Health: Joint Public-Private Responsibility in an Era of New Threats

Paul R. Torrens

CHAPTER TOPICS

🔹 Levels of Prevention

🔹 Historical Evolution of Health Promotion and Disease Prevention in the United States

🔹 The Structure of Organized Public Health Efforts in the United States

🔹 The Role of the Private Sector in Health Promotion and Disease Prevention

🔹 Public Health in an Era of Terrorism and Emerging Diseases

LEARNING OBJECTIVES

Upon completing this chapter, the reader should be able to

1. Understand the role of public health services in protecting the health of populations.

2. Differentiate the various levels of prevention.

3. Appreciate the history of public health in the United States.

4. Understand the roles and duties of each level of government in providing public health services.

5. Appreciate the increasingly important role of the private sector in public health.

6. View public health services as a collective requirement of all participants in the health care system.

Lester Breslow contributed to previous editions of this chapter.

In the past, if one were discussing the organization of health services in the United States, that discussion would most likely not include a great deal of detail with regard to health promotion or disease prevention. It would probably not cover in very great detail the organization of governmental public health services either. *Health services* in the past meant curative and treatment services for the most part, and health promotion or disease prevention services were considered only peripherally, if at all.

This is not to suggest that the providers of health care services in the past were uninterested in keeping their patients healthy over a long period of time. Rather, it is meant to suggest that the model of health care in the past was focused around acute treatment of short-term illnesses (with some notable exceptions). Public health was the job for governmental agencies and was seen as something quite distinct and very rarely overlapping with curative and treatment services.

In recent years, fortunately, a new paradigm for health promotion and disease prevention has emerged that is based on a public-private partnership to protect and preserve the health of the American public. The newer challenges of terrorism and emerging diseases have further enhanced the urgency of this relationship. This chapter will examine this new paradigm of health promotion and disease prevention and will provide the modern health care practitioner with a better framework for understanding and dealing with the major health problems of the public.

LEVELS OF PREVENTION

To understand the new framework for health promotion and disease prevention, it is important first to provide background information about the levels of prevention, as included in the terms *primary, secondary,* and *tertiary prevention.* Without a clear understanding of the levels of prevention, it would be difficult to understand the relative roles of the public and the private sectors with regard to the enhancement of the health of the public.

Primary prevention means averting the occurrence of disease. It includes those measures that are applied or brought into effect *before* disease is present. These may include general attempts to promote better health by efforts to educate the public, to establish standards of appropriate sanitation, to apply specific methods of protection such as immunizations, to remove occupational hazards, and to protect from known carcinogens. Primary prevention focuses on the promotion of healthy lifestyles and specific protections from known hazards.

Secondary prevention means halting the progression of disease from its early, unrecognized stage to a more severe one and preventing the complication or sequelae of disease. It focuses on early diagnosis and/or prompt treatment of a health problem that would otherwise have serious impacts on the health of individuals. This means identifying the presence of a problem before it breaks the clinical horizon and before it becomes symptomatic in most cases, although it also includes attempts to discover disease early while it is still effectively treatable. In the case of coronary artery disease, for example, secondary prevention would focus on identifying individuals at high risk for disease— people, for example, who have a strong family history of heart disease, a history of heavy smoking, a lack of exercise, or a blood lipid profile that is abnormal. These early screening efforts can lead to more specific and focused tests and examinations that might further establish the early diagnosis of potential disease while it can still be constructively handled.

Tertiary prevention involves the prevention (or at least, the limitation) of the effects of disease once it has been identified. This level of prevention operates on the premise that simply because disease is present does not mean that its course should be allowed to run unhindered. In the case of coronary artery disease, for example, tertiary prevention would include efforts at cardiac rehabilitation and exercise programs, control of stress, maintenance of optimum weight and diet, and possibly adherence to a medical regimen that might reduce the future risk of further worsening of the disease.

In the new paradigm of public/private partnership in health promotion and disease prevention, there is a role for both the public and the private sectors at each level of prevention. Sometimes the roles are quite different and separate; other times the roles are similar, and perhaps overlapping, requiring some collaboration and coordination. The important message, however, is that there are several different levels on which health promotion and disease prevention can focus and a wide variety of interventions that can be sponsored by both public and private sectors.

HISTORICAL EVOLUTION OF HEALTH PROMOTION AND DISEASE PREVENTION IN THE UNITED STATES

To understand the present circumstances in the United States with regard to health promotion and disease prevention, it is important to review the history of public health activities in the United States. Much of our tradition and organizational framework for public health activities in the United States today is the product of the thinking and actions of previous generations (Brockington, 1956; Rosen, 1993). Therefore, it is important to know these developments and to understand how they affect our current thinking.

In the eighteenth century in the United States, public health activities were, for the most part, limited to individual cities and were focused on protection of the public in those cities from diseases introduced by travelers arriving from elsewhere. Early public health efforts in the United States in the eighteenth century focused on inspection of ships arriving in harbors along the eastern sea coast and included laws for the isolation and

quarantine of persons suspected to be carrying diseases that might be spread to the general population. In some of these cases, local governments established institutions (pest houses) to voluntarily (or involuntarily) contain suspected disease carriers until they either became noninfectious or, more likely, expired from their illness. During this period, the focus of public health activity in the United States was carried out by local governments and was limited to preventing the introduction of disease into the populations of port cities.

The nineteenth century marked a great advance in public health and was described by C.E.A. Winslow as "the great sanitary awakening" (Winslow, 1923). In this period, problems of sanitation were identified as a cause of disease, and public health efforts were focused on the improvement of social and environmental conditions. Housing, water supply, and sewage disposal were all the focus of organized public health activities, with the intent of reducing the disease burden on the public by improving the physical environment. As in the eighteenth century, these activities in the nineteenth century were generally carried out by cities and local governments, with the thrust of organized public health services being carried out on a local level, not necessarily on a state or national one.

In Massachusetts, Lemuel Shattuck published a landmark report in 1850 (*Report of the Sanitary Commission of Massachusetts*) that, for the first time, collected vital statistics on the population of Massachusetts, pointing out the variable threats to health throughout the state as a result of variable sanitary conditions (Shattuck, 1850). His report recommended, among other things, new census schedules, regular surveys of local health conditions, supervision of water supplies and waste disposal, and special studies on specific diseases such as tuberculosis and alcoholism. Probably most important was the recommendation of the establishment of a State Board of Health to enforce sanitary regulations. Massachusetts did set up such a State Board of Health in 1869, becoming the first state in the United States to do so.

From the late nineteenth century to the early twentieth century, many of the sanitary threats to public health were brought under control, and emphasis shifted to the prevention of acute illnesses by use of increasingly available immunizations and vaccinations. This shift of emphasis from sanitary and environmental threats toward individual bacteriological threats to health signaled a major change in the role of health departments. In previous years, organized public health services focused more on problems that were sanitary and environmental in nature and did not necessarily involve individual people; the efforts were more engineering in nature than they were directly clinical. After the turn of the century, public health activities began to turn more directly toward the prevention of disease in individual people. Organized public health activities moved away from structural protections of food, water, sewage, and housing toward more personal and individual protection through immunization of children. Organized public health activities remained largely local government activities, but there now began to be increasing state government activity in public health as well.

As the twentieth century began to progress, federal government activities grew with regard to specific health problems related to children. The United States Children's Bureau was formed in 1912, and the first White House conference on child health was held in 1919. The Sheppard-Towner Act of 1922 established the federal Board of Maternity and Infant Hygiene; this act provided administrative funds to the Children's Bureau and also provided funds to the states to establish programs in maternal and child health. It also established a pattern of federal-state relationship that was to become standard in later years, with the federal government requiring individual states to develop a plan for providing services, to designate a state agency to administer the program, and to report on operations and expenditures of the program to the federal government. States that did not wish to comply with these regulations were deemed ineligible to receive federal funding, thereby setting the model of the federal practice for establishing guidelines for public health programs and providing funds to the state to implement programs meeting these guidelines.

The Social Security Act of 1935 further expanded the federal government's leadership role in setting national directions for public health; it also further solidified the federal-state partnership with regard to the delivery of public health services in the United States. Under the terms of the Social Security Act of 1935, grants were provided to the states for aiding state and local health departments to provide maternal and child health services as well as the expansion of the work of state and local governments. This marked the first major effort of the federal government to see that a nationwide system of state and local government public health organizations were put into place. By the time that Joseph Moutin issued his landmark report on local public health services in 1946, almost 80 percent of the total United States population had some access to organized local public health services. These services may not have always been of great depth, but at least a national framework of organized local public health services had been established (Moutin, Hankela, & Druzin, 1947).

The period of the New Deal in the 1930s also had a profound effect on the development of governmental public health services, but this effect was unfortunately somewhat negative with regard to the leadership of state and federal government activities. During these times, there was considerable pressure to expand the delivery of personal health services, both curative and preventive, more broadly to the public at large, and there was even some consideration by Franklin Roosevelt's administration of a mandatory, universal health insurance program that would cover the entire population. Because the role of the federal government in so many other areas was aggressively expanding, it was believed that perhaps there might be a similar expansion of governmental role with regard to the direct provision of health services.

Unfortunately, the political backlash against the expansion of the role of the federal government in the direct provision of health services—led primarily by the American Medical Association—was successful in forcing public health officials to assume a more cautious attitude toward the role of government assistance. It became quite clear that there was no strong political support for the expansion of governmental health services, at least in the curative area, and many public health officials limited their activities to those programs and functions that were of a more traditional nature (i.e., sanitation, immunization, early detection, and confinement of communicable diseases) rather than risk the wrath of organized medicine. This did not mean that the organized public health efforts of local, state, and federal government were reduced in volume, but it did mean that the governments were much more cautious in expanding the scope of their services, being careful to keep them within the confines of prevention and not venturing into treatment.

Indeed, it should be pointed out that the feeling in the United States was so conservative with regard to the federal government's role in health care that a cabinet-level department focusing on the health of the United States' people was not established until 1953, almost 180 years after the establishment of the republic! Various public health activities had been initiated by the federal government over the years, but it was not deemed necessary, or possibly, politically feasible, to have a federal "department of health," as health was seen as a personal matter involving private physicians and their patients. It should be pointed out that this same type of thinking governed our nation's thoughts with regard to education and social welfare: these also were seen as local matters in which the federal government should not be involved, at least not directly. The creation in 1953 of a federal Department of Health, Education, and Welfare (HEW) provided a national focus for developing and implementing federal government policy with regard to these three important areas.

In the period of 1953 to the present, there has been a great expansion of governmental activity focused on the public's health, much of it in the traditional public health areas, but much more in

programs and functions related to the provision of personal health services. The passage of the Medicare and Medicaid programs in the mid-1960s is generally not seen as an expansion of the federal government's traditional public health role, but in retrospect, the passage of these financing mechanisms for the expansion of personal health services probably has had as major an impact as any of the previous, more traditional public health activities.

One further important development in public health thinking and theory was the passage of the federal Health Planning and Resource Development Act of 1974 (PL 93-641). Under this law, the federal government provided the funds to individual states for the establishment of a State Health Planning and Development Agency whose purpose was to plan and control the future development of health services—primarily hospitals—in the United States. The thinking behind the passage of this law was that there needed to be a coordinated planning effort to ensure that the proper type and volume of health services were available in equitable fashion throughout the United States, and that this could be carried out only by some type of publicly mandated planning effort to coordinate and regulate the development of these services. Although this national health planning effort was really a public health effort in the broadest sense, it was never fully connected to the already existing public health structures in the country and was never fully accepted as a legitimate public health activity by many formal public health professionals. The implementation of the Health Planning and Resource Development Act of 1974 was complicated and filled with significant controversy throughout the country; the law has since been allowed to lapse on both federal and state levels, and there is presently no direct attempt, by either federal or state governments, to plan the distribution of personal health services.

Lessons from History

What can be learned from this review of the evolution of organized public health efforts in the United

States? What important political, social, and cultural trends can be identified that will tell us more about the current and future status of public health in the United States? There are several major points to emphasize.

First, it should be pointed out that organized public health activities in the United States began in local, seaport communities and only gradually expanded to state and federal government agencies. Indeed, the Constitution of the United States reserves to the states all functions (such as health) not specifically earmarked to the federal government. For most of our country's history, public health was an activity that was primarily carried out by a local or state governmental agency, and it was only after World War II that it was perceived as necessary or appropriate to have a federal cabinet-level Department of Health, Education, and Welfare.

In many ways, this development would suggest that our country views public health activities (and perhaps health activities in general) as a local and state matter; federal government involvement developed mostly after World War I, and mostly because of the abundance of federal tax revenues to be redistributed to states and local governments. The continuing efforts to reduce the size and scope of the federal government and to return basic functions (and funds) to local and state governments in recent years may be seen as a continuation of this general idea.

Organized public health activities in the United States began with the quarantine and isolation of potential disease carriers, moved on to the improvement of sanitation in the environment, then went on to focus on immunization of children and control of individuals with contagious infectious disease. Almost all these activities focused on acute infectious diseases, regardless of their origins. This has given rise to an unofficial and generally unspoken agreement that the primary mission of organized public health efforts in the United States should be toward the prevention and control of acute illness rather than chronic disease.

Organized public health efforts in the United States have focused on outbreaks of illnesses such as diphtheria and polio because of the suddenness and the severity of any outbreaks of these illnesses. In reality, however, the much more serious and major public health problems of the United States are no longer acute infectious diseases but rather are chronic long-term degenerative conditions such as heart disease, cancer, and stroke. Organized public health efforts throughout the United States have a well-recognized role in protecting the public from outbreaks of infections, but they spend considerably less time and energy on problems of a much more serious and long-term nature, such as cancer, alcoholism, and mental illness. By default, organized public health agencies in the United States have accepted an acute illness prevention role as being appropriate, but they have not accepted a chronic disease prevention role to the same degree of intensity.

Because of the unfortunate political controversies of the 1930s around a possible national health insurance program, it would have to be admitted that there has been a relatively guarded relationship between the private medical sector and organized public health agencies throughout the country. As long as the organized public health agencies kept to the more traditional public health roles of sanitation, immunization, and infectious disease control, their activities were generally supported by the private sector. However, whenever the public health sector became more active in the provision of general health services or in the governance or planning of facilities and personnel in the private sector, considerable opposition arose. As a result of this opposition, organized public health agencies have been rather cautious about expanding their efforts beyond the boundaries of what were perceived as "traditional" public health activities.

This is probably most marked and most obvious in reviewing organized public health's unwillingness or inability to assert any major role in the planning or regulation of the provision of health services in the United States. Although a broad definition of *public health* would certainly include the necessity of ensuring that the public has adequate access to personal health services, this planning or regulatory role has not been one that public health agencies have been willing to assume, or been allowed to assume by other forces in society. As a result, the health care system of the United States is a relatively unplanned and poorly coordinated system compared to most other major industrialized countries throughout the world. In these countries, it is assumed that public health must protect the interest of the public in obtaining access to appropriate health services of high quality, but that has not been an accepted role for organized public health in the United States until now.

THE STRUCTURE OF ORGANIZED PUBLIC HEALTH EFFORTS IN THE UNITED STATES

The United States utilizes a very intricate combination of local, state, and federal government public health agencies to accomplish the public sector's responsibilities to the American public (Scutchfield & Keck, 2002). Compared to other countries of the world, the United States has one of the most complex sets of relationships between different levels of government of any country in the world, a set of relationships that reflects the unique social and political values of the people of the United States. To understand how public sector activities in health promotion and disease prevention accomplish their objectives, it is important to understand each of the three elements in the public sector—the local, state, and federal government efforts—and then, after understanding how each segment works, understand the relationships between and among them.

In its important 1988 review of public health in the United States, *The Future of Public Health,* the Institute of Medicine stated that the mission of public health was to assure conditions in which people can be healthy; it further stated that the governmental

role in public health was made up of three functions: assessment, policy development, and assurance (Institute of Medicine, 1988). Looked at in another way, these functions could be described as identification of the major public health problems, mobilization of necessary effort and resources, and assurance that vital conditions are in place so that crucial services are received.

With regard to assessment, this heading includes all of the activities involved in community diagnosis, such as surveillance, identifying needs, analyzing the causes of problems, collecting and interpreting data, case finding, monitoring and forecasting trends, research, and evaluation of outcomes. Assessment was seen by the Institute of Medicine committee as inherently a public function because policy formation, in order to be legitimate, is expected to take in all relevant information and to be based on neutral and objective factors. Moreover, public decisions take place in the context of limited resources so that a function of government is to provide a central mechanism by means of which competing proposals can be evaluated with only the best interest of society in mind. A fully developed assessment function is absolutely essential for an ideal public health system: without it, a society's real problems cannot be accurately measured, nor can alternative solutions be objectively evaluated (Fallon & Zgodzinski, 2005).

Policy development is the process by which a society makes decisions about public health problems, chooses goals and the proper means to reach them, handles conflicting views about what should be done, and allocates resources. The Institute of Medicine asserted that government provides overall guidance in this process, as it alone has the power to give answers that are binding on the entire society. In order to maintain its credibility in this policy development role, the governmental public health agency must pay attention to the quality of the policy development process itself and must raise crucial questions that no one else can raise. To carry out this function effectively, the governmental public health agency must be equipped for its policy role with technical knowledge and professional expertise; this knowledge base of public health can therefore temper the excesses of partisan politics and make for fair social decisions.

The assurance function of governmental public health agencies makes sure that necessary services are provided to reach agreed-upon goals, either by encouraging private sector action, by requiring it, or by providing services directly. The assurance function in public health involves the implementation of legislative mandates as well as the maintenance of statutory responsibilities. It includes regulation of services and products provided in both the public and private sectors, as well as maintenance of accountability to the people by setting objectives and reporting on progress. Carrying out the assurance function requires the exercise of social authority; therefore, this is not a responsibility that can be delegated to the private sector. Members of society expect the government to make certain that they enjoy at least adequate safety and security.

In reviewing the activities of the various governmental levels with regard to public health functions, it will be clear that some levels carry out more of one function than another. For example, the federal government level of public health in the United States has more of an assessment and policy development function than it does an assurance function, whereas state and local government public health activities have more of an assurance and assessment function than they do of policy development.

Federal Government Public Health Activities

The federal government's role in public health was relatively limited until the passage in 1913 of the Sixteenth Amendment to the United States Constitution, which authorized a national income tax. Prior to that time, the federal government's role in much of public life in the United States was relatively limited, particularly with regard to public health because the government had neither statutory nor regulatory authority, nor did it have financial resources available to carry out its will. After

the passage of a national income tax in 1913, the resources of the federal government in the United States became so overwhelming that federal government authority in all aspects of life, including public health, became the dominant aspect of governmental activity in the United States. Although local and state governments actually have more formal and official responsibilities placed upon them to carry out public health functions than does the federal government, the federal government has by far the greater financial resources and power to make possible implementation of laws and regulations throughout the country. The federal government, therefore, has the predominant role in public health activities in the United States, not necessarily because of its explicitly assigned public health functions under the United States Constitution, but rather because it has more financial power and authority available to it because of the national income tax.

The federal government's activities in public health in the United States are carried out through the Department of Health and Human Services, a cabinet-level department in the federal government. Although the exact internal organization of the Department of Health and Human Services varies somewhat from Congress to Congress and president to president, there is one descriptive characteristic that seems to remain: The Department of Health and Human Services is composed of a series of relatively separate superagencies that have comparatively little interaction with each other and that relate to quite different specialized constituencies, both public and professional. The Department of Health and Human Services is not a carefully designed and well-integrated organization that was intentionally put together to accomplish very specific functions of the whole organization; rather, it is an historical collection of powerful, individual, specialized agencies that at various times in their history were added into an already-existing federation of superagencies. As a result, the Department of Health and Human Services cannot be seen as functioning as a single, well-coordinated organization with a clear operating agenda that governs all of its parts; rather, the agendas of the individual separate superagencies, taken together, make up the policy of the department itself.

The federal Department of Health and Human Services can most easily be understood as having two major subdivisions, one related to health activities and the other related to human services activities. On the human services side of the department would be organizations such as the Administration on Aging; the Administration for Children, Youth, and Families; and the Social Security Administration (the agency that administers the Social Security program). On the health services side of the department would be health-related organizations such as the Centers for Disease Control and Prevention; the Food and Drug Administration; the Health Resources and Services Administration; the National Institutes of Health; the Alcohol/Drug Abuse/Mental Health Administration; and the Centers for Medicare and Medicaid Services. Approximately two-thirds of the total budget of the entire Department of Health and Human Services is devoted to human services activities (and the vast bulk of that is specifically devoted to the Social Security Administration), while approximately one-third of the total Department of Health and Human Services budget goes to health-related activities (and the vast majority of that goes to the Medicare and Medicaid programs).

The major activities of the federal Department of Health and Human Services with regard to public health can be described through its eight primary functions: (1) documenting the health status and health situation in the United States through the gathering and analysis of statistical data; (2) sponsoring research in both basic and applied sciences; (3) formulating national objectives and policy; (4) setting standards for performance of services and protection of the public; (5) providing financial assistance to state and local governments to carry out predetermined programs; (6) ensuring that personnel, facilities, and other technical resources are available to carry out national policies and goals through support for training, construction, and program development; (7) ensuring public ac-

cess to health care services by the provision of special health insurance programs; and (8) providing limited direct services to certain subgroups of the population.

The major portion of the federal government's health activities are conducted through contracts and grants to states, localities, and private providers and organizations. The federal government acts through financing intergovernmental and interorganizational contracts to encourage various public health initiatives, convening participants around an issue, coordinating activities, and developing state and local provider coalitions. In return for federal funds, states, localities, and private organizations must follow the federal standards and policies set in the contract. In most of its activities, the federal government takes an oversight, policy-setting, and technical assistance role, rather than a direct-provider role.

Most contracts to states and localities were initially offered as categorical grants, focusing on particular health issues or populations (such as research training grants for education, nutrition information programs, substance abuse and mental health programs, and family planning programs). In the early 1980s, the federal government grouped numerous categorical grants to states into four major block grants: one in preventive health, one in maternal and child health, one in primary care, and one in alcohol/drug abuse/mental health. The more traditional public health functions of the Department of Health and Human Services have generally been channeled through the Health Resources and Services Administration and the Centers for Disease Control and Prevention, but these are by no means the only channels by which federal public health finances and resources are channeled to state and local governments.

It should be noted that one of the federal government's major health activities, the provision of a large volume of direct patient care through the Veterans Administration, has no formal or organizational connection with the Department of Health and Human Services. The Veterans Administration and its extensive network of hospitals and clinics throughout the United States does not operate under the authority or jurisdiction of the Department of Health and Human Services at all.

State Government Public Health Activities

States are the principal governmental entity responsible for protecting the public's health in the United States. In the Tenth Amendment to the United States Constitution, states are designated as the repository of all government powers not specifically granted to the federal government. States carry out most of their responsibilities through their police power—the power to enact and enforce laws to protect and promote the health and safety of the people.

There are 55 state health agencies in the United States (the 50 states plus the District of Columbia, Guam, Puerto Rico, American Samoa, and the Virgin Islands). It is probably safe to say that each state agency is somewhat different from all the rest, as there is wide variation in the exact way in which state health agencies are organized. In general, each state agency is directed by a health commissioner or a secretary of health. Each agency also has a state health officer (required to be a licensed physician) who is the top public health medical authority in the state; in many states, the state health officer is the director of the state agency, but in some states, the state health officer works for a non-physician director who is the administrator of a larger agency or department. In approximately half the states, there is also some type of state Board of Health or similar appointive body that is charged with the responsibility for approving policy in the public health area and for reviewing the use of public funds. Approximately half the states do not have Boards of Health and operate their public health agencies as administrative units of state government without any outside appointive oversight.

Earlier we described the federal Department of Health and Human Services as a somewhat loose collection of superagencies, each of which operated in a semiautonomous fashion from all the rest.

State public health agencies, on the other hand, are relatively compact in the organization of their public health services and function as a single operational unit that is usually fairly well integrated within itself. The variation among state public health agencies, however, is that the public health function may be gathered together with a wide variety of other health-related agencies under some type of superagency or department. In some states, the traditional public health functions, usually gathered together in a single operational unit, are housed in a superagency that also contains organizations that deal with environmental issues, mental health services, services for retarded or disabled individuals, as well as the state Medicaid program. There is no uniform arrangement for these state-level superagencies; thus, the public health unit may stand alone as an organizational unit or may be associated with up to four or five other health-related units in a superagency.

Regardless of the organizational arrangement, there are certain functions and activities that seem to be common throughout the 55 state public health agencies in the United States. These include the following general functions: (1) collect and analyze health statistics to determine the health status and general health situation of the public; (2) provide general education to the public on matters of public health importance; (3) maintain state laboratories to conduct certain specialized tests that are required by state public health law; (4) establish and police public health standards for the state as a whole; (5) grant licenses to health care professionals and institutions throughout the state and monitor and inspect the performance of personnel and institutions as appropriate; and (6) establish general policy for local government public health units and provide them with financial support as may be appropriate.

In general, state public health agencies nationwide receive half of their financial resources from state taxes, approximately one-third from federal government grants and contracts, and the remainder from special sources such as licensing fees and reimbursements. In discussing federal public health agencies, we pointed out that the financial resources of the federal public health activities draw on the very large national income tax for the financing of their operations, and at the same time, the federal government agencies have relatively few mandated responsibilities that must be carried out. By contrast, state governments must depend on a less robust (as evidenced by the 2000–2003 fiscal era) state income tax for approximately half of their funding and, at the same time, have many more mandated services that they must provide. In general, state health departments are moderately well funded for the services that they are required to provide but considerably underfunded in terms of the potential health promotion and disease prevention services that they could provide.

If it can be said that the federal government public health agencies focus their energies on the identification of major health problems in the country and the establishment of national policies to attack these problems, state public health departments concentrate their energies on translating national health goals and objectives into state policy and spend a considerable bit of their time seeing that that policy is carried out. Many of these policies are carried out by the state public health agencies themselves, and many of them are carried out by local public health agencies under the direction and supervision of state health departments.

Local Government Public Health Activities

Local health departments are the front line of public health services in the United States. It is here in the local government agencies that the actual daily work of public health takes place, and it is here that the policies and strategies decided upon by federal and state public health agencies must be carried out. It is here where the stress of meeting public health challenges is greatest and where deficiencies or shortfalls are most visible and obvious (Levy & Sidel, 2005).

Local health departments carry out their activities under the authority delegated by either their state or their local jurisdictions. Depending upon the interests and the resources of the local government, the local government public health function may either be very broad and energetic or very narrow and restricted. Some local health departments serve a single city or county, while others cover a group of counties. In about one-third of the states, the local health units are actually district offices of state health agencies, and in another one-third, the local health agencies are responsible to both local governments and the state public health agency.

The organization of the local public health agency is generally relatively simple, with the local public health agency responding directly to the local elected authority—either a mayor, county administrator, or board of supervisors. In its operations, however, the local public health authority must depend on state or federal funds for approximately half of its operating budget, so the leaders of the local public health agencies must continuously maintain a dual reporting function, one to their local government and the other to the state and/or federal government that provides them with the bulk of their operating revenues.

A special committee of the American Public Health Association, chaired by Haven Emerson in 1945, defined the six basic functions of a local health department as follows (Emerson, 1945):

1. Vital statistics—recording, tabulating, interpreting, and publishing of essential facts of births, deaths, and reportable diseases

2. Communicable disease control—tuberculosis, venereal disease, measles, hepatitis, and AIDS

3. Sanitation—supervision of milk, water, and eating places

4. Laboratory services

5. Maternal and child health services, including supervision of the health of children in schools

6. Health education of the public

For the most part, local public health departments continue to carry out the vital statistics, communicable disease control, environmental sanitation, and maternal and child health functions even up to the present time. They also, for the most part, maintain active public health education programs, although these efforts have become increasingly endangered by budgetary deficiencies. For the most part, laboratory services are no longer provided by local public health departments but are now provided by state health departments. And for the most part, the local public health department's functions are very immediate and in direct contact with the public: recording births and deaths, trying to maintain control or contact of individual people with serious communicable diseases, inspecting restaurants and other public gathering places to identify sanitary problems, and making sure that newborn infants receive their immunizations for infectious diseases and that children in school have some degree of health supervision. If the federal government's functions can be described as distant, nationwide, impersonal, and related to policy, the local government's public health function can be described as immediate, individual, pragmatic, and personal. The basic operating unit of local government public health only serves to enhance this sense of immediate contact with the public because it is usually represented by the local health center or local public health office; this is usually situated in areas of the greatest public health problems and at locations that provide the easiest access to the most susceptible segments of the population.

Unfortunately, the disconnection between mandated required services and financial resources becomes most apparent at the local public health level. In the United States, local governments are usually the least well financed of the three levels of government, and it is no different for local public health agencies.

Integrating Public Health Services

From this description, it can be seen that the public portion of our nation's health promotion and disease prevention activities depends on an intricate collaboration and cooperation between three levels of governmental agencies: federal, state, and local.

It involves elaborate transfer of financial resources from the federal government (where the resources are most abundant) to state governments (where resources are less abundant but still sufficient) and through to local public health agencies (where resources are scarcest and responsibilities most intense). The public portion of our nation's health promotion and disease prevention activities is, for the most part, focused first on the protection of the public from potential threats to health and only secondarily on the active promotion of healthier lifestyles (Novick & Mays, 2001).

Although the public health professionals in governmental health agencies know very well that the greatest long-term impact on the health of our nation's people probably depends on changes in styles of living, those same public health professionals very often find themselves limited in their ability to engage in activities that are directly focused on lifestyle change. Federal, state, and local government public health agencies can create policies and goals to encourage individual personal lifestyle change, but for the most part, the actual implementation of those changes probably rests with the private sector, with the providers of medical care. Governmental public health agencies can go only so far with the resources available to them in creating an atmosphere for major lifestyle change and improvement and, therefore, must depend upon their private-sector colleagues to carry the effort more directly into the homes of individual people. Nevertheless, governmental public health agencies have played a vital role in the protection of the public, in setting strategies and goals for the improvement of the health status of the public, and in motivating the public to move to an even higher level of healthful living.

For that next level of health promotion and disease prevention, however, the full involvement and participation of the private sector is necessary. The importance of the private-sector clinical role was originally stressed in the United States Preventive Services Task Force Report in 1989 and was reinforced by the United States Public Health Service's major reports, *Healthy People 2000* and *Healthy People 2010,* which set national health promotion and disease prevention objectives for the country (U.S. Department of Health and Human Services, 2000; U.S. Preventive Services Task Force, 1989; U.S. Public Health Service, 1990).

THE ROLE OF THE PRIVATE SECTOR IN HEALTH PROMOTION AND DISEASE PREVENTION

It is comparatively easy to discuss the role of governmental public health agencies: usually they have been in existence for some time, have clearly defined roles, and have well-documented track records extending over many years. When one approaches the role of the private sector in health promotion and disease prevention, however, discussion becomes more difficult and more diffuse, if no less important. Indeed, in the minds of many individuals, the role of the private sector, particularly the physician in private practice, is increasingly central in creating the major lifestyle changes that are viewed as being so important to the prevention of disease over the long term.

Many deaths in the United States are attributable to lifestyle and personal actions on the part of individuals, such as tobacco use, improper diet and activity patterns, overuse of alcohol and firearms, unsafe sexual behavior, and vehicular accidents while under the influence of alcohol. Most of these causes of death are only partially amenable to change by broad social or legislative actions, and only individual behavior change will really affect many of them. The physician in medical practice is in a key position to influence behavior change because research has shown that individuals are more likely to follow improved health habits if they are encouraged to do so by their usual medical practitioner. The central role of the practicing physician in encouraging and enhancing improved personal life habits has long been acknowledged and must be central to any future

national plan of health promotion and disease prevention.

There are two major barriers to the individual physician's assuming the central role in health promotion and disease prevention: (1) the individual physician's willingness and ability to perform these health promotion and disease prevention activities, and (2) the ability of the population to access the services of a private physician.

With regard to the physician's interest in, and ability to perform, health promotion and disease prevention activities, it has long been noted that physicians are generally more interested and more competent in matters related to curative and treatment activities than they are in matters related to health promotion and disease prevention. This may be a reflection of their early medical training, which may have lacked emphasis on health promotion and disease prevention, or it may be related to the physician's natural human tendency to see curative treatment as "doing something" while seeing health promotion and disease prevention as "not doing something." Physicians are by nature activists and are more naturally drawn to the interventions where they are likely to see results in a relatively short period of time as opposed to events where the consequences of their actions will be known only, if at all, many years later.

It should also be pointed out that in the previous era of fee-for-service medicine, physicians were only reimbursed for treatment activities and were usually not reimbursed, either by insurance companies or by individuals paying their own bills, for prevention services. The former methods of payment for medical services encouraged increased active treatment of illness but did not encourage its active prevention. It is only natural, therefore, that physicians in the past should have responded to obvious incentives by spending more of their time and energies on treatment and less on prevention.

Probably a greater barrier to enhancing the role of the private physician in health promotion and disease prevention is the limited access that a significant portion of our population has to medical care. A significant portion of the United States population is uninsured or has very limited insurance, with relatively large financial burdens still resting with the individual patient who is unlikely to visit a physician on a regular basis. If individual people in the United States discover that their insurance plans do not cover health promotion and disease prevention and that they must pay for such tests themselves, they are less likely to use such tests and procedures and to visit a physician on a regular basis to obtain the counseling and encouragement that might be possible there.

It would seem natural to suggest, therefore, that if our nation wishes to involve the private sector in extensive health promotion and disease prevention activities that reach our entire population, it must be arranged in some fashion for the entire population to have health insurance coverage that ensures adequate access to medical care (Levy & Sidel, 2005). Without universal health insurance coverage of some kind, it is an illusion to talk about a nationwide health promotion and disease prevention effort, as a significant percentage of the population (and, perhaps, those at highest risk) cannot access the one place where the most influential health promotion and disease prevention counseling might take place—the office of a private medical practitioner. Universal health insurance coverage, therefore, is central to any nationwide effort of health promotion and disease prevention.

Merely having universal health insurance coverage, however, is not enough if that health insurance coverage does not include financing for health promotion and disease prevention tests, procedures, and counseling. Many of the health insurance plans issued at the present time do not include reimbursement for health promotion and disease prevention, and as a result, individuals who may actually have health insurance coverage of a general nature are not covered for health promotion and disease prevention services. Therefore, it is essential that the design of future health insurance packages include financing for these services. Without such financing, individuals may be actively discouraged from seeking health promotion and disease prevention

tests and procedures, as well as advice and counseling, from their primary physician.

The Role of Managed Care in Health Promotion and Disease Prevention

The advent of managed-care health insurance coverage around the United States may present an opportunity to accomplish some of these health promotion and disease prevention objectives, particularly if the specific managed-care plans are those of the health maintenance organization (HMO) type, which reimburse physician groups on a *per capita* basis. The advent of managed care of the HMO type presents opportunities for the expansion of health promotion and disease prevention in ways that have not been previously available (Breslow, 1996; Koplan & Harris, 2000).

It is important to note two essential elements of the HMO type of managed-care plan: (1) the official assignment of the long-term responsibility for supervising all aspects of an individual's care to a specific physician or medical group, and (2) the reimbursement of that physician or medical group on a *per capita* basis. Each of these specific aspects of HMO managed care is very supportive of the general long-term thrust in health promotion and disease prevention.

With regard to the first (i.e., the assignment of long-term responsibility for an individual's care to a specific physician), HMO managed-care plans require the identification of a specific primary care physician for each person covered by that type of insurance. This puts a particular physician on notice that this individual patient (or family unit) is his or her long-term responsibility. This identification of the individual physician as having an official long-term and continuing responsibility for an individual or a family changes the perspective of the individual physician away from the provision of specific individual services and toward the long-term health of the individual or the family. The designation of an individual physician as a patient's primary care doctor further solidifies the long-term role of that physician in managing the entire health-related set of activities in the minds of both the physician and the patient.

The use of *per capita* reimbursement to the primary care physician further reinforces the long-term nature of the relationship and particularly emphasizes the long-term role of attempting to reach maximum health outcomes, not just providing individual fee-for-service interactions. The HMO *per capita* reimbursement method serves as a reminder to the physician that his or her financial rewards are dependent upon keeping the individual patient as healthy as possible, rather than simply providing a series of individual services to a sick person. The dynamics in the HMO managed-care plan thereby provide more incentives for keeping people healthy.

Managed-care insurance coverage of the HMO type also has a great advantage over the previous fee-for-service type of coverage in that it not only assigns official responsibility to an individual physician or medical group, but it also holds that physician or medical group accountable for what happens to the patient. In the past, no physician or medical group was responsible for reporting to any insurance plan or purchaser of health care about the long-term pattern of services and their results. The individual physician merely provided one service after another on an individual and relatively unconnected basis, and no accountability was ever really required as to how the pattern of individual services eventually affected the overall health of an individual patient.

Under the new forms of HMO managed care, not only is it possible to assign individual long-term responsibility to a specific physician or medical group, but it is also possible, and, indeed, increasingly the rule, to designate specific actions that the physician or group must take during the course of a particular year. It is increasingly common for HMO managed-care plans to outline certain specific services or practices that a physician must follow and also to require documentation of the completion of those services.

For example, many HMO managed-care plans require that physicians provide certain health promotion and disease prevention services (such as immunizations for children, provision of mammograms for women over a certain age, blood cholesterol measurements, and the like). Not only are the HMO managed-care plans able to require physicians to provide these services, but they are also able to require the physicians to report that these services have actually been completed.

What this means for the encouragement of health promotion and disease prevention activities on the part of the physician should be obvious. In the future, if it is judged that a certain pattern of health promotion and disease prevention services or activities should be provided to an individual patient during the course of a particular year, that requirement can be written into the contract with the individual physician before he or she is allowed to assume long-term responsibility for the patient. Unwillingness to perform these health promotion and disease prevention actions would bar the physician from being able to contract with the HMO managed-care plan in the first place. The contract language can also ensure that the physician agrees to provide information that will allow the plan to determine whether the services have actually been delivered to the patient as agreed upon.

Many aspects of managed care are cause for concern among thoughtful observers of health care in the United States, but the enhancement of health promotion and disease prevention activities is not one of them. Indeed, one of the major positive aspects of managed care is its potential ability to install an organized, well-financed, and well-documented system of care that emphasizes health promotion and disease prevention. Despite whatever other concerns may exist about managed care, it is clear that the growth of managed-care health insurance coverage offers an opportunity for an entirely new era with regard to the promotion of better health and prevention of future disease in the United States.

PUBLIC HEALTH IN AN ERA OF TERRORISM AND EMERGING DISEASES

Public health services received tremendous new attention following September 11, 2001, from both the increased threat of terrorist attacks and the emergence of new diseases (Table 6.1) (Shadel et al., 2004). Preparation for potential terror events has been funded in varying degrees by federal and state sources. The focus on such preparation has encompassed a wide range of public health activities including monitoring, planning, mobilization, coordination with other entities, and prepared response. Public health services are integral to any response to external attack, and the expertise of public health agencies and officials has been expanded through training, expansion of capabilities, acquisition of equipment, and a more prepared workforce.

Table 6.1. Illustrative Twenty-First Century Emerging Public Health Threats

Terror	Natural Disasters	Disease
Active attacks on commerce	Earthquakes	Anthrax
Economic attacks including those on banking	Extreme heat	Avian influenza
	Floods	Botulism
	Hurricanes	Ebola hemorrhagic fever
Interference with food, water, utilities, supplies	Landslides and mudslides	Hantavirus
	Power outages	Lassa fever
Internet attacks	Tornadoes	Plague
	Tsunamis	Ricin toxin
	Volcanoes	Viral encephalitis
	Wildfires	
	Winter weather	

As with terror threats, in recent years the advent of emerging new disease challenges, including SARS, hemorrhagic fevers, avian flu, and other potential illnesses, has led to increased surveillance and preparation. The potential impact of these threats could be huge in the United States and internationally, such that public health agencies are expected to be prepared to respond, and indeed, to anticipate potential threats (Merson, Black, & Mills, 2005). Combined with possible terrorist use of infectious agents such as anthrax, reliance on public health agencies may be greater than funding and staffing would suggest is realistic.

Finally, of course, natural disasters also pose tremendous challenges for public health agencies. Hurricanes, earthquakes, fires, and floods have all demonstrated their impact on human populations nationally and internationally. The prospective preparation for these events has clearly been grossly inadequate. Most local public health agencies remain underfunded and understaffed if the expectation is that they will be capable of mounting a full and appropriate response (Rowitz, 2003).

In addition to natural disaster and terrorism, accidents, the impact of crowding, certain effects of population aging, chemical infringements, drug misuse, and many other concerns affect the public health arena as well. And public health-related events can lead to other complications such as displacement of people, disruptions in the food and water supplies, lack of access to health care, impacts on utilities, and separation of family members. The scope of direct and indirect effects of many events on the public's health is huge, perhaps much greater today than in past years.

Clearly the role of public health in protecting our nation has greatly expanded over the past few years. The traditional threats facing the nation's public health are now clearly augmented by expectations for a broader array of capabilities to respond to newly strengthen challenges on many more fronts. Recognizing the importance of public health services to the nation, further development of this capability is not only essential, but it is also cost effective and beneficial to our nation's future survival.

SUMMARY

It should be clear from this discussion of health promotion and disease prevention in the United States that this is a shared responsibility between the public (governmental) and the private sectors of health care (Institute of Medicine, 2003). Neither sector can do what the other can do, and neither sector can do it alone. For the people of this country to reach their maximum health status, it will be necessary to forge an even stronger public-private partnership that allows both sectors to use their unique roles and advantages to advance the health of the public in ways that have never before been possible.

REVIEW QUESTIONS

1. What are the various levels of prevention?
2. Discuss the historical evolution of health promotion and disease prevention in the United States.
3. What are the lessons from history of public health development in the United States?
4. Describe and discuss the structure of organized public health in the United States.
5. Discuss the role of the private sector in health promotion and disease prevention in the United States.
6. Discuss the role of managed care in health promotion and disease prevention in the United States.
7. List some of the major public health threats that have recently emerged in the twenty-first century.
8. Summarize the future of public health in the United States.

REFERENCES & ADDITIONAL READINGS

Aaron, H. J. (1993/94). Paying for health care. *Domestic Affairs, 2,* 23–78.

Anderson, G. F., Hussey, P. S., Frogner, B. K., & Waters, H. R. (2005). Health spending in the United States and the rest of the industrialized world. *Health Affairs, 24*(4), 903–914.

Breslow, L. (1996). Public health and managed care: A California perspective. *Health Affairs, 15,* 92–99.

Brockington, C. (1956). *A short history of public health.* London: J & A Churchill.

DesHarnais, S., Kobrinski, E., Chesney, J., et al. (1987). The early effects of the Prospective Payment System on inpatient utilization and the quality of care. *Inquiry, 24,* 7–16.

Diagnosis-related groups (DRGs) and the prospective payment system. (1984). American Medical Association: Chicago.

Emerson, H. (1945). *Local health units for the nation.* New York: Commonwealth Fund.

Enthoven, A. (1981). The competition strategy; status and prospects. *New England Journal of Medicine, 304,* 109–112.

Fallon, F. L., & Zgodzinski, E. J. (2005). *Essentials of Public Health Management.* Sudbury, MA: Jones and Bartlett.

Fuchs, V. R. (1984). "Though much is taken": Reflictions on aging, health, and medical care. *Milbank Memorial Fund Quarterly, 62,* 143–166.

Gornick, M., Greenberg, N. J., Eggers, P. W., et al. (1985, December). Twenty years of Medicare and Medicaid: Covered populations, use of benefits, and program expenditures. *Health Care Financing Review,* (Annual Suppl.), 13–59.

Guterman, S., & Dobson, A. (1986). Impact of the Medicare Prospective payment system for hospitals. *Health Care Financing Review, 7,* 97–114.

Guterman, S., Eggers, P. W., Riley, G., Greene, T. F., & Terrell, S. A. (1988). The first 3 years of Medicare prospective payment: An overview. *Health Care Financing Review, 9*(3), 67–77.

Hillman, A. L., Welch, W. P., & Pauly, M. V. (1992). Contractual arrangements between HMOs and primary care physicians: Three-tiered HMOs and risk pools. *Medical Care, 30*(2), 136–148.

Hsiao, W. C., Braun, P., Becker, E. R., et al. (1992). Results and impacts of the resource-based relative value scale. *Medical Care, 30*(11), NS61–NS79.

Hsaio, W. C., Bruan, P., Dunn, D., Becker, E. R., DeNicola, M., Ketcham, T. R. (1988). Results and policy implications of the resource-based relative-value study. *New England Journal of Medicine, 319*(13), 881–888.

Hsiao, W. C., Bruan, P., Yntema, D., & Becker, E. R. (1988). Estimating physicians' work for a resource-based relative-value scale. *New England Journal of Medicine, 319*(13), 835–841.

Institute of Medicine of the U.S. National Academy of Sciences (1988). *The future of public health.* Washington, DC: National Academy Press.

Institute of Medicine. (2003). *The future of the public's health in the 21st century.* Washington, DC: National Academy Press.

Koplan, J. P., & Harris, J. R. (2000). Not-so-strange bedfellows: Public health and managed care. *American Journal of Public Health, 90*(12), 1824–1826.

Levy, B. S., & Sidel, V. S. (2005). *Social injustice and public health.* New York: Oxford University Press.

Lubitz, J., & Prihoda, R. (1984). Use and costs of Medicare services in the last two years of life. *Health Care Financing Review, 5,* 117–131.

Lundberg, G. D. (1991). National health care reform: An aura of inevitability is upon us. *Journal of the American Medical Association, 265*(19), 2566–2567.

Merson, M., Black, R., & Mills, A. (2005). *International public health: Diseases, programs, systems, and policies.* Sudbury, MA: Jones and Bartlett, 2005.

Moutin, J., Hankela, E., & Druzin, G. (1947). *Ten years of federal grants-in-aid for public health, 1936–1946* (Bull. No. 300). Washington, DC: Public Health Service.

Neuschler, E. (1990). *Canadian health care: The implications of public health insurance.* Wasington, DC: Health Insurance Association of America.

Novick, L., & Mays, G. (2001). *Public health administration: Principles for population-based management.* Sudbury, MA: Jones and Bartlett.

Reinhardt, U. E. (1985). The compensation of physicians: Approaches used in foreign countries. *Quality Review Bulletin, 11,* 366–377.

Reinhardt, U. E., Hussey, P. S., & Anderson, G. F. (2004). U.S. health care spending in an international context. *Health Affairs, 23*(3), 10–25.

Rice, T. (1992). Containing health care costs in the United States. *Medical Care Research and Review, 49*(1), 19–65.

Roemer, M. I. (1977). *Comparative national policies on health care.* New York: Marcel Dekker.

Roemer, M. I. (1978). *Social medicine: The advance of organized health services in America.* New York: Springer.

Rosen, G. (1993). *A History of Public Health* (expanded ed.). Baltimore: The Johns Hopkins University Press.

Rowitz, L. (2003). *Public health leadership: Putting principles into practice.* Sudbury, MA: Jones and Bartlett.

Scutchfield, F., & Keck, W. (2002). *Principles of public health practice* (2nd ed). Albany, NY: Delmar.

Shadel, B. N., Chen, J. J., Newkirk, R. W., Lawrence, S. J., et al. (2004). Bioterrorism risk perceptions and educational needs of public health professionals before and after September 11th: A national needs assessment survey. *Journal of Public Health Management and Practice, 10*(4), 282–289.

Shattuck, L. (1850). *Report of the sanitary commission of massachusetts.* Boston: Dutton & Wentworth, 1850. (Reprinted by Harvard University Press, Cambridge, MA, 1948.)

Smith, C., Cowan, C., Heffler, S., Catlin, A., & National Accounts Team (2006). National health spending in 2004: Recent slowdown led by prescription drug spending. *Health Affairs, 25*(1), 186–196.

U.S. Preventive Services Task Force. (1989). *Guide to clinical preventive services: An assessment of the effectiveness of 169 interventions.* Baltimore: Williams & Wilkins.

U.S. Public Health Service. (1990). *Healthy people 2000: National health promotion and disease prevention objectives* (DHHS Pub. No. PHS 91-50212). Washington, DC: Department of Health and Human Services.

Waldo, M. O. (1990). Addendum: A brief summary of the Medicaid program. *Health Care Financing Review, 12,* 171–172.

Winslow, C. E. A. (1923). The evolution and significance of the modern public health campaign. Reprinted in *Journal of Public Health Policy, 1*(1), 15–24.

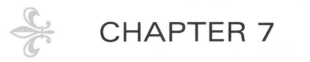

CHAPTER 7

Ambulatory Health Care Services and Organizations

Stephen J. Williams

CHAPTER TOPICS

- Historical Perspectives and Types of Care
- Use of Ambulatory Care Services
- Ambulatory Practice Settings
- Institutionally Based Ambulatory Services
- Government Programs
- Noninstitutional and Public Health Services
- The Role of Ambulatory Services
- Managing a Medical Practice
- Professional Practice Organizations

LEARNING OBJECTIVES

Upon completing this chapter, the reader should be able to

1. Understand the role of ambulatory care services.
2. Appreciate the evolution of ambulatory care as a distribution system.
3. Review the primary ambulatory care providers.
4. Outline the organizational role and control mechanisms of ambulatory care services.
5. Assess the allocation of responsibility for coordination, integration, appropriateness, and rationalization between ambulatory care and other sectors.
6. Understand how practices are managed.

This chapter addresses the array of services that provide care in communities to noninstitutionalized patients. The chapter addresses the multitude of service distribution channels, practices, and patterns utilized in the provision of physician, dental, and other professional services. Some services related to institutionalized patients such as those admitted to hospitals or nursing homes are also mentioned as they pertain to ambulatory care, recognizing the increasing connection between various types and levels of health care services.

Ambulatory care has increased dramatically in status in the health care system over the past three decades as the system has moved toward increasingly integrated and, ultimately ideally, seamless provision of care. The trend toward providing services in less expensive and less intensive surroundings and facilities, encouraged by the march of technology and by pricing and reimbursement pressures, is further accelerating these trends.

The ambulatory arena, which encompasses a very broad array of services as exemplified by the partial listing in Table 7.1, serves two principal roles in the health care system. First, these services provide an increasingly greater percentage of all direct patient care in the form of personal and preventive health services. Second, ambulatory care is increasingly serving the role of care manager in allocating resources to meet patient needs in clinical decision making. Because of the increasingly complex nature of ambulatory care services, this chapter will discuss the historical and current nature of these services but will also delve into the managerial considerations involved in organizing, developing, and controlling this segment of the health care system.

The role of ambulatory care services in organizing and delivering physician, dental, and other professional services is continuing to evolve. But the fundamental realignment of the nation's health care system, driven by technology, quality concerns, cost and reimbursement imperatives, and by the desires of consumers, is now set in place and is irreversible.

Table 7.1. Illustrative Ambulatory Care Services

Solo practice
Group practice
Hospital clinics
Hospital emergency rooms
Ambulatory surgery centers (hospital-based and freestanding)
Community-wide emergency medical systems
Poison control centers
Community hotlines
Neighborhood (community) health centers
Migrant health centers
Community mental health centers
Federal systems—Veterans Administration, Indian Health Service, military health services
Home health services
School health services
Prison health services
Public health services and clinics
Family planning and other specialized clinics
Industrial clinics
Pharmacies
Vision care
Medical laboratories
Indigenous practitioners

HISTORICAL PERSPECTIVES AND TYPES OF CARE

Traditionally, ambulatory care services have been viewed as the primary source of contact that most people have with the health care system. Although there are few concise definitions of ambulatory care, these services can be defined as care provided to noninstitutionalized patients. Sometimes ambulatory care is termed care for the "walking patient." Ambulatory care includes a wide range of services, from simple, routine treatment to surprisingly complex tests and therapies.

Ambulatory care originated with the healing arts themselves. In primitive societies and for many years thereafter, until the advent of institutional care, all care was provided on what might today be referred to as an ambulatory care basis. Of course, the types of care given then bear little resemblance to today's health care, but the history of civilization demonstrates a consistent commitment to caring for the sick using whatever knowledge had been available at the time. Remarkable forms of medical practice occurred in Greece, Rome, and other relatively sophisticated societies. In fact, many primitive societies even had their own indigenous practitioners such as religious healers and medicine men.

In more recent times, ambulatory care was provided in many new settings by a variety of more advanced practitioners. In Europe, and later in the United Sates, many of these services were given to wealthy patients in their homes; poor people were cared for in dispensaries and public clinics. With improvements in hospital care, more patients of all social classes received both inpatient and outpatient care in hospital settings. In the United States, the poor have always been more likely than the wealthy to obtain care from the hospital than from private physicians.

In the United States, ambulatory care services were traditionally provided by individual medical practitioners working in their offices and in patients' homes and by public clinics operating primarily for poor and indigent patients. The limited technological armament that physicians required allowed them to travel easily, carrying with them their principal equipment and supplies. Thus, home care was common, especially among wealthier patients. Physicians' offices were frequently located in their homes or in other small buildings, as opposed to today's medical office buildings or large medical centers. The general practitioner who made house calls, provided guidance, and offered available treatments was typical of the primary care provided before and somewhat after World War II.

For the poor in both Europe and the Untied States, care—when available—was often limited to public or philanthropic clinics or dispensaries. Private practitioners may have given their time to serve the poor, but their devotion to the patient was probably limited, as was the availability of care and the facilities in which services were provided.

Early efforts to link ambulatory care services and integrate them formally with inpatient care were promoted in this country and in Europe, in part, through the concept of regionalization. In Great Britain, the concept was presented in the Dawson Report, which eventually led to the National Health Service (United Kingdom Ministry of Health, 1920).

Since World War II, an explosion of medical knowledge has led to increasing specialization, more complex technology, and rapid changes in the settings and nature of services. Fewer physicians are able or willing to travel to the patient's home, and many can no longer carry with them either the equipment and supplies or the specialized personnel available in an office. The growth of technical specialization, in particular, has led to the rapid expansion of new settings for providing care, such as group practices and, more recently, a profusion of specialized facilities. Increased knowledge has also led to the partial phasing out of the traditional general practitioner, replaced by the broadly trained family practitioner, a specialty whose development was encouraged by managed care and by concerns over the comprehensiveness of care.

The increasing sophistication of insurance mechanisms and the use of ambulatory care services as a control mechanism on the use of all services have led to an increase in the degree of structure of the health care system. This increasing structure has primarily occurred in the private, nongovernmental sector. The concept of social and economic regulation of the system through governmental intervention, carried to a high level of sophistication in the Dawson Report, has largely been abandoned, at least for the foreseeable future. Integration of services now focuses largely on multiple, independently organized systems of care that are competitive with one another.

Levels of Ambulatory Care Services

The diversity of services, providers, and facilities involved in ambulatory care today is truly amazing and growing all the time. Ambulatory care services can be differentiated by, as contrasted to public health, discussed in the previous chapters, levels of care. Primary prevention reduces the risks of morbidity by removing or reducing disease-causing agents and opportunities from our society. These activities include efforts to eliminate environmental pollutants that are suspected of causing diseases such as cancer. Other examples of primary prevention include encouraging people to use automobile seat belts, treatment of water and sewage, and sanitation inspections in restaurants. Preventive health services are more direct personal interventions to detect and prevent disease. Examples of these services include hypertension, diabetes, and cancer-screening and immunization programs. The combination of primary prevention and preventive services is our first line of defense against disease.

Medical care that is oriented toward the daily, routine needs of patients, such as initial diagnosis and continuing treatment of common illness, is termed primary care. This care is not necessarily highly complex and does not generally require sophisticated technology and personnel. The vision of the general practitioner of bygone days, traveling from house to house ministering to the sick, represents the traditional role of primary care, which is replaced in today's society by considerably more skilled practitioners in relatively more complex facilities.

In addition to providing services directly, the primary care professional should serve the role of patient advisor, advocate, and system gatekeeper. In this coordinating role, the provider refers patients to sources of specialized care, gives advice regarding various diagnoses and therapies, and provides continuing care for chronic conditions. In many organized systems of care, such as managed-care programs, this role is also very important in controlling costs, utilization, and the rational allocation of resources.

The evolution of technology and medicine's increasing ability to intervene in illness have led to greater specialization of health care services. These more specialized services, termed secondary and tertiary care, are provided in both ambulatory and inpatient settings. The content of secondary and tertiary care practices is usually more narrowly defined than that of the primary care provider. Subspecialists, who provide the bulk of secondary and tertiary care, also often require more complex equipment and more highly trained support personnel than do primary care providers.

In recent years, the evolution of health care services has led to greatly expanded provision of secondary care on an outpatient, or ambulatory care, basis. Numerous diagnostic and surgical services of increasing complexity have been shifted to the ambulatory arena. Recent advances in the use of fiber optics and other technologies suggest that this trend will continue.

There are no clear dividing lines for primary versus secondary and secondary versus tertiary care. Secondary services include routine hospitalization and specialized outpatient care. These services are more complex than those of primary care and include many diagnostic procedures as well as more complex therapies. Tertiary care includes the most complex services, such as open-heart surgery, burn treatment, and transplantation, and is provided in inpatient hospital facilities.

USE OF AMBULATORY CARE SERVICES

Historically, and at the present time, most ambulatory care services are provided in solo and group practice office-based settings. Institutional settings for care, primarily the hospital, although an important component of the health care system, remain less prominent. Overlap between office-based practice and institutional settings is increasingly common, however, as the dividing lines between various components of the health care system continue to blur. Managed-care programs especially tend to integrate these services. The development of increasingly sophisticated information systems and reimbursement mechanisms increasingly facilitate the integration of services across all levels of care.

Measures of the use of ambulatory care services are contained in Tables 7.2, and 7.3, which present survey results on utilization patterns based on national data that are representative of the entire United States population. These data are taken from the *National Health Interview Survey* (Adams, Dey, & Vickerie, 2007), a national survey of Americans' use of health care services, and they complement the utilization data presented in other chapters.

Tables 7.2 and 7.3 describe doctor visits experienced by Americans in various demographic categories. The very young and the very old report higher utilization of ambulatory services, and females generally experience higher utilization than males. The lowest income groups in our population, not coincidentally those of lower health status as well, experience the highest utilization of ambulatory services when the data are examined by income groups. In examining the data by health status, ambulatory services utilization is highest for the less healthy, as would be expected.

Table 7.2. **Health Care Visits to Doctors' Offices, Emergency Departments, and Home Visits within the Past 12 Months: United States, 2003**

Characteristic	Number of Health Care Visits			
	None	1–3 Visits	4–9 Visits	10 or More Visits
			Percent Distribution	
All persons	15.8	45.8	24.8	13.6
Age				
Under 18 years	11.3	54.5	26.7	7.5
18–44 years	22.4	46.7	19.1	11.8
45–64 years	14.7	42.2	26.6	16.5
65 years and over	6.3	31.5	35.8	26.4
Sex				
Male	20.6	46.8	21.9	10.7
Female	11.1	44.9	27.7	16.3
Race				
White only	15.7	45.6	25.1	13.6
Black or African				
American only	14.7	45.8	25.2	14.3
Hispanic or Latino	25.3	42.9	20.3	11.5
Poverty status				
Poor	20.9	37.8	23.7	17.6
Near poor	19.8	41.5	23.6	15.1
Nonpoor	13.7	48.4	25.4	12.6

Table 7.3. Visits to Physician Offices and Hospital Outpatient and Emergency Departments by Selected Characteristics: United States, 2003

Age, Sex, and Race	All Places	Physician Offices
	Number of visits in thousands	
Total	1,114,504	906,023
	Number of visits per 100 persons	
Under 18 years	307	232
18–44 years	300	229
45–64 years	442	377
65 years and over	754	664
Sex		
Male, age adjusted	338	273
Female, age adjusted	442	360
Race and age		
White, age adjusted	399	332
Black or African American, age adjusted	391	261

Table 7.4, also based on data from the *National Health Interview Survey*, indicates dental visit use. Such use is more dependent on financial access and the data clearly show lower use by lower income people and by the older population. Dental use would seem to fall short of preventive recommendations for various population groups also.

Use of Office Setting Services

Most utilization data are available from survey research results. To obtain more detailed information on health care use in physician office settings, the federal government has conducted periodic surveys of private, office-based physicians—the *National Ambulatory Medical Care Survey* (Hing, Cherry, & Woodwell, 2006). The National Ambulatory Medical Care Survey (NAMCS) is based on a sampling of visits to nonfederal office-based physicians. The survey has been performed annually since 1989.

Table 7.4. Dental Visits During the Prior Year According to Selected Characteristics: United States, 2003

Characteristic	2 Years of Age and Over	2–17 Years of Age	18–64 Years of Age	65 Years of Age and Over
	Percent of persons with a dental visit in the prior year			
Total	66.3	75.0	64.8	58.0
Sex				
Male	63.6	74.1	60.9	58.4
Female	68.9	75.9	68.6	57.7
Race				
White only	67.5	76.0	65.9	59.8
Black or African American only	58.4	70.5	58.1	38.7
Hispanic or Latino	52.4	64.5	48.3	46.0
Poverty Status				
Poor	48.2	65.8	44.5	37.1
Near poor	52.3	66.6	49.1	43.6
Nonpoor	73.4	80.8	72.0	67.8

Table 7.5. Number and Percent Distribution by Sex of Office Visits for the Top 10 Principal Reasons for Visits: United States, 2004

Principal Reason for Visit	Number of Visits in Thousands	Patient's Sex	
		Female	Male
All visits	910,857	100.0	100.0
General medical examination	56,703	5.2	7.7
Progress visit, not otherwise specified	48,302	5.3	5.3
Postoperative visit	26,299	2.9	2.8
Cough	25,951	2.5	3.3
Prenatal examination, routine	24,816	4.6	—
Medication, other and unspecified kinds	16,483	1.7	2.0
Hypertension	14,510	1.4	1.8
Symptoms referable to throat	14,470	1.7	1.5
Knee symptoms	14,241	1.5	1.7
Well-baby examination	11,023	1.0	1.6

SOURCE: From *National Ambulatory Medical Care Survey: 2004 Summary. Advance Data from Vital and Health Statistics,* no. 374, by E. Hing, D. K. Cherry, and D. A. Woodwell, 2006, Hyattsville, MD: National Center for Health Statistics.

Data collection is based on the physician, who is randomly assigned to a one-week reporting period during which an encounter form is used to record symptoms.

Table 7.5 lists the most common reasons for all office visits. The relative prominence of routine care, of follow-up or ongoing care, and of relatively simple primary care is striking and reflects the predominance of the routine, day-to-day needs of patients seeking ambulatory care services.

Further understanding of the nature of the visits is obtainable from additional data regarding the services provided to patients and the interactions shared between patients and physicians. The principal sources of payment for patient office visits are private and commercial insurance, Medicare, HMOs, and other managed-care arrangements. The percentage of visits included in this last category likely will increase in future years while managed care grows in popularity.

The most common drug categories prescribed during the physician office visits are classified in Table 7.6. The most prevalent categories of drugs

Table 7.6. Therapeutic Classification for the 10 Drugs Most Frequently Prescribed at Office Visits: United States, 2004

Therapeutic Classification	Number of Prescriptions
Antidepressants	81,185
NSAID	73,737
Antiasthmatics/bronchodilators	69,507
Antihypertensive agents	69,113
Hyperlipidemia	63,996
Antihistamines	58,163
Acid or peptic disorders	56,906
Antiarthritics	54,783
Blood glucose regulators	53,069
Nonnarcotic analgesics	51,918

SOURCE: From *National Ambulatory Medical Care Survey: 2004 Summary. Advance Data from Vital and Health Statistics,* no. 374, by E. Hing, D. K. Cherry, and D. A. Woodwell, 2006, Hyattsville, MD: National Center for Health Statistics.

Table 7.7. Percent Distribution of Office Visits, by Time Spent with Physicians: United States, 2004

Time Spent with Physician	Percent Distribution
All visits	100.0
Visits at which no physician was seen	4.9
Visits at which a physician was seen	95.1
Time (with a physician)	100.0
1–5 minutes	3.6
6–10 minutes	18.7
11–15 minutes	40.1
16–30 minutes	31.2
31 minutes and over	6.4

SOURCE: From *National Ambulatory Medical Care Survey: 2004 Summary. Advance Data from Vital and Health Statistics,* no. 374, by E. Hing, D. K. Cherry, and D. A. Woodwell, 2006, Hyattsville, MD: National Center for Health Statistics.

include cardiovascular and renal, antimicrobial, and pain-relief agents. As technology changes, the classification distribution of various drug categories will likely change in prevalence as well.

The distribution of office visits by the duration of the visit (Table 7.7) indicates that relatively few visits require either very short or very long physician contacts. The typical physician office visit requires only about 5 to 15 minutes of time; nearly three-fourths of all visits require 15 minutes or less. A high percentage of visits conclude with the recommendation that the patient return at a specified time interval for a follow-up visit. An interesting issue in resource utilization is the impact of physician assistants, nurse practitioners, and other professionals on the time allocation of physicians in clinical care.

The *National Ambulatory Medical Care Survey* provides some insight into the nature of office-based ambulatory care. Much more extensive documentation of the survey and results for various types of services, providers, and patient characteristics is available from the federal government.

The survey data are an aid to planning health services in the ambulatory care setting and provide perspectives on national patterns of utilization. The applicability of the data to setting standards of performance in managed-care settings or under contracted agreements for service, however, is limited because of the many variables that could not be adequately measured.

AMBULATORY PRACTICE SETTINGS

Significant differences exist among physician practice settings. The two primary noninstitutional settings for the provision of ambulatory care are solo and group practice. Each of these settings may be a component of larger systems of care through such integrating mechanisms as referral arrangements, insurance contracts, and direct ownership of practices, especially in vertically integrated health care delivery systems.

Although the solo practice of medicine has traditionally attracted the greatest number of practitioners, group practice and institutionally based services have expanded dramatically, continuing a trend that has been building over the past 30 years. Changing lifestyles, the cost of establishing a practice, personal financial pressures on practitioners, contracting and affiliation opportunities under managed care, and the burdens of running a business have enhanced the attractiveness of group practice for many physicians. With sharp increases in the number of physicians beginning practice, the growth of alternative settings, and especially of group practice, has been dramatic. Although solo practice remains a viable avenue for providing ambulatory care services, these other settings have rapidly assumed a more prominent and visible role in the health care system, particularly as they provide a further mechanism for the integration, management, and control of health care services.

Solo Practice

Solo practitioners are difficult to uniformly characterize. Early sociological studies focused on specific questions, such as referral patterns or quality of care, and they did not provide a comprehensive picture of what the solo practitioner did. Studies that did contribute to a more complete understanding of the activities of solo practitioners were based on physicians in one geographic area or a particular specialty, and the results of these studies, although interesting and useful, may not be applicable to other practices or areas. In addition, solo practitioners are heterogeneous; they include many types of health care professionals who provide an immense array of services.

Most solo practitioners perform a number of functions in the office, including patient care, consultations, and administration and supervision of office staff. The requirements for administration, for supervision of personnel and for insurance paperwork have been increasing in recent years. Solo practitioners are also affiliating with managed-care networks that help ensure a viable patient population.

Solo practice is often associated with an increased feeling that the provider cares about the welfare of the patient, possibly resulting in a stronger patient-provider relationship that occurs in other settings. There is some evidence that this situation, where it occurs, is a result of the lower level of bureaucracy or organizational complexity in solo practice. Because there is also some evidence that the relationship between patient and physician is related to patient compliance with medical regimens, patients who perceive that they are receiving more personalized care may respond to the care process more positively.

Solo practitioners may not be as restricted in referrals to specialists as providers in some other settings, such as group practice, where organizational loyalties intervene. Managed-care contracts, however, may limit referral options.

From the provider's perspective, solo practice offers an opportunity to avoid organizational dependence and to be self-employed; there is also no need to share resources or income with other providers. Philosophically, solo practice is most closely aligned with the traditional economic and political organizations that used to characterize medicine; younger physicians faced with discounting, contracting, and networks for care, however, may no longer identify with the more traditional perspectives.

All the increasingly complex problems of administering a practice must be dealt with in solo practice unless a professional manager is hired. Furthermore, competitive pressures in the health care industry are leading many practitioners to question the feasibility and desirability of going it alone. Many solo practitioners are now affiliated with larger entities such as independent practice associations, practice management companies, and other organizations. Thus, solo practice offers distinct opportunities and has philosophical and emotional appeal but is far from devoid of problems and constraints, especially in light of the realities of medical practice today.

Group Practice

Office-based practice includes, in addition to solo practice, group practice. This form of practice has been growing in popularity in recent years, especially as the increasing pressures of practice have led many providers to seek alternative settings in which to work.

Group practice is an affiliation of three or more providers, usually physicians, who share income, expenses, facilities, equipment, medical records, and support personnel in the provision of services through a formal, legally constituted organization. The definition of group practice, developed by the American Medical Association and the Medical Group Management Association, is three or more physicians formally organized to provide medical care, consultation, diagnosis, and/or treatment through the joint use of equipment and personnel, and with income from medical practice distributed in accordance with methods previously determined by members of the group. Although definitions of a group practice vary somewhat, the essential element is formal sharing of resources and income.

History of Group Practice

Some of the earliest group practices in the United States were started by companies that needed to provide care to employees in rural sites where medical care was unobtainable. For example, the Northern Pacific Railroad organized a practice in 1883 to provide care to employees building the transcontinental railroad. This industrial clinic was one of a number of such clinics founded in the nineteenth century.

Even more significant, however, was the establishment of the Mayo Clinic in Rochester, Minnesota—the first successful nonindustrial group practice. The Mayo Clinic, originally organized as a single-specialty group practice in 1887 and later broadened into a multispecialty group, demonstrated that group practice was feasible in the private sector. The Mayo Clinic also represented a reputable model for group practice in a national atmosphere of fierce independence where group practice was viewed with skepticism and distrust. By the early 1930s, there were about 150 medical groups throughout the country, many of which were located in the Midwest (Rorem, 1931). Most included or were started by someone who had practiced or trained at the Mayo Clinic.

In 1932, the Committee on the Costs of Medical Care was established to assess health care needs for the nation. It issued a report that suggested a major role for group practice in the provision of medical care. The committee recommended that these groups be associated with hospitals to provide comprehensive care and that there be prepayment for all services. The report strongly supported the concept of regionalization that eventually gained wide recognition in the establishment of the British National Health Service, our own military health care systems, and other national models of organized health service systems.

Other constituencies, including some unions, also developed group practices. After World War II, a number of pioneering groups were established. In New York City, the Health Insurance Plan of New York was organized to provide prepaid medical care to the employees of the city—an idea promoted by Mayor Fiorello LaGuardia. On the West Coast, the Kaiser Foundation Health Plan was established to provide health care to employees of Kaiser Industries; Kaiser is an affiliation of plans and providers that is now serving millions of Americans across the nation. In Seattle, a revolutionary development was the establishment of the Group Health Cooperative of Puget Sound, a consumer-owned cooperative prepaid group practice. It was founded by progressive individuals who were dissatisfied with the private medical care available to them in the late 1940s.

Developments in medical practice also spurred the group practice movement. Perhaps most notable was the increasing specialization of medicine and the rapid expansion of technology. This increasing sophistication meant that no individual practitioner could provide all the expertise that patients would require. It also meant that more complex and expensive facilities, equipment, and personnel were needed to care for patients. Group practice provided a formal structure for sharing these costs among providers. Many people believed that resources would be used more efficiently in groups. In addition, multispecialty groups, encompassing more than one specialty, could provide patients with more of their health care under one roof and, hence, reduce problems of physical access to care and coordination of services.

Group practice was also thought to promote higher quality care. Most of the different specialists that a person required would be practicing together and would thus have the opportunity to discuss patient problems among themselves, share a common medical record, and be more able to ensure the quality and continuity of care. Therefore, group practice was viewed by many as being advantageous for the physician—offering opportunities such as easily developed referral arrangements, sharing of after-hours coverage, greater flexibility in working hours, and less financial risk—while also benefiting the patient.

Opposition to group practice occurred mostly for political and philosophical reasons. The American Medical Association and local medical societies have, at times, opposed group practice. Many early group practices had difficulties when physicians were denied admitting privileges in local hospitals. Community-based specialists sometimes refused to treat patients referred by group-practice physicians. In more recent years, however, opposition to group practice has disappeared, and restrictive laws no longer exist. The need to form affiliations for contracting under reimbursement programs and for achieving efficiencies in organizing health services more generally has also driven the growth of group practice.

The American Medical Association has conducted surveys of physician-oriented medical group practices in the United States on a periodic basis (Havlicek, 1999). The dramatic increase in popularity of practices is reflected in Table 7.8. The number of reporting group practices has more than doubled since 1975. There are more than 20,000 group practices in the United States, the majority of which are single-specialty groups. Even more dramatic is the growth in the number of physicians in a group-

practice setting. The average size of all group practices in the United States is about nine physicians. Most group practices are professional corporations or partnerships. Managed care has led to group practices in contracting arrangements such as the independent practice associations (IPAs).

Group practices may be formed by, or affiliated with, larger organizations such as hospitals or health systems. The larger entity may provide capital, management services, patient flows, and contracting assistance to the smaller group. Groups may be affiliated with one another through various mechanisms that may provide management services and contracting potential for solo and smaller group practitioners while preserving a degree of independence for these practitioners. A group practice without walls has been another avenue utilized to affiliate practitioners. In essence, practices are merged but are able to maintain their existing locations with administrative services carried out in a central office or through a contract with a management services organization. There are for-profit management companies and some not-for-profit entities providing these services to physician groups and, in some instances, actually purchasing groups outright, as well. In the past, some of these companies collapsed due to overpaying for groups and other financial miscues.

A critical assessment of group practice yields distinct advantages and disadvantages for both patients and providers as compared to other modalities for providing ambulatory services. Some of these are summarized in Table 7.9. Some of the topics listed under patient or provider perspectives could readily pertain to both.

Advantages of Group Practice

The advantages of group practice from the perspective of the provider include shared operation of the practice, joint ownership of facilities and equipment, centralized administrative functions, and, in larger groups, a professional manager. The professional manager can provide expertise in areas often lacking among the providers such as billing, personnel management, patient scheduling, ordering of supplies, negotiating, and contracting.

Table 7.8. Number of Medical Groups and Number of Physicians in Group Practice, United States, Selected Years

Year	Total Number of Groups	Number of Physician Positions in Group Practice
1969	6,371	40,093
1975	8,488	66,842
1980	10,762	88,290
1984	15,186	139,127
1988	16,495	155,628
1991	16,576	184,358
1996	19,820	206,557
2006 (est.)	25,000	300,000

Adapted from *Medical Groups in the U.S., 1999 Edition. A Survey of Practice Considerations* by P. L. Havlicek, 1999, Chicago: American Medical Association.

Table 7.9. Some Advantages and Disadvantages of Group Practice

Advantages	Disadvantages
From perspective of the provider	
Availability of professional manager	Less individual freedom
Organizational responsibility for patient	Possible excessive use of specialists
Less physician administrative time	Fewer outside consultants
Shared capital expense	Possible reduced identity with patient and community
Shared financial risk	Group rather than individual decision making
Improved contracting and negotiating ability	Sharing of all problems
Better coverage and shared on-call shifts	Necessity of working with others
More flexible working hours	Less individual incentive and more orientation toward security
More peer interaction	Income limitations
Increased access to specialists	Income distribution arguments
Broader array of ancillary services	
Stable income for providers	
No direct financial concerns with patient	
Lower initial investment	
More time for continuing education	
More flexible vacation time	
Generally excellent benefits	
Possible efficiencies of scale	
Use of nonphysician practitioners	
From perspective of the patient	
Care under one roof	Possible lessening of provider-patient relationship
Availability of specialists, laboratories, and so on	Possible overuse of ancillary services
Improved coverage and emergency care	Possible high provider turnover
Central location of medical and administrative records	Heavy patient loads and possible increase in waiting time
Simplified referrals	Less provider incentive for care
Peer interaction among providers	More bureaucracy
Better administration of group	
Possible promotion of efficiency in patient care	

Financially, the group relieves the provider of the heavy initial investment often required to establish a practice. In most groups, however, co-ownership requires that new members buy into the group through the purchase of a share of the group's capital assets over a period of time. Rather than having to independently absorb the ups and downs of a practice, as solo practitioners do, those involved in a group practice share income and expenses within the group, allowing for moderation of those fluctuations experienced in individual practices.

The participation of physicians in group practice has also a significant advantage in facilitating the development of arrangements for contracting and negotiating. The group can support increased levels of participation, has a knowledgeable group-practice administrator to manage the contracts, and can respond to the market with a wider range of services. Having a professional manager to negotiate on behalf of the group further enhances the relative attractiveness of group practice, particularly for physicians who lack experience in interpreting and negotiating contracts.

Patient-care responsibilities are also shared in group practice. This sharing results in greater flexibility of working hours for the provider, as well as more time for vacation and continuing education, without sacrificing the quality of care for the patient. For example, providers cover for each other during vacations and after normal working hours. Although most practitioners in solo practice arrange for patient-care coverage, the continuity of care and the extent of coverage are probably greater in group practice, as patients' medical records and the full resources of the group are always available, even if specific providers are not working.

The use of certain personnel may be more advantageous in group than solo practice. Receptionists, medical records and information systems specialists, laboratory and radiology technicians, and nurses may be used more efficiently and in the specialized areas of their training in many medium- and larger-sized groups. In addition, there is some question about whether any savings that are achieved will be returned to payors or simply represent higher incomes for providers.

The effect of groups on patient care, especially on the quality of care, is an important issue. Sharing of medical records, computer-assisted quality assurance, peer interaction, easy referrals and consultations with specialists, more sophisticated and accessible ancillary services, and more skilled and diversified support personnel are all arguments suggested in support of higher-quality care in group practice. For the patient, the group offers a wide range of services under one roof so that travel between providers is reduced and access increased. A unified computerized medical record can contribute to continuity of care and less duplication in diagnosis and treatment. Managed-care contracts in groups can be more comprehensive and promote integrated care.

Group practices usually offer more accessible care after normal working hours. Some groups also

offer emergency services through their own emergency rooms or clinics. Groups with a broader community perspective may even be involved in programs such as school health services and community immunization efforts, and the use of a professional manager should benefit the patient through more efficient scheduling and patient flow and improved overall management of the practice.

There are also some distinct disadvantages to group practice for providers, patients, and communities. From the perspective of the provider, practicing in a group implies less individual freedom, with a variety of restrictions imposed through the sharing of a practice. Managed-care contracts may require a higher level of monitoring of clinical care as well. In addition to reduced freedom, group practice entails sharing responsibilities and problems with others. The interpersonal requirements for working out these responsibilities may not appeal to all practitioners. Older individuals who have been working in solo practice may especially be unlikely to adapt readily to group practice.

The financial advantages for group practice are a trade-off against some restrictions on income generation and the necessity of complying with the group's income distribution and practice pattern requirements. Thus, there is often more security and fewer risks, but also less incentive and reward for individual initiative and production.

INSTITUTIONALLY BASED AMBULATORY SERVICES

In addition to solo and group practice in the traditional private sector, many institutions have expanded their involvement in ambulatory care. These institutionally based settings, especially those associated with hospitals, are discussed next.

The hospital has evolved from an institution for poor people who could not be cared for at home to a provider of a full range of health services from primary to tertiary care. As technological advances have brought more services into the hospital and expanded the scope of care provided, the hospital has assumed an especially important role in the provision of highly complex health services. At the same time, an increasing number of people have sought primary care from hospitals, sometimes as a result of the lack of access to other sources of care. Most hospitals now operate outpatient services.

Traditional hospital outpatient services have been provided in clinics and emergency rooms. In many hospitals, clinics used to have second-class status as compared to complex and expensive inpatient services. However, as hospitals have recognized the important role of primary care, especially in managed-care contracting and are seeking to expand the base of patients who are potential users of inpatient and ancillary services, more attention has been directed toward improving clinic operations and services.

Hospital clinics include both primary care and specialty clinics. Many hospitals differentiate between clinics for walk-in patients without appointments and those for scheduled visits. Triage is an important function of hospital clinics and emergency services. Specialty clinics are usually organized by department and provide services such as ophthalmology, neurology, and allergy care. In teaching hospitals, and especially academic medical centers, clinics serve as important settings in which house staff members provide ongoing care to patients and follow-up after hospitalization. Clinics also provide an opportunity to expose medical students and house staff to ambulatory care services in order to complement the traditionally more extensive experience with inpatient care.

Many hospital primary-care clinics evolved from an orientation of service to the poor and were staffed by physicians who served without reimbursement in exchange for staff privileges. The level of commitment to the patient under such circumstances was—not surprisingly—less than desirable. Many hospitals now employ physicians and other practitioners as full-time clinic staff. Some hospitals have established primary-care group practices to com-

plement other outpatient services and to assume the burden of providing primary care to patients who seek most of their care from the hospital or as a component of a vertically integrated health care delivery system. Hospitals are also increasingly employing hospitalists and intensivists physicians who are stationed at a hospital full time to care for inpatient and sometimes critical clients. Hospitals with ambulatory care resources can negotiate contracts for providing a wide range of both inpatient and outpatient services. Enhanced preparation for coping with major community emergencies such as terrorism and natural disasters is another expanded function of hospital-based ambulatory care.

Ambulatory Surgery Centers

A further innovation in hospital-based care has been the development of ambulatory surgery centers. Originating in hospitals in Washington, D.C., Los Angeles, and elsewhere, these organized hospital units provide one-day surgical care. Patients are usually screened for acceptability by their personal surgeons and then report at an assigned date and time for surgery. The surgeon is supported by the unit's facilities, equipment, and personnel, and the patient is discharged 1 to 3 hours after surgery when recovery from anesthesia is sufficiently complete.

In the early 1970s, freestanding ambulatory surgery centers were opened; one of the first was in Phoenix, Arizona. These facilities are independent of hospitals and usually provide a full range of services for the types of surgery that can be performed on an outpatient basis. Community surgeons are granted operating privileges and can perform surgery in these facilities when the patient agrees and when there are no medical contraindications.

Other facilities are also used for ambulatory or outpatient surgery. Many physicians informally performed surgery in their offices, although this practice has declined in some specialties as a result of malpractice concerns and the increasing availability of better-equipped and -staffed alternative facilities. Some specialties, such as oral surgery, plastic surgery, and ophthalmology extensively use formal office-based surgical facilities.

Emergency Medical Services

The emergency room, like other hospital departments, has undergone transformation in recent years. The emergency room has expanded in the range of services offered and in complexity. Preparation for possible terrorist attacks and for discussion has also increased. An especially important long-term trend has been the increasing use of the emergency room for primary care. Because the emergency room requires sophisticated facilities and highly trained personnel and must be accessible 24 hours a day, costs are high and services are not designed for nonurgent care. To reduce the burden on the emergency room and to meet patient need more effectively, many hospitals treat patients on a triage basis. In this process, often performed by a nurse, the patient's health care needs are determined and the patient is referred to a more appropriate source of care within the hospital.

Emergency medical services have also been increasingly integrated with other community resources. Included are drug and alcohol treatment programs, mental health centers, and voluntary agencies. Most major urban centers have developed formal emergency medical systems that incorporate hospital emergency rooms as well as transportation (ambulance and possibly aircraft) and communication systems (landline and cell phones).

GOVERNMENT PROGRAMS

In addition to private-sector and institutionally initiated efforts, government programs have been used to increase the availability of health care resources in many communities. These programs have adapted some of the concepts of private institutional settings, especially those of group practice.

Neighborhood health centers were funded starting in 1965. Originally intended to serve approximately 25 million people, this federal program never reached its initial objectives. The program was designed to provide primary medical care with a family orientation. It was targeted for population groups in need of services, as reflected by such indicators as disease prevalence and income level. At the same time, the centers were intended to employ people from the communities they served in positions that would offer opportunities for training and advancement.

Although these health centers were originally intended to serve the poor, changes in federal policy that encouraged them to collect fees from patients and from third-party insurers have broadened the socioeconomic mixture of patients obtaining care. A related category of provider, the free clinic, evolved from a strong social commitment but has had to face similar financial realities. In some communities, the combination of former free clinics, neighborhood health centers, public agency clinics, and some hospital clinics and groups now forms an informal safety net of providers for individuals who lack private insurance or access to other sources of care, or who simply need care from an available, sympathetic provider.

Other community health centers that have been funded by the federal government include migrant health centers serving transient farm workers in agricultural areas and rural health centers. The National Health Service Corps has supported practitioners who were placed in urban and rural areas with shortages of medical resources. The Community Mental Health Center program was established to provide ambulatory mental health services in underserved areas.

The federal government directly operates many health facilities. The Veterans Administration includes the largest health services system under a unified management structure in the United States. The Indian Health Service is charged with ensuring access to medical care on Indian reservations and in certain other locations.

NONINSTITUTIONAL AND PUBLIC HEALTH SERVICES

As noted in the introduction to this chapter, there are many ways in which ambulatory and community health services are provided. Home health services are provided by visiting nurse associations, proprietary companies, some hospitals (especially those in vertically integrated systems), public health departments, and other agencies. These services allow people to remain in their homes and yet receive essential health services, thereby reducing costs and increasing the quality of life for many.

Rural health care has required unique and innovative solutions in many communities, especially in the absence of adequate supplies of physicians and facilities. In rural Alaska, many towns are served by physicians and other professionals who regularly fly in to treat patients. Satellites and the Internet are used to facilitate communications with subspecialists in urban medical centers.

Other community health services not discussed in detail here include, but are not limited to, school health services; prison health services; vision care; dental care provided by solo, group, and institutionally based practitioners; foot care from podiatrists; and drug dispensing from pharmacists, who often also extensively advise and educate consumers—a mandate now under many state laws. Voluntary agencies also provide health care services such as cancer screening clinics and health education. Finally, many indigenous health practitioners offer their services in this country and abroad. These practitioners include chiropractors, "medicine men," naturopaths, and others. The supportive and sometimes curative role of these individuals is often underestimated.

THE ROLE OF AMBULATORY SERVICES

Ambulatory care services, and particularly physician-related care, provide a service distribution network for most noninstitutional health care services. How that network distributes services throughout the community and to various population groups is of critical importance to ensuring access and availability of services in the community. In many contexts, the distribution network serves as the delivery vehicle for specific insurance products, particularly under managed-care plans. This distribution system is typically tied into other related care such as inpatient and laboratory services.

The distribution network is critical to ensuring the availability of services for at-risk population groups such as traditionally underserved minority populations, the poor, and individuals with unique needs such as pregnant women, children, and the elderly. Distribution networks must be energized by appropriate management structures and by the availability of adequate funding to assure that they deliver needed care. These services may be funded, or provided directly, by government programs for certain populations.

The distribution network is further defined by the composition of primary and specialty providers and services, supportive technology such as imaging capacity and laboratory services, and other needed health care resources. The management, monitoring, and evaluation of these distribution networks is typically the principle function of health care managers in delivery organizations, increasingly influenced by contractual demands from insurers, employers, and other payors and influenced by patient expectations and attitudes.

The delivery network can be evaluated by measures of effectiveness and efficiency, quality of care, and services provided. The satisfaction of payors, patients, and providers is also integral to assessing the success of the networks and delivery mechanisms.

Many complex factors affect the success of delivery systems in providing the care needed by populations. Patient, provider, payor, and system issues must be carefully weighed in assessing how all services are delivered to the client population and potential areas for improving this effort. For example, patients need the appropriate mix of primary care and specialty services, access to appropriate technology, and, at the same time, need to be treated ethically, humanely, and in a manner that promotes patient compliance and satisfaction.

Patients are the clients and in a typical retail setting would be respected as such. In the health care system, provider organizations and individual professionals do not always adapt to the service model embodied by the retail sector of the economy. Overall, however, the nation's health care system has greatly improved its customer perspective during the past couple of decades. The interjection of third-party payors into the transaction process leads some to adopt the philosophy that the payor rather than the patient is the true customer, leading to distortions in the patient-provider relationship. This is a particularly significant problem when the payor is a government program, especially Medicaid or other safety net programs. It is imperative for the nation's health care delivery network to view each patient as a valued customer regardless of source of payment, racial or ethnic group, age, or other intervening characteristic.

The management of these complex enterprises requires sophisticated business skills and the availability of adequate information. Increasingly sophisticated management practices and the development of state-of-the-art management information systems are now enhancing the capability of health services administrators to run the health care system and its component organizations. Medical practices have generally not reached the level of sophistication seen in the institutional setting except that many larger groups have significant resources available for sophisticated management capabilities.

MANAGING A MEDICAL PRACTICE

This section of the chapter is designed to convey the flavor of managing medical practices in the highly competitive environment within which the nation's health care system operates today. The professional manager in the ambulatory care arena must be a jack-of-all-trades with extensive skill capabilities in a variety of technical areas (Keagy & Thomas, 2004).

The Medical Group Management Association, the national organization of group-practice administrators, has outlined the technical areas of professional knowledge that convey the broad array of expertise and skills required in this arena today. These areas include financial management, human resource management, planning and marketing, information systems, risk management, governance and organizational dynamics, business and clinical operations, and professional responsibility. Each of these skill and expertise domains encompasses a broad array of topics and specific technical capabilities.

Today's manager must be knowledgeable and adept at a huge range of activities from strategic planning to contract negotiations to the expanse of personnel management. In addition, professional managers in this arena, unlike many other institutional settings, typically deal with not only strategic concepts and issues, but also the minutia of day-to-day management. Interacting with various constituencies including payors, physicians and other providers, and patients is a daily requirement.

Administrators in ambulatory care are now expected to provide organizational leadership and direction to a much greater extent than in the past. Strategic planning, budgeting, financial decision making, physician and staff recruitment, retention, evaluation, cash-flow analysis, capital expense planning, development and application of information systems for financial reporting, quality evaluation, and legal compliance are other examples of the broad spectrum of responsibilities and duties.

Managed-care contracts, the lifeblood of many medical practices today, have become increasingly complex and demanding. Administrators in many regions of the country must negotiate sophisticated contractual arrangements with various managed-care payors. These contracts often contain stipulations with regard to practice patterns, fee discounts, reporting requirements, quality assessment and credentialing, dispute resolution through arbitration, and many other complex provisions. Contracting with multiple payors, each with its own set of contract requirements, further complicates the administrative role. And, of course, many of the insurance provisions discussed elsewhere in this book apply to these contracts and are subject to interpretation and negotiation.

The increasing array of interdependencies between the ambulatory care arena and inpatient and other services must also be considered, particularly in contract arrangements where the group is assuming a broad array of risks. For example, groups that are moving to employ hospitalists will need to clarify work assignments for physicians serving in this role versus other members of the group and will have to coordinate care for patients who are in an inpatient setting being treated by the physicians within the group. The increased role of such quality and utilization-related mechanisms as utilization management, clinical protocols, disease management, and various contracting arrangements for selective subspecialty contracts must all be considered as well.

PROFESSIONAL PRACTICE ORGANIZATIONS

Medical practices can be organized from a variety of legal perspectives. Determination of the appropriate structure in an individual group will be determined by tax, organizational and governance, and

liability issues. Groups can be organized as for-profit or non-profit entities depending on ownership considerations. For-profit entities can include traditional for-profit corporations, partnerships, or limited liability companies. In certain instances, the physician practice and the operational and physical assets of the group may be organized separately, depending on state physician practice acts.

Compliance with a variety of state and federal laws, particularly regulations related to Medicare, Medicaid, and Health Insurance Portability and Accountability Act (HIPAA), as well as the Stark law provisions and various other practice parameters must also be considered in organizing and operating medical groups. Tax law is a further important consideration, particularly as it pertains to control over physician after-tax income and the ability to maximize, where appropriate, retirement plan funding. Tax-exempt practices must comply with a variety of federal and state legal and tax considerations as well and will have certain income tax and charitable donation advantages.

In most instances, physician compensation and other payment arrangements must be carefully designed to comply with federal and state laws, especially those related to Medicare fraud and abuse. Payments between groups and other organizations such as hospitals or ambulatory surgery centers and laboratories must be designed to strictly adhere to these regulations to avoid conflicts of interest and other illegal arrangements.

Physician practices can be organized as a component of physician-hospital relationships under various forms of vertical integration. Physicians practicing in these arrangements sell their practices to hospital entities as a means to access capital and clinical distribution networks. The hospital network then invests in computerized information systems, marketing, and managed-care contracting to utilize the distribution networks created as a mechanism for providing services to patients under managed-care contracts. However, under these arrangements, physicians lose control and are subject to clinical monitoring and accountability. The substantial capital investments required from hospital systems also sometimes result in unprofitable arrangements, particularly when managed-care contracts pressure payment levels. Managing hospitals and managing physician practices also requires vastly different skills and approaches that some hospital administrators lack awareness of.

Many other hospital-physician relationships have been developed or are currently under development. Joint ventures such as for imaging centers or other services that allow physician participation in economic product development with associated financial rewards are popular in some areas of the country. These arrangements can present a minefield with regard to compliance with federal and state regulations such as those mentioned previously.

A variety of other contractual relationships and organizational forms can be used to relate physician practices with other components of the health care system and to organize physician delivery systems themselves. As discussed elsewhere in this book, a number of these contractual arrangements form portions of managed-care systems. For example, independent practice associations, or IPAs, are a form of health maintenance organization utilizing community-based physician practices as contractual organizations to provide managed-care physician services. The IPA allows for independent physician practice while providing a mechanism to form a health maintenance organization and to offer a contracting approach to such organizations.

The physician-hospital organization, or PHO, is another arrangement based on contracts between hospitals and medical staffs that allow for a health care delivery and distribution system that integrates a range of health services. As with all other contractual relationships in the health care environment, there are numerous legal and regulatory issues associated with all of these arrangements. In addition, complex financial concerns are also faced by participants in these systems. Many of the newer forms of organizing ambulatory services have had difficulty in many parts of the country for a variety of reasons, some of which relate to financial, governance, and control factors.

Another organizational and contractual development in the industry, alluded to previously, relating physician practices to hospital organizations and systems has been the management services organization, or MSO, and the related physician practice management company, or PPMC. These organizations perform a management function organizing and managing services and may be a joint venture between physician practices and hospitals. Other forms of contractual relationships and management arrangements, such as physician-hospital organizations or PHOs and medical foundations, also exist in various locations throughout the country.

Especially complex are arrangements that may infer physician financial gain as a result of various incentive or contractual arrangements that could potentially be interpreted as violations of federal (Stark) Medicare law or other potentially prohibited situations. Particularly complex are arrangements that involve physician equity ownership in joint ventures or ancillary services and other arrangements that could represent a conflict of interest, potentially in violation of federal law. Physician practices need to be particularly careful in structuring arrangements such as physician payments for hospital administrative services, hospital or other entity reimbursement of practice expenses, physician pay for performance, quality of care, and productivity incentives, contracting-related bonuses and incentives, compensation schemes, and payments for participation in marketing and other auxiliary services.

Physician Practice Management

Medical practices are complex organisms that require an array of management skills. Among the most important of these skills is financial management.

Financial Management

Financial management of medical practices and especially larger physician practices requires corporate-style accounting and financial systems including, but not limited to, balance sheet and income and revenue statements, flow of funds analysis, capital budgeting for major expenditures, and cash management (Wolper, 2005). Monitoring and controlling the flow of funds within a practice is particularly important for providers involved in managed-care contractual arrangements, especially those involving capitation payments where budgeting and control of expenditures can be critical to profitability. The development of a business plan using financial models allows practices to determine in advance which services are appropriate to provide from a financial perspective. Overall control of financial parameters is a key function of the management staff.

Another critical concern in the area of financial management for most medical practices is taxation. Because most practices are for-profit entities, the taxes accrued at the practice or individual provider level can be an important determinant of the amount of profit taken home by the owners of the practice, typically physicians. Federal and some state tax changes since the mid-1980s have reduced the flexibility of many individuals and entities in controlling the amount of taxes paid. Therefore, it is important for medical groups to determine those areas of their operations that have a linkage to taxation. For example, where appropriate, tax advantaged corporate retirement plans may offer an unusual ability to reduce current taxation. The legal structure of the practices and many other complex considerations will impinge on the exact nature of such a plan.

Ultimately, as for any other business entity, increasing revenue and decreasing expenses is the key to profitability. For practices that are in a nonprofit or not-for-profit setting, these issues are still critical to ensuring financial viability and to generating excess revenues over expenses that can be invested into the practice. Controlling expenditures is often integrally tied to capital investment decisions and to personnel issues and staffing. Effective negotiation of managed-care contracts and, where appropriate, budgeting, especially for managed care and nonprofit entities, are also vital considerations.

Reimbursement and Other Issues

Another interesting aspect of practice management involves provider reimbursement issues, particularly those pertaining to physicians. Physician practices, and especially group practices, use a variety of models for distributing income to physicians who are, in many instances, the owners of the practice. Physician reimbursement and income distribution formulas can affect or, in turn, be affected by productivity, specialty, reputation, and many other factors. Physician reimbursement is generally designed to incentivize providers in a variety of ways depending on the ownership and nature of the practice.

Practices often will incentivize providers to promote productivity as measured by revenue generated or services provided. In some practices, physicians and other professional providers may be paid a straight salary although this is not typical. Salary plus incentive compensation based on such factors as productivity is more common, where the underlying salary is a guaranteed minimum income level. Some practices have quite complex reimbursement formulas considering such factors as specialty differentials, research activities, involvement in marketing, tenure in the group, hours worked, administrative duties assumed, and so forth. Compensation is a complex and typically proprietary issue that is the subject of considerable discussion and sometimes intense debate in many practices.

Sometimes reimbursement issues in multispecialty groups are a focal point for internal medicine and family practice specialists who argue that they bring in the patients, use the laboratory, and generate demand for other referral services. Surgeons, on the other hand, claim that they generate a greater percentage of total revenue and place less of a burden on some of the physical facilities and staff. Providers under managed-care contracts may value their ability to control utilization and costs, while providers under preferred provider plans and fee-for-service arrangements may argue that they bring in more revenue for their efforts. Blending the diversity of providers, patient payment sources, and services offered in a practice and implementing a reimbursement structure that appropriately incentivizes the providers while ensuring good quality care, is a continuing struggle in the ambulatory care arena.

Other complex responsibilities for managers in medical practices include a broad range of issues related to human resources. Personnel costs represent the largest single expenditure in many medical settings and managing that resource is extremely important to the financial viability of a practice. In addition, numerous and complex federal and state regulations impinge on employment in any setting. Maintaining appropriate personnel, recruiting, hiring, evaluation, promotion, and termination policies and procedures requires an increasingly high level of sophistication. Individuals working within a medical practice typically experience workplace stress and require sensitive supervision. Employee compensation and incentives are other areas of complexity as well.

No practice would be successful without solid leadership by both the practice manager and the medical staff. Practice management requires rallying all the employees around the goals and objectives of the practice and constantly assuring a high level of enthusiasm, consumer sensitivity, awareness of privacy, and many other considerations on the part of the employees. Federal law now requires compliance with a variety of rules and regulations pertaining to patient privacy and all payors now expect practices to comply with contractual agreements and claims reimbursement procedures.

A revolution in management of medical practices is under way with the implementation of new information systems technology. The holy grail of the application of computer systems in health care practices is the computerized medical record. Many larger and some medium- and smaller-sized practices are in the process of implementing a partially or completely automated computerized medical record. Although the technology has taken an unusually long time to be developed and prepared for implementation, the hardware and software capability for automated medical records now appears to be available.

Automated medical records allow for many advances in managing clinical care and the practices themselves. By capturing the details of interactions between patients and health care providers in an increasingly cost-effective manner, computerized medical records are paving the way for a revolution in health care management and quality assurance.

Automated medical records are also being implemented with associated technologies such as computerized drug and laboratory test ordering. Increasingly, integrated components of information technologies not only allow for such valuable quality checks as drug interactions but also provide for a more comprehensive collection of clinical and managerial data overall.

The traditional applications of automated information technologies have long included numerous administrative functions including determination of eligibility under insurance plans, billing (including credit and collections), insurance billing, appointment scheduling, and physician and other resource monitoring. The integration of computerized medical records into legacy systems has tremendous implications for much more comprehensive and interaction-specific tracking of patient resource use, quality assessment, referral and follow-up tracking, and other more advanced applications. Among other applications for computerized medical records are the use of patient-specific clinical protocols and guidelines and other clinical decision support systems; tracking patients to ensure appropriateness of care and to reduce duplication of services; automated quality reporting; advanced decision support information for management of practices, including provider-specific utilization data, revenue and expense accounting, and other management relevant information.

Of considerable concern in the application of many of these automated and computerized systems is patient privacy. Federal privacy laws, particularly under recently implemented requirements, complicate the collection, dissemination, and analysis of information where patient identifiers are still attached and available. In addition, interchange of data among providers, provider organizations, insurers, and other entities requires sophisticated protection for assuring patient privacy.

SUMMARY

Ultimately, the costs and quality of health care services are directly related to the success of the system's management. In ambulatory care, where resources are often stretched thin, this concept is even more valid. The ability to provide more and better care to more people will depend on improved management, integrated information systems, more efficient services, and a commitment to enhancing the operations side of delivery organizations. This is no small task and is the challenge for the future in ambulatory and community health care.

REVIEW QUESTIONS

1. What services are incorporated within ambulatory care services?
2. Describe the evolution of ambulatory care in terms or its role in the operation and rationalization of the health care system.
3. How has the organization of ambulatory care been changed by the development and growth of managed care?
4. Describe the most prominent settings for ambulatory practice in the United States.
5. Describe the general types of institutionally based ambulatory health care services.
6. What managerial attributes enhance ambulatory care organizations?
7. Describe the challenges ambulatory care will encounter in the future and its role in the U.S. health care system.

REFERENCES & ADDITIONAL READINGS

Adams, P. F., Dey, A. N., & Vickerie, J. L. (2007). *Summary health statistics for the U.S. population: National Health Interview Survey, 2005.* National Center for Health Statistics. Vital Health Stat. 10(233). Washington, DC: U.S. Government Printing Office.

Havlicek, P. L. (1999). *Medical groups in the U.S., 1999 edition. A survey of practice characteristics.* Chicago: American Medical Association.

Hing E., Cherry D. K., & Woodwell, D. A. (2006). *National ambulatory medical care survey: 2004 summary. Advance data from vital and health statistics.* No. 374. Hyattsville, MD: National Center for Health Statistics.

Keagy, B. A., & Thomas, M. S. (Eds.). (2004). *Essentials of physician practice management.* San Francisco: Jossey-Bass.

Rorem, R. (1931). *Private group clinics.* Chicago: University of Chicago Press.

United Kingdom Ministry of Health. (1920). *Dawson report, interim report on the future provision of medical and allied services.* London: His Majesty's Stationery Office.

Wolper, L. F. (2005). *Physician practice management. Essential operational and financial knowledge.* Sudbury, MA: Jones and Bartlett.

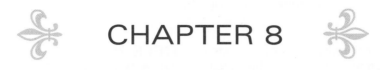

CHAPTER 8

Hospitals and Health Systems

Stephen J. Williams and Paul R. Torrens

CHAPTER TOPICS

- History of the Hospital
- The Scope of the Industry
- Structure of Hospitals and Health Systems
- Hospital Organization
- The Hospital and Medical Staff
- Key Issues Facing the Hospital Industry

LEARNING OBJECTIVES

Upon completing this chapter, the reader should be able to

1. Understand the role of the hospital in today's health care system.
2. Appreciate the historical trends that have shaped the hospital industry.
3. Understand the types of hospitals, ownership patterns, and differentiating characteristics of various hospitals.
4. Comprehend the development of health systems and the role of hospitals in such systems.
5. Follow the impact of competitive pressures and other developments on the structure and operation of hospitals and health systems.
6. Understand the internal organizational structure of hospitals.

The hospital's role in the nation's health care system has changed dramatically over the years. The hospital originated as an institution for the poor, offering little in the way of therapy, and then evolved into the center of the system and the primary technology focus of health care. Now the hospital is a provider of highly specialized services and the hub of an assortment of other activities. The traditional independence of each hospital has been dramatically altered by horizontal and vertical integration within the health care system such that today few hospitals are truly freestanding entities. The technology to manage hospitals has likewise changed with an information systems focus and the application of complex parameters of performance measurement.

Expectations of consumers, providers, and payers have also changed dramatically over the years with the anticipation of more effective interventions at more efficient and competitive pricing. Finally, as has always been the case in the past, the hospital industry continues to face immense challenges, opportunities, and expectations for the future.

The hospital has also changed from an island of care to an institutional octopus, with tentacles springing out throughout the community, affiliating with other institutions and providers, and providing outreach services for consumers. On the inpatient side, hospitals are increasingly providing the most complex of care to the most critically ill patients. On the outpatient side, most hospitals are broadening the array of services that they offer to better compete.

Hospitals face the challenges of sick and dying patients, demanding payers, government officials seeking accountability, physicians demanding the availability of the latest equipment and support, and many other crosscurrents. Some hospitals are for-profit entities, while others are not-for-profit. Some hospitals are highly specialized while others offer a broad range of services. Hospitals are often major employers in their communities and many provide the bulk of indigent care for low-income and disenfranchised citizens. Through it all, the backbone of hospital management has increasingly adopted the managerial principles of commercial industry, seeking to provide services in an efficient, but cost-effective manner, and to offer competitive pricing to third-party and governmental payers. The challenges of this industry are immense and unlikely to recede in the decades that follow.

HISTORY OF THE HOSPITAL

Although the hospital today is in the forefront of technology and clinical medicine, the history of the nation's hospitals actually began as facilities for housing the poor and the ill. These institutional warehouses for human suffering were the almshouses, the pest houses, the poor houses, and the workhouses that sheltered the homeless, the poor, the mentally ill, those with serious degenerative diseases, and others for whom there was little to offer in the era before modern medicine. Isolation of individuals during epidemics of cholera and typhoid, among other diseases, also led to the utilization of these institutions. Little medical knowledge was available and few individuals received any significant treatment.

The middle class avoided these institutions and received their care at home. Not until the 1700s and 1800s did hospitals emerge with a mission of providing some form of clinical medical care. Many of these early hospitals were supported by philanthropic efforts and religious organizations. Also during this period, many public hospitals were established in various cities to provide for the social needs of local populations, laying the groundwork for our modern acceptance of local government as the provider of last resort.

Finally, by the early 1900s, with the introduction of scientific method in medical practice and the recognition that hospitals and clinical medicine must adhere to a stricter formulation of practice focused on scientific discovery, was the era of the truly modern hospital established.

Throughout the twentieth century, the escalating advance of knowledge accelerated the focus of the hospital as a center for medical technology. After World War II, the hospital's role as a center of technology and innovation became firmly established. At this point, the practice of medicine itself was increasingly dependent on scientifically valid knowledge and training. Finally, over the past 30 years the degree of rigor of clinical practice and the scope of scientific knowledge has escalated greatly, and the hospital has become a center of high standards, scientific applications, and advanced technological capability.

At the same time, the increasing shift of services to an ambulatory care arena facilitated by technological advancement itself has left the hospital with an ever-more complex base of patient care, higher acuity, and higher costs. In addition, pressure from payers, as noted previously, has escalated greatly as has the expectation of providers and consumers alike. Industry consolidation, vertical and horizontal integration, public policy concerns, and quality assessment and assurance have placed the operation of the nation's hospitals under tremendous scrutiny. Yet, through it all, the nation's hospitals have risen to the challenge of providing superlative care overall in a high-intensity, stressful atmosphere that has significantly contributed to our improved health status and well-being. This is a remarkable achievement in light of countervailing financial and political pressures that have always buffeted the hospital industry. We owe a great debt of gratitude to the nation's hospitals and to those dedicated individuals who work within these institutional walls for achieving so much in an environment that started as a warehouse for the poor and sick, left to die without care and concern.

THE SCOPE OF THE INDUSTRY

Although the hospital industry has seen its share of the nation's health care dollar decline somewhat, hospital systems are still immense segments of the industry and of our nation's economy. (See Table 8.1.)

Table 8.1. Hospital Expenditures by Source of Funds: United States, Selected Years

Source of Funds	1960	1990	2003
	Amount in billions		
Hospital care expenditures	$9.2	$253.9	$515.9
	Percent Distribution		
All sources of funds	100.0	100.0	100.0
Out-of-pocket payments	20.8	4.4	3.2
Private health insurance	35.8	38.3	34.4
Other private funds	1.2	4.1	4.1
Government	42.2	53.2	58.3
Medicaid	—	10.9	16.9
Medicare	—	26.7	30.3

In 2003, the hospital industry alone accounted for more than $500 billion of expenditures. In 1960, the industry counted for only $9.2 billion of economic activity annually.

The growth of private health insurance and government entitlement programs, particularly Medicare, has shifted the burden of paying for hospital care to third parties. In 1960, more than 20 percent of the hospital bill was paid by people out of their own pockets; by 2003, this percentage had dropped to 3.2 percent. Private health insurance now accounts for a little more than one-third of all hospital expenditures while government programs account for nearly 60 percent. Medicare alone counts for nearly a third of all hospital expenditures; in many facilities the Medicare program pays about half the bill overall. Certainly, for the nation's seniors, Medicare is a critical source of support for paying for the enormous costs of hospitalization.

The number of hospitals in the United States has decreased dramatically. Table 8.2 illustrates this decline with the total number of hospital in 1975 at 7,156 dropping by 2003 to 5,764. A small number of the nation's hospitals are owned and operated by the federal government. These include the Veteran's Administration Hospitals and military facilities. The vast majority of hospitals are nonfederal and are nonprofit, for-profit, or owned by state and local governments. The information in this table

Table 8.2. Hospital and Beds by Ownership and Hospital Size: United States, Selected Years

Type of Ownership and Size of Hospital	1975	1995	2003
Hospitals		Number	
All hospitals	7,156	6,291	5,764
Federal	382	299	239
Nonfederal	6,774	5,992	5,525
Community	5,875	5,194	4,895
Nonprofit	3,339	3,092	2,984
For profit	775	752	790
State-local government	1,761	1,350	1,121
Bed size			
6–24 beds	299	278	327
25–49 beds	1,155	922	965
50–99 beds	1,481	1,139	1,031
100–199 beds	1,363	1,324	1,168
200–299 beds	678	718	624
300–399 beds	378	354	349
400–499 beds	230	195	172
500 beds or more	291	264	256

reflects hospital ownership, and it should be noted that some hospitals, while owned by one type of entity, may be operated under contract by another entity, such as a hospital management company.

The largest grouping of hospitals in the nation are nonprofit community hospitals. Although their numbers have declined overall, they remain the primary source of hospital care for most Americans. These hospitals are owned by nonprofit entities, although they are sometimes operated under contract by for-profit or other nonprofit corporations that specialize in managing hospitals and health systems.

Nonprofit entities, including hospitals, function under special provisions of corporation law in each state, and under federal and state tax provisions that recognize their community service function. The nation has approximately 1 million nonprofit entities of various sorts and hospitals have long been a traditional service provider in the nonprofit sector.

Nonprofit entities serve a community service and have special recognition under the law due to their role in our society. Nonprofit entities do not have owners and are governed by a community-based board that has ultimate authority for operation of the entity. Nonprofit entities are generally exempt from most taxes at the federal, state, and local levels including income and property taxes. Many nonprofit entities have tax exempt status under Section 501C(3) of the federal tax code, allowing individuals to make potentially tax deductible donations to these organizations. Nonprofit entities are able to raise funds through donations, retained earnings, and debt obligations, often on favorable terms.

Nonprofit entities may be "sponsored" by various types of organizations. Many hospitals have traditions of religious sponsorship. However, they are not owned by such sponsors. Nonprofit entities may also affiliate with each other through various organizational arrangements. Most nonprofit hospitals operate in a manner similar to other types of hospitals by employing modern management techniques, sophisticated information systems, and other principles of twenty-first-century management. Non-profit entities are generally expected to provide some indigent care and serve the community in a variety of ways as well.

A much smaller percentage of the nation's hospitals are operated as for-profit businesses. For-profit entities have owners and issue stock to those owners to reflect their equity position. For-profit entities, including hospitals, may be publicly or privately held. Publicly held for-profit entities have stock that is available for purchase by anyone, typically through the nation's various stock exchanges. A variety of accountability and registration rules and regulations affect publicly owned for-profit entities, generally administered by the Securities and Exchange Commission at the federal level and similar entities at the state level. Privately held for-profit entities also issue stock, but that stock is not available to the general public for purchase. Accountability and other regulatory oversight are much less for privately held entities.

For-profit hospitals may be independent and historically in this country and throughout the world today many for-profit hospitals have been owned by the physicians who practiced in them. Today, however, due to the tremendous capital costs of building, maintaining, and operating a hospital, most hospitals in the United States that are for profit are part of large multihospital chains, most of which are publicly traded. For-profit hospitals are not just accountable to the community but must also provide a return on investment to the shareholders; therefore they expect to generate a profit to pay a return to the equity investors for their capital. For-profit hospital companies may also manage not-for-profit and governmental hospitals as a separate line of business.

The third category of ownership in Table 8.2 is state and local government hospitals. These are hospitals that are owned by state or local governments, but again, may be managed under contract by other entities, either for-profit or not-for-profit management companies. Many local government hospitals are owned by counties or other local government units. They are often the providers of last resort, bearing the burden of indigent care in their communities.

In the western United States, hospital districts were created much like water districts to provide infrastructure for communities as populations moved West. These local taxing districts were responsible for the construction and operation of hospitals for their communities. In recent years the taxing authority of these districts has accounted for a very small percentage of total hospital operational costs.

As reflected in Table 8.2, the majority of the nation's hospitals are relatively modest in size as measured by licensed hospital beds. The very large institutions are typically teaching hospitals, often associated with medical schools, and have a range of residency programs for postgraduate medical education. The small hospitals are typically in rural areas, raising particularly complex issues regarding financial viability.

Broadly speaking, large hospitals are more prevalent in the East as the trend over time has been to build smaller rather than larger facilities. Significant numbers of smaller hospitals, particularly in urban areas, have closed over the past 25 years due to financial and competitive pressures, and to the difficulty of efficiently operating a small number of hospital beds. Specifying the optimal side of a hospital is particularly difficult given the complexity of services now offered on an inpatient basis. Most likely, the very small and very large hospitals are the least efficient.

As reflected in Table 8.3, the total number of hospital beds has dropped from just under 1.5 million to just less than 1 million since 1975. This trend reflects a combination of closures and reductions in operating licensed beds among those hospitals still in operation. Large hospitals, because of their size, account for a disproportionate share of the total number of hospital beds. About 70 percent of the nation's hospital beds are in nonprofit facilities.

As reflected in Table 8.4, there are approximately 36 million admissions to the nation's hospitals every year, of which 25 million are to nonprofit hospitals. The number of admissions has been remarkably

Table 8.3. Hospital Beds by Ownership and Hospital Size: United States, Selected Years

Type of Ownership and Size of Hospital	1975	1995	2003
Beds by Ownership		Number	
All hospitals	1,465,828	1,080,601	965,256
Federal	131,946	77,079	47,456
Nonfederal	1,333,882	1,003,522	917,800
Community	941,844	872,736	813,307
Nonprofit	658,195	609,729	574,587
For profit	73,495	105,737	109,671
State-local government	210,154	157,270	129,049
Bed size			
6–24 beds	5,615	5,085	5,635
25–49 beds	41,783	34,352	33,613
50–99 beds	106,776	82,024	74,025
100–199 beds	192,438	187,381	167,451
200–299 beds	164,405	175,240	152,487
300–399 beds	127,728	121,136	119,903
400–499 beds	101,278	86,459	76,333
500 beds or more	201,821	181,059	183,860

Table 8.4. Hospital Admissions by Ownership and Hospital Size: United States, Selected Years

Type of Ownership and Size of Hospital	1975	1995	2003
Beds by Ownership		Number in thousands	
All hospitals	36,157	33,282	36,611
Federal	1,913	1,559	973
Nonfederal	34,243	31,723	35,637
Community	33,435	30,945	34,783
Nonprofit	23,722	22,557	25,668
For profit	2,646	3,428	4,481
State-local government	7,067	4,961	4,634
By hospital bed size			
6–24 beds	174	124	162
25–49 beds	1,431	944	1,098
50–99 beds	3,675	2,299	2,464
100–199 beds	7,017	6,288	6,817
200–299 beds	6,174	6,495	6,887
300–399 beds	4,739	4,693	5,590
400–499 beds	3,689	3,413	3,591
500 beds or more	6,537	6,690	8,174

stable over the years, but the total number of hospital days has declined dramatically due to sharp reductions in the average length of stay. A relatively small proportion of admissions to hospitals are accounted for by the smaller hospitals.

Examining hospital utilization based on population data illustrates a significant decline in discharges per thousand U.S. population as reflected in Table 8.5. Overall explanation of this trend lies in changes in the number of Americans, which

Table 8.5. **Discharges and Days of Care, Nonfederal Short-Stay Hospitals: United States, Selected Years**

Characteristic	1980	2003
	Discharges per 1,000 population	
Total	173.4	119.5
Age		
Under 18 years	75.6	43.6
18–44 years	155.3	91.3
45–54 years	174.8	99.5
55–64 years	215.4	145.7
65 years and over	383.7	367.9
Sex		
Male	153.2	104.4
Female	195.0	135.1
Geographic Region		
Northeast	162.0	127.6
Midwest	192.1	117.1
South	179.7	125.8
West	150.5	103.9
	Days of care per 1,000 population	
Total	1,297.0	574.6
Age		
Under 18 years	341.4	195.5
18–44 years	818.6	339.7
45–54 years	1,314.9	477.2
55–64 years	1,889.4	735.9
65 years and over	4,098.3	2,088.3
Sex		
Male	1,239.7	546.7
Female	1,365.2	605.2
Geographic Region		
Northeast	1,400.6	694.4
Midwest	1,484.8	507.9
South	1,262.3	609.8
West	956.9	476.4

has led to a larger denominator. Declines in discharges are much more moderate for higher-age individuals.

Overall, changes in technological innovation combined with financial pressures from payers has led to an increasing proportion of medical care being provided on an ambulatory basis, and to much shorter lengths of stay for equivalent diagnoses for those patients who are admitted to the hospital. The impact of these trends is to yield a much higher intensity or complexity of care for hospitalized patients.

Table 8.6 presents hospital occupancy rates since 1975 for the nation's hospitals. Even with shorter lengths of stay, the closure of many hospitals, and an overall reduction in the number of hospital beds, occupancy rates remain on the decline. On average, today, only about two-thirds of the nation's hospital beds are filled with patients each night. This trend is evident in virtually every category of hospital ownership.

In the days since September 11, 2001, and more recently since various epidemics and natural disasters, the issue of ideal targets for hospital occupancy rates has become much more complex. How much capacity should be maintained for potential utilization in emergency situations is a complex policy issue. Maintaining unused capacity costs money. As a result, the industry has some reluctance to do so. On the other hand, operating at a more efficient level of occupancy, say 85 or 90 percent, not only restrains the ability to respond to normal fluctuations in utilization but also significantly impacts the ability of hospitals to respond to a critical community emergency situation. Alternatives for providing reserve back-up capacity for community-based emergencies have become an important priority as communities prepare for

Table 8.6. Hospital Occupancy Rates by Ownership and Hospital Size: United States, Selected Years

Type of Ownership and Size of Hospital	1975	1995	2003
Occupancy Rates by Ownership		Percent	
All hospitals	76.7	65.7	68.1
Federal	80.7	72.6	64.8
Nonfederal	76.3	65.1	68.3
Community	75.0	62.8	66.2
Nonprofit	77.5	64.5	67.7
For profit	65.9	51.8	59.6
State-local government	70.4	63.7	65.3
By hospital size			
6–24 beds	48.0	36.9	31.9
25–49 beds	56.7	42.6	44.6
50–99 beds	64.7	54.1	57.2
100–199 beds	71.2	58.8	62.6
200–299 beds	77.1	63.1	67.0
300–399 beds	79.7	64.8	68.5
400–499 beds	81.1	68.1	70.7
500 beds or more	80.9	71.4	74.2

unforeseen events without significantly impacting hospital cost structures.

STRUCTURE OF HOSPITAL AND HEALTH SYSTEMS

Although technological advancement and reimbursement policy are among the key factors affecting the development of the hospital industry over the past half century, other dramatic changes in the corporate environment of health care and particularly of the hospital sector have served a prominent role in affecting hospital management. Horizontal and vertical integration and the affiliation of hospitals with each other and with other sectors of the health care system have been extremely important developments in the organizational structure in governance and in the operational management of the hospital industry. These changes in the legal and organizational environment have profoundly affected how the hospital industry is structured and lines of accountability. The introduction of an increasingly typical corporate environment for the hospital industry has, to an extent, changed the roles for the key players, affected the organizational design, and facilitated other related changes within the industry such as closures and consolidations.

Horizontal and Vertical Integration

The development of organizational and financial efficiency in the hospital industry has been most accelerated by both vertical and horizontal integration. Because both of these forms of integration have been occurring, it is certainly fair to say that this is an industry in transition still seeking a level of equilibrium that can respond to changes in the health care marketplace and pricing as well as providing an adequate response to the invested community. Along with horizontal and vertical integration, the industry has experienced a tremendous

phase of closures and consolidations, particularly affecting smaller institutions. The dramatic changes in the number of operating hospital beds and hospitals in the United States are a result of this process as the industry seeks to provide more competitive products and pricing, an increasingly market-driven health care economy dictated by such payers as the government programs and various forms of managed care.

Both horizontal and vertical integration have experienced ebbs and flows over the past decades. The objectives of integration of resources have also varied depending on the participants involved and local market conditions. National integration of various types, particularly for horizontal integration, has also been driven in part by the behavior of for-profit entities. To this day, the success of both vertical and horizontal integration varies tremendously across the country, and changing economic and market conditions suggest that such integration is a dynamic rather than static process with players possibly assessing their assets and adding and subtracting from their portfolios.

In horizontal integration, similar units of production affiliate with each other. For example, for-profit and not-for-profit chains of hospitals under common ownership operating in different geographic locations all providing similar hospital-based services would be a horizontally integrated system. Horizontal integration occurs in the for-profit and not-for-profit sectors and can involve various levels of organizational affiliation from direct ownership to looser affiliation arrangements. Horizontal integration, designed to provide an enhanced level of efficiency of scale across multiple institutions and in related geographic areas, may serve to reduce duplication of services and marketplace competition. In a form of horizontal integration associated with regionalization of health services, smaller hospitals may feed into larger tertiary care facilities. Horizontal integration may also facilitate operational efficiency such as purchasing, information systems, quality assurance, and management capacity. Horizontally integrated multihospital networks may establish contractual arrangements with other types of health care providers and participate in larger health care delivery systems.

Vertical integration implies the establishment of integrated health care delivery systems that incorporate all or most aspects of the health care process. In this form of integration, inpatient hospital services, ambulatory care services, mental health, long-term care services, and other related health care products are incorporated into a comprehensive delivery system. Vertical integration, in many respects, is more complicated than horizontal integration because it involves a range of highly diverse and not always easily integrated services. Vertical integration was prompted by the objective of negotiating with insurers and managed-care providers such that the full range of services could be provided in a contractual arrangement. In addition, vertical integration provides for feeding patient flows into hospital inpatient services and other critical delivery components to ensure the financial viability of these institutions. Vertical integration allows for greater capture of patients within integrated systems and a more established institutionally based relationship with physicians. Vertically integrated systems in managed-care settings typically contract for a broad range of services rather than just for inpatient or other discrete care. Vertically integrated services provide a delivery chain for a range of health services rather than specializing in only one product. Vertically integrated systems have greater capture of premium dollars but at the same time, assume a greater degree of financial risk. This increased risk has represented a significant challenge in recent years. Some vertically integrated systems have also established their own health plans independently or in conjunction with insurance entities. However, this trend has faced significant challenges from financial and legal perspectives and they increase the risk to the institutional provider.

Both horizontally and vertically integrated systems of care need to align physician interests with institutional objectives. This has always been a challenge in health care and continues to be so, particularly with today's more competitive markets and

pricing pressures. Vertically integrated systems may have a greater likelihood of success in this regard because they can control a broader range of delivery systems and capture more of the health care dollar. Physician ownership initiatives such as for ambulatory, surgery centers, or even specialty hospitals are an additional threat to hospital delivery systems.

HOSPITAL ORGANIZATION

The traditional organization of hospitals is centered around three sources of power. These are the governing entity, the medical staff, and the administration.

Traditional hospital governance was predicated on independent institutions each with its own corporate-style board. Legally and structurally, the governing body has ultimate authority for all activities and decision making within the organization, delegating certain tasks among administration and the medical staff. Among nonprofit entities, these boards were historically composed of well-to-do individuals who could provide a platform for fundraising. Over time demands for accountability resulted in substantially ramped-up professional representation on these governing bodies. Physicians, accountants, attorneys, and others with a knowledge base relevant to institutional governance were elected to membership. Although frequently a volunteer activity with minimal, at least by corporate standards, pay and fringe benefits, public service was the key motivation. For-profit entities have typically been components of larger corporations with advisory rather than legally binding governing boards.

Hospital governing entities have delegated day-to-day management of the institution to hospital administration and the clinical medical affairs to the medical staff, which itself is typically formally organized with by-laws, elected officials, and specific duties and responsibilities.

In recent years, considerable effort has been directed toward educating members of governing entities and hospitals to better understand the principals and legal responsibilities of hospital management and to more critically assess decision-making activities, particularly pertaining to large capital investments, organizational mission, the role and management of medical staff, and contractual arrangements with other entities.

With both horizontal and vertical integration, the ultimate governance responsibility is typically shifted to the highest level of organizational structure. Depending on corporation status of components within the larger organization separate boards may exist with statutory authority or may serve primarily in an advisory capacity. In the for-profit sector, a parent organization governing board serves a corporate role analogous to that of any public or privately held for-profit corporation. In the publicly held environment, the corporate board has an additional legal responsibility attributable to securities; regulation and corporate governance are defined by state and federal laws.

For all governing entities, specific duties and responsibilities are specified in the legal charter or other documents creating the organization and defining the duties, responsibilities, and membership of the board. With increased accountability for individual and collective acts of governance, board members must assume that they do have personal and professional liability to perform their corporate duties in an appropriate fiduciary manner.

Hospital administration has also changed appreciably over the years moving toward a more traditional corporate operational approach. In addition, hospital management increasingly incorporates the delegation of responsibility to an array of other managers including, on the front lines, departmental administrators. Specific technical expertise is typically incorporated into the management structure in such areas as information systems, finance, legal environment, quality assurance, marketing, and contracting. Traditional roles such as patient care, including the hotel function, physical plant, admissions, discharge, other operational responsibilities, and various other key functions, are also represented.

Today's hospital administrators are often defined by traditional corporate titles and attractive pay packages. In the not-for-profit sector, senior-level hospital managers typically earn from the $100,000s to more than $500,000 per year. In the for-profit sector, these managers may also receive stock and stock options and other equity-related benefits. In both nonprofit and for-profit sectors, managers typically receive valuable benefit packages and in some instances, pay for performance and other types of bonuses. Hospital administrators usually have a management-related background or have clinical training and have worked their way into a management position or some combination of both. Hospital managers, like their employees, work in a relatively high-stress and demanding environment, answering not only to their formal bosses, but also to the public, consumers, physicians, and other constituencies.

THE HOSPITAL AND MEDICAL STAFF

With authority delegated from the governing entity, the hospital medical staff has specific responsibilities related to the clinical care provided in the facility and regulation of those individuals who practice clinically. Hospital and medical staffs are typically organized with elected officials, various committees, and with a leadership role represented by the president of the medical staff.

State medical practice laws generally prohibit direct employment of physicians by hospitals. As a consequence, and due to historical independence of physician practices, physicians and other health care professionals have affiliated with institutions such as hospitals in a variety of other ways. Historically, these affiliations have primarily been through membership in hospital medical staffs. More recently, hospitals and physicians have affiliated through joint ventures such as physician/hospital organizations, indirect employment of practitioners in other contractual arrangements, hospital purchases of group practices, and a variety of other models.

Hospital medical staff membership has generally followed a model whereby physicians apply for hospital privileges in their area of specialty and are vetted by a committee of the hospital medical staff supported by administration. If found to be of good character and having a reputable clinical reputation, physicians are granted privileges, which is, in essence, the ability to admit and discharge patients, provide care within the hospital facilities, and serve as a participating member of the medical staff. Although the governing entity is ultimately responsible for granting privileges, this responsibility is usually delegated to the medical staff in recognition of their knowledge of clinical practice and ability to assess professional skills. The evaluation of individuals for the granting of privileges is one of the key and most important roles of the medical staff. Physicians, for example, are evaluated on their medical and specialty residency training, their track record of clinical care as reflected in medical malpractice and other quality assurance indicators, and their reputation in other respects.

When a physician is granted privileges, he or she remains subject to surveillance by the medical staff to ensure continued maintenance of a minimum level of quality of care. This surveillance typically consists of monitoring cases to assess any instances for patterns of poor quality of care as well as other indicators of difficulty such as being associated with a physician impaired with alcohol or drug or other abuse. Hospitals and their medical staffs also serve a regulatory role in reporting violations of clinical practice standards by physicians and other practitioners to state licensing agencies and other entities.

Physicians, as members of the medical staff, may participate in various committee assignments and historically were expected to provide some level of indigent care although this requirement in many instances has largely dissipated. In most hospitals physicians are also expected to utilize their clinical privileges only in those areas in which they have proper training and credentialing.

Physicians and other professionals who are less frequently utilizing a specific hospital may be granted a separate category of privileges for occasional use with less expected participation and fewer responsibilities. Physicians who are interested in clinical leadership positions may assume responsibility for medical staff committees or seek to be a leader in the medical staff hierarchy. Increasingly, physicians who are interested in managerial roles may also be employed for that purpose by the hospital on the administration side, typically a position such as vice president for medical affairs.

In addition to credentialing physicians for hospital privileges, the medical staff is typically responsible for ensuring the quality of care provided in the hospital under delegated authority from the governing entity. Various committees may be formed for this purpose, including a quality assurance committee or other peer review committee. The medical staff will seek to provide feedback to physicians and other clinicians who are not meeting expected standards of the quality of care in their clinical practices within the institution. This feedback can take many forms, including quantitative data assessment comparing each individual to the norms of other practitioners in their specialties, or even informal feedback from the medical staff president or a clinical department chief. Ultimately, hospital privileges may be revoked in extreme situations where clinical standards are clearly not met. In this instance, appropriate due process must be followed utilizing specified procedures as outlined in the medical staff bylaws.

The increasing utilization of computerized information systems and a more interested younger generation of clinicians have greatly accelerated the attention to data-based assessments of quality of care. National voluntary organizations have worked hard to promote these efforts so as to elevate the overall quality of care provided in the nation's hospitals. Voluntary accrediting agencies, in particular, have also increasingly pressured institutional providers to incorporate quality assurance mechanisms in their ongoing production methods. Many types of approaches have been developed in this regard, including a range of processes designed to encourage the use of clinical approaches that are validated from scientific and evidence-based research. Many clinical quality assurance and quality improvement techniques have been adapted from the corporate environment, particularly industrial settings as well. Payers are also demanding enhanced quality surveillance and improvement.

In contrast to a typical corporate environment, hospitals do not directly employ most physicians, who are key decision makers and decide resource allocation and utilization. Thus, the medical staff serves an important role in aligning physician behavior and objectives with institutional needs. Medical leadership is particularly important in today's complex environment to facilitate this relationship. Ultimately, the traditional hospital structure, particularly with regard to the medical staff, is inconsistent with managing an organization that faces numerous competitive and pricing pressures. Some medical staff organizations, such as those in group practice, model HMOs that directly own all resources in their systems, and certain governmental entities such as the military and veteran's administration hospitals, have more direct control over the medical staff.

KEY ISSUES FACING THE HOSPITAL INDUSTRY

The hospital industry almost continuously faces key critical issues that challenge its structure, viability, and roles in health care. This section discusses many of these issues.

Specialty Hospitals

In recent years, the development of highly specialized hospitals has gained considerable traction.

Although not a new concept by any means, the more rapid recent development of these specialty hospitals poses a threat to community general hospitals to a much greater extent than in past years. The new specialty hospitals include those focused on cancer and heart disease and other highly discrete areas of practice in lucrative fields such as orthopedic surgery.

To further complicate the controversy over specialty hospitals, these institutions are increasingly partially owned by the physicians who practice within them. Ironically, in the early days of the modern development of hospitals, physician ownership was not unusual. However, the popularity of physician-owned proprietary hospitals today has been challenged by two ramifications. The first is that these hospitals draw profitable patients from community hospitals, and the second potential conflict of interest is represented by physicians admitting patients to hospitals in which they have an ownership interest.

Of course, our quality of care data suggest that high volumes of discrete services can enhance quality. From some perspectives, highly specialized institutions may in fact provide the best care. On the other hand, many of these specialty hospitals may siphon off insured and relatively healthier patients, leaving the less profitable and more complicated cases to community general hospitals.

Physician ownership of specialty hospitals raises concerns that financial incentives will affect the treatment decisions, such as the use of specialty and diagnostic services. In addition to providing care to the less complex and more profitable cases, these hospitals may also leave the uninsured and underinsured to community and public hospitals for treatment. The combination of adverse selection and less private insurance and public coverage for community general hospitals and government facilities does raise significant policy concerns.

Federal policy development has been slow to respond to this trend. Medicare has complex rules regarding physician ownership of health care resources and potential conflicts of interest. And both the Medicare and Medicaid programs have a valid concern with respect to the distribution of health care costs across all facilities and patient groups. The impact of specialty hospitals on community general hospitals and governmental hospitals has yet to be fully assessed, but this development is potentially significant clinically and financially.

Changes in Technology

The hospital industry is all about technology. Although the hotel function of a hospital is in a way primary to its purpose, it is the provision of technology that is its true mission. Technology has shaped the physical and operational structures of hospitals, has affected the lives of patients and families, and has provided a delivery vehicle for physicians in clinical practice.

From its earliest days as a modern institution, the availability of technological resources has defined the services provided in hospitals. The discovery of anesthesia and of antisepsis clearly established the early stages of the provision of surgical care. The vast array of imaging technologies has had tremendous impact on effective intervention for patients seeking care in the hospital setting. Laboratory, diagnostic, and other technological innovations have also greatly facilitated clinical medicine. Successful intervention is dependent on the technology of innovative therapies including pharmacological interventions and surgical techniques.

More recently, the huge range of technological advancements that have vaulted to the forefront of the tertiary care role of inpatient services within hospitals have included organ transplantation, a vast array of minimally invasive surgical technologies, advanced cardiac treatments, primarily through a variety of surgical interventions, an impressive range of successes in advanced emergency and trauma care, and vast improvements in the underlying technologies related to information systems, medical records, and other aspects of hospital and health care operations to facilitate the delivery of services to patients. Technological advances have affected obstetric patients, pediatric care needs, patients with terminal illnesses, and a range of other problems that present to the inpatient side of hospital operations.

Technological advancement has led to the development of increased specialization and clinical practice, expansion of specialized services, new medical and surgical specialties, and treatments for many diseases for which little curative or other care could be provided in the past. Advanced technologies including the many applications of lasers, the use of ultrasonic technology for treatment, and more recently, the development of automated surgical assistant or robot technologies have all been revolutionary.

Hospitals operate in competitive markets and the pressure to provide a full range of technology, and to keep that technology current, yields significant cost pressures and even potential conflicts with medical staff members. Insurers and employers as well as government entities seek to pay for the latest technologies, but at efficient pricing.

The continuing advancement of technology is a double-edged sword providing us with tremendous new capabilities, but at the same time, many challenges. The hospital, perhaps more than any other sector of the health care system, faces these opportunities and challenges in the most dramatic ways. And, ultimately, it is their customers, their patients, and their physicians who utilize these hospitals and health care systems, who have the highest expectations and often the least sensitivity about costs.

Clinical Practice Patterns

Hospital design and operations are significantly affected by accepted clinical patterns of practice. The increasing attention to best practices and practice norms of various types, particularly under quality assurance programs, requires institutional adherence to various protocols and guidelines. Information systems and other operational requirements must also be compliant with the need to provide evaluative information to assess and report on physician clinical patterns of practice. Medicare and many managed-care contracts require such reporting. Accreditation by the Joint Commission for Accreditation of Health Care Organizations and other specialty accreditation bodies also requires the availability and interpretation of data.

In addition to the availability of appropriate information to monitor and evaluate clinical protocols and practice guidelines, institutions are increasingly expected to offer a governance structure that assigns responsibility for these activities. Typically, in most community hospitals, that responsibility is delegated from the governing body to the medical staff. The governing board and institutional administration, however, retain responsibility for successful compliance with these requirements. Individual practitioners are likewise increasingly being held accountable for their practice patterns and behavior through a variety of monitoring and feedback mechanisms.

The complexity of integrating all the requirements pertaining to clinical practice is of itself a significant burden on institutional operations. Legal and ethical expectations, combined with reporting requirements contained in various contractual arrangements, further enhance the depth and complexity of this obligation. Physician independence has been significantly weakened by the introduction of various external regulatory requirements.

Reimbursement Mechanisms

Hospitals and hospital systems are heavily constrained by the reimbursement mechanisms that pay their bills. The most significant source of funds for most hospitals is the federal Medicare program. As discussed elsewhere in detail in this book, financial mechanisms for reimbursement under the Medicare program have become increasingly complex. Medicare has moved to reward efficiency and specialization while increasingly squeezing institutional cash flow. Medicare, being a federal program, also has significant regulatory and force of law powers unknown to third-party insurers in the private sector. Medicare has imposed an array of requirements to reduce fraud and abuse, but these efforts have had secondary

effects in complicating organizational administration and financial arrangements.

Nongovernmental sources of payment, primarily from managed-care organizations, have themselves become fraught with complexity and cost pressures. Most payers now seek a competitive market advantage in pricing in an attempt to drive down the cost of health care, while at the same time shifting an increased burden of cost to the consumer. The negotiated per diem rates are heavily discounted and many insurers exclude a range of reimbursements for various specific services.

Many third parties also require reporting from institutional providers on utilization patterns, use of resources and services, and other parameters of the care process. Hospitals are generally expected by payers to provide extensive oversight of practitioners through aggressive credentialing efforts and other responsibilities. All these developments have resulted in pressure to improve efficiency, reduce waste and duplication, and provide care as quickly as possible and at the lowest possible cost.

While payers are increasingly squeezing payments to all providers, hospitals in particular are susceptible to financial pressures. Hospitals provide services that require a high degree of capital investment, have limited control over the cost of many of their products due to such considerations as shortages of nursing and other specialized personnel and the high cost of innovative products, and finally, the expectations on the part of both consumers and individual practitioners for reasonable ambience and excellent outcomes.

Academic Medical Centers

Academic medical centers typically consist of medical schools and their primary teaching hospitals. Academic medical centers provide tertiary, secondary, and primary care but have a principal focus on biomedical research, teaching of medical residents and medical students, and often an array of other professional training, research, and service activities. These organizations are highly complex with a multitude of power structures, funding sources, and sometimes conflicting missions.

Hospitals that are part of academic medical centers are operationally constrained by the demands of the teaching mission, particularly with regard to medical students and postgraduate medical education, and a mandate to conduct both basic biomedical and applied clinical research. Financial efficiency and consumer satisfaction are not typically the top priorities. Physicians and researchers place considerable demands on these organizations to provide the latest technology and staffing and to allow for teaching and clinical investigation.

The success of academic medical centers in achieving their missions should be a national priority. The long-term strengths and successes of our health care system depend on this. Although not necessarily widely acknowledged, financial efficiency in fact should probably not be a top priority from a national health policy perspective. Unfortunately reimbursement policies by Medicare and other government and private payers typically do not overtly allow enough latitude for academic medical centers. In addition, academic medical centers are frequently the providers of last resort, further restraining cash flows and viability. Local government and, to an extent, private insurers through cost shifting, pick up part of the tab.

A lot of attention has been directed toward academic medical centers in recent years. The challenge is to reconcile the needs for medical education and research with the fiscal realities of available resources in a manner that will meet our nation's educational and clinical needs. This remains a huge challenge for the nation's health care system.

SUMMARY

The hospital industry has faced numerous challenges over the years and will continue to do so in the future. Markets have changed, pricing pressures have increased, and consumer and payer expectations have evolved. Yet, through it all, our nation's hospitals have continued to provide the best hospital-based care in the world, delivering a technology that is second to none with top-notch staff dedicated to patient care.

REVIEW QUESTIONS

1. Describe the historical development of hospitals in the United States.
2. Describe the differences between nonprofit and for-profit hospitals.
3. List the major trends that have occurred within the hospital sector.
4. What is horizontal integration, and why is it used?
5. What is vertical integration, and why is it used?
6. Describe the internal organization of community hospitals.
7. Describe the key issues facing the hospital industry.

REFERENCES & ADDITIONAL READINGS

Birkmeyer, J. D., Siewers, A. E., Finlayson, E. V. A., Stukel, T. A., Lucas, F. L., Batista, I., Welch, H. G., & Wennberg, D. E. (2002). Hospital volume and surgical mortality in the United States. *New England Journal of Medicine, 346,* 1137–1144.

Davis, M., & Heineke, J. (2003). *Managing services: Using technology to create value.* Boston: McGraw-Hill/Irwin.

Gapenski, L. (2004). *Healthcare finance: An introduction to accounting and financial management* (3rd ed.). Chicago: AUPHA Press/Health Administration Press.

Halm, E. A., Lee, C., & Chassin, M. R. (2000). *How is volume related to quality in health care? A systematic review of the research literature.* Prepared for National Academy of Sciences, Interpreting the volume-outcome relationship in the context of health care quality workshop. Washington, DC.

Kelly, D. L. (2003). *Applying quality management in healthcare: A process for Improvement.* Chicago: AUPHA/Health Administration Press.

Martin, L. L., & Sage, R. (Eds.). (1993). *Total quality management in human service organizations.* New York: Sage Publications.

CHAPTER 9

The Continuum of Long-Term Care

Connie J. Evashwick

CHAPTER TOPICS

- Definition of Long-Term Care
- Clients of Long-Term Care
- How Long-Term Care Is Organized
- Service Categories
- Integrating Mechanisms
- Long-Term Care Policy

LEARNING OBJECTIVES

Upon completing this chapter, the reader should be able to

1. Describe who uses long-term care and under what circumstances.
2. Explain the role and scope of services included in long-term care.
3. Articulate how long-term care services are organized, operated, financed, and integrated.
4. Evaluate model delivery system approaches to long-term care for the future.
5. Articulate national policy issues pertinent to long-term care.

WHAT IS LONG-TERM CARE?

- A child with cerebral palsy attends a special needs classroom in a public school, with therapy available on-site, and her parents care for her when she is at home.

- An 85-year old recovering from a broken hip receives meals on wheels during the week and relies on her daughter for meals over the weekend.

- A young man with schizophrenia lives in sheltered housing, with financial assistance provided through a public housing voucher program and medication or counseling assistance available from an on-site staff when needed.

- An elderly couple, one of whom is blind from advanced glaucoma and one of whom is crippled with severe arthritis, uses a money-management service from a local community agency to pay their bills, since neither can write a check.

- A middle-aged woman with multiple sclerosis has a live-in attendant to assist her with the activities of daily living.

All these are examples of long-term care provided by formal or informal sources. Long-term care is defined as health, mental health, residential or social support provided to a person with functional disabilities on an informal or formal basis over an extended period of time with the goal of maximizing the person's independence. Services change over time as the person's and caregivers' needs change.

The goal of long-term care is to help people achieve functional independence, in contrast to the goal of acute care, which is to cure. People of all ages and a wide range of clinical diagnoses need long-term care. The vast majority of long-term care (80 to 90 percent) is provided by friends and family. However, formal services are essential to enable

the informal system to be sustained. The formal services that provide long-term care are described in this chapter using a conceptual framework referred to as "the continuum of long-term care." The ideal is an integrated set of services that provides continuity of care over time and across settings. In reality, services are highly fragmented due to financial drivers, local community variation, and a lack of uniform federal and state policies. This chapter provides an overview of the ideal continuum of care juxtaposed with the reality of existing services, structure, and policies.

WHO NEEDS LONG-TERM CARE?

The clients of long-term care are growing rapidly. They represent a mosaic of population segments of those with functional disabilities. Three intersecting concepts warrant explanation to understand the users of long-term care.

The fundamental reason that a person needs long-term care is because they suffer from one or more functional disabilities. *Functional ability* is a person's ability to perform the basic activities of daily living (ADLs) or instrumental activities of daily living (IADLs). ADLs include the ability to bathe, dress, perform personal care and grooming, walk, transfer from bed to chair, maintain bowel and bladder continence, and eat. ADLs were initially defined by Katz and colleagues through research (Katz et al., 1963), and years of study have produced commonly accepted measures and scales of functioning. ADLs tend to involve large motor skills, and they are lost in a predictable order. IADLs are more loosely defined (Lawton & Brody, 1969) but typically involve cognitive reasoning and finer motor skills. IADLs include telephoning, managing money, taking medications, grocery shopping, housekeeping, doing chores, and using transportation.

The conditions that underlie the need for long-term care may be physical health, mental health,

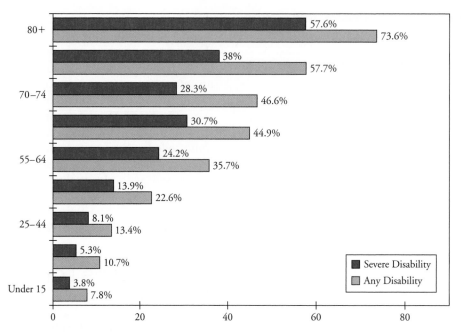

Figure 9.1. Disability Prevalence by Age, 1997

SOURCE: From *Health, United States, 2005* (Special Excerpt), *Trend Tables on 65 and Older Population* (DHHS Pub. No. 2006-0152) (Table 58, p. 243), National Center for Health Statistics.

or a combination, as well as family situation and environmental context. Of the 288 million people in the United States in 2005, more than 12 percent, or more than 35 million people suffered from some type of disability that limited their ability to perform basic activities of daily living (National Center for Health Statistics, 2005). Limitations in functional ability affect people of all ages but increase with age and the concomitant chronic conditions that accumulate with aging. Figure 9.1 shows the estimated number of people with disabilities. How a person manages a functional disability depends on several factors, including other health conditions, age, family and social support, economic status, housing, and personal preference.

Chronic is defined by the *National Health Interview Survey* as any condition that lasts 3 months (or 90 days) or more (National Center for Health Statistics, 2007). Chronic conditions may derive from physical or mental conditions. Over the

progression of a disease, both may occur. Chronic conditions may be as life-threatening as coronary artery disease or as harmless as mild arthritis. In 2005, an estimated 133 million people had some type of chronic condition (Hoffman, Rice, & Sung, 1996). Chronic conditions often (although not always) result in functional disabilities.

An *impairment* as used by the *National Health Interview Survey* is defined as "a chronic or permanent defect, usually static in nature, that results from disease, injury, or congenital malformation. It often represents a decrease in or loss of ability to perform various functions." Permanent impairments, such as limb amputation or blindness, may require an initial adjustment and are then more or less stable. People may attain a level of independence by learning special skills to overcome the disability or by using adaptive devices. For example, a person with myopia can have their vision corrected by wearing glasses or contact lenses and thus suffer no disability as a result of their impairment. Nonetheless, impairments are closely associated with functional disability.

Impairment, chronic condition, and functional ability are intertwined. For example, a person who is blind, who lives with a supportive family, learns Braille, and masters the immediate environment, may achieve a fair degree of independence on a daily basis. However, if that person ages and becomes cognitively diminished, he or she may no longer be able to remember the environment, and without the ability to use the visual clues (or just simple notes or lists) that a person with sight can use to help overcome cognitive weaknesses, is less able to function independently. If that person then slips and breaks a hip, suffers a permanent impairment, and has to use a walker, they will lose more functional ability than a sighted person or a person without cognitive impairment who is able to understand rehabilitation routines.

In addition to a person's health and mental health, social situation, finances, housing, and community context all affect the extent to which a person can perform ADLs and IADLs independently and the type of assistance they may need. Contrast a male veteran in a wheelchair who lives with a spouse, can afford a personal caregiver, resides in a one-story home, and lives in a large urban community served by a community-based agency coordinating services for the disabled and a Veterans Affairs hospital that provides a full range of health care for people with disabilities with an elderly widow who breaks her hip, has no family nearby, has no income except Social Security, resides in a two-story walk-up in a small rural town, and must travel 30 miles to reach a hospital with an orthopedic service. The man will maintain his independence by working with a multifaceted support system; the older woman will most likely end up moving to a relative's home or an assisted living facility for those with low income and be forced to move away from her friendship network.

The United States makes no single, constant, routine count of people needing long-term care

that factors in all the variables that determine if, what type, and how much care a person needs to perform ADLs and IADLs. Rather, subsets are counted, and each subset of the total population has a segment that may require long-term care at some point from formal or informal sources. Population segments at high risk of needing long-term care are growing steadily. They include the aged (especially those age 75 and older), those with certain chronic conditions (such as stroke, mental illness, degenerative neurological conditions, Alzheimer's disease), people positive for HIV/AIDS, and children with special health care needs, to mention just a few. For each group, and each individual, the care needed will vary and will be some combination of informal care provided by family and friends and formal care provided by external organizations. The rationale for structuring the long-term care system for specific segments of the population rather than a single encompassing system is based on the differing needs of each segment and the multiple factors that shape service delivery, particularly financing.

Users of long-term care services are called by differing terms, depending on the service. Table 9.1 shows the terms used by various services.

Table 9.1. Terminology for Users of Select Services

Service	Term for Clients
Nursing homes	Residents
Hospitals	Patients
Adult day services	Participants
Home care	Clients
Hospice	Patients
Outreach	Consumers
Wellness programs	Clients
Disease management programs	Enrollees
Durable medical equipment	Customers
Assisted living	Residents

HOW IS LONG-TERM CARE ORGANIZED?

One of the greatest challenges of long-term care is that there is no single organized formal delivery system. As noted earlier, the vast majority of long-term care is provided by friends and family. Care is orchestrated around the unique needs of each individual and family, as well as the resources of the particular community. A person may require multiple services, provided in a range of settings, and by professionals representing a broad spectrum of disciplines. Moreover, services can be expected to change over time as the client's and family's needs change or as new technologies arise. Thus patterns of care vary, for population segments as well as individuals.

To analyze long-term care service delivery, the conceptual framework of an ideal continuum of long-term care is used. The continuum of care is defined as

> A client-oriented system composed of both services and integrating mechanisms that guides and tracks clients over time through a comprehensive array of health, mental health, and social services spanning all levels of intensity of care. (Evashwick, 1987)

The ideal continuum of care is the formal care system that complements the informal services provided by friends and family. The ideal continuum of care is a comprehensive, coordinated system of care designed to meet the multifaceted needs of persons with complex and/or ongoing problems efficiently and effectively. A continuum is more than a collection of fragmented services. It includes mechanisms for organizing those services and operating them as an integrated system.

The purpose is to facilitate the client's access to the appropriate services at the appropriate time, quickly and efficiently. Ideally, a continuum of care does the following:

- Matches resources to the client's health and family circumstance.
- Monitors the client's condition and changes services as needs change.
- Coordinates the care of many professionals and disciplines.
- Integrates care provided in a range of settings.
- Enhances efficiency, reduces duplication, and streamlines client flow.
- Pools or otherwise arranges financing so that services are based on need rather than narrow eligibility criteria.
- Maintains a comprehensive record incorporating clinical, financial, and utilization data.

A true continuum should serve three major goals: (1) Provide the health and related support services that foster independence, for the client as well as the family, (2) achieve cost-effectiveness by maximizing the use of resources, and (3) enhance quality through appropriateness and continuity of care. Some clients may use only select components of the system and may remain involved with the organized system of care for a relatively short period of time; others may use only a limited and stable set of services over a prolonged period of time.

Continuum Overview

More than 60 distinct services can be identified in the complete continuum of care. For simplicity, the services are grouped into seven categories, as shown in the schematic and in Table 9.2. The seven categories represent the basic types of health care and related services that a person could need over time, through periods of both wellness and illness. Table 9.2 lists select services within each category but should not be interpreted as the complete list of all health and mental health services. The table does not include social support services, which also comprise a lengthy list.

By definition, the continuum of care is more than a collection of fragmented services; it is an integrated system of care. The United States health care delivery system has evolved historically as highly fragmented. Integration of services does not happen automatically. For providers, payers, and clients to gain the system benefits of efficiencies of

Table 9.2. Categories and Services of the Continuum of Care*

Extended
Skilled nursing facility
Step-down unit
Swing bed
Nursing home follow-up
Intermediate care facility for the mentally retarded
Long-term care hospital
Psychiatric hospital (residential model)

Acute
Medical/surgical inpatient services
Psychiatric acute inpatient services
Rehabilitation short-term inpatient services
Interdisciplinary assessment team
Consultation service

Ambulatory
Physician's office
Outpatient clinics
▪ Primary care
▪ Specialty medical care
▪ Rehabilitation
▪ Mental health
▪ Surgery
Psychological counseling
Day hospital
Adult day services

Home Care
Home health—Medicare
Home health—Private
Hospice
High-technology home therapy
Durable medical equipment
Home visitors
Homemaker and personal care
In-home caregiver

Outreach and Linkage
Screening
Information and referral
Telephone contact
Emergency response system
Transportation
Senior services program
Meals on Wheels
Mail order pharmacy

Wellness and Health Promotion
Educational programs
Exercise programs
Recreational and social groups
Senior volunteers
Congregate meals
Support groups
Disease management

Housing
Continuing care retirement community
Independent senior housing
Assisted living
Congregate care facility
Adult family home
Group home
Board and care facility
Alcohol and substance abused facility

*Lists of services within each category are not exhaustive.

From "Definition of the Continuum of Care," by C. Evashwick, 2005, in *The Continuum of Long-Term Care*, C. Evashwick (Ed.), Albany, NY: Delmar.

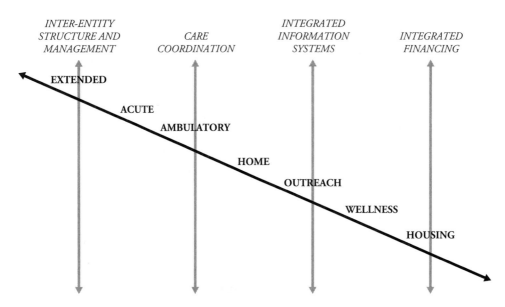

Figure 9.2. Services and Integrating Mechanisms of the Continuum of Care

SOURCE: From "Definition of the Continuum of Care." by C. Evashwick, 1987, in *Managing the Continuum of Care,* by C. Evashwick and L. Weiss (Eds.), Gaithersburg, MD: Aspen Publishers.

operation, smooth client flow, and quality of service, formal structural integrating mechanisms are essential. Four integrating management systems are required: inter-entity structure and management, care coordination, integrated information systems, and integrated financing (Figure 9.2).

SERVICE CATEGORIES

This section briefly describes each of the seven service categories and presents data, when available, on major or select services within each category. Not every client will use every service. However, the ideal is that the services are available and accessible if a person should need them. There is no set order for the services, since each client will use ones appropriate for his or her individual and unique needs.

A significant aspect of the services is that each has its own operating characteristics, even within the same category. Services vary according to intensity of care offered, professional and support staffing, predominant financing, licensing, certification, accreditation, equipment, space, and significant other management dimensions. This variation poses a challenge to managers trying to coordinate services, as well as to payers and clients who are trying to achieve continuity of care.

Extended Inpatient Care

Extended inpatient care is for people who are so sick or functionally disabled that they require on-going nursing and support services provided in a formal health care institution, but who are not so acutely ill that they require the technological and professional intensity of a hospital. The majority of extended inpatient care facilities are referred to "nursing facilities" or "nursing homes," although this is a broad term that includes many levels and types of programs. Specialty facilities range from subacute units in hospitals to intermediate care facilities for the mentally retarded or developmentally disabled to psychiatric hospitals caring for the severely mentally ill on an indefinite basis. Nursing facilities in the nation number about 16,100, with about 1.4 million residents at any given time (American Association of Homes and Services for the Aging, 2007).

The cost of a nursing facility ranges from $4,000–7,000 per month, depending on location and scope of services rendered. Medicaid pays for about 47 percent of all nursing facility care, and residents and their families pay for about one-third (Center for Medicare and Medicaid Services, 2007).

The lifetime probability of ever being admitted to a nursing home (under the present U.S. standard of care) is about 50 percent. However, average length of stay has decreased dramatically over the past 30 years, just as likelihood of admission has increased. Both reflect the trend for nursing facilities to become technologically more sophisticated and to function as short-term stopping places in between home and hospital rather than as permanent residential settings.

Nursing facilities can be accredited by the Joint Commission and can be certified by Medicare and Medicaid to participate as providers to those enrolled in these government programs.

Two excellent sources of information about nursing home are the trade associations that represent for-profit and not-for-profit nursing homes, respectively: http://www.ahca.org, http://www.aahsa.org, and the Federal Centers for Medicare and Medicaid Services, http://cms.nhs.gov

Hospitals

The nation's hospitals are a broad array of institutions that provide care for those with acute problems and emergencies, but that also care for many people with chronic conditions and long-term health problems. The most current information can be found on the website of the American Hospital Association at http://www.aha.org. Community general hospitals are the most prevalent type, numbering about 4,936 of the 5,756 total U.S. hospitals existing in 2005 (American Hospital Association, 2007a). However, various types of hospitals specialize in long-term care, including categories of psychiatric, rehabilitation, chronic disease, orthopedics, and long-term (defined as average length of stay of 23 days or more). Hospitals also provide extensive outpatient services, including many used by those needing long-term care, ranging from rehabilitation to mental health counseling to outpatient surgery. Hospitals have evolved from a focus on strictly acute care to promoting health with disease management and health education programs.

Hospitals admit more than 37 million people each year, but this number includes those who are readmitted who are those most likely to be long-term care users. Average length of stay is 4 to 5 days for adults under the age of 65 and about 6 days for those age 65 and older. The leading causes of hospital admissions are chronic conditions: heart problems, cancer, mental illness, stroke, respiratory conditions, and fractures derived from osteoporosis.

Medicare and private insurance are the primary payers for hospital services, with individuals paying relatively little from out-of-pocket. However, hospital costs are the largest single category of expenditure for Medicare, other government health programs, and private insurance. Hospitals are accredited by the Joint Commission.

Ambulatory Care

Ambulatory care services are provided in a formal health care facility, whether a physician's office or the outpatient clinic of a hospital or an adult day program. They include a wide spectrum of preventive, maintenance, diagnostic, and recuperative services for people who manifest a variety of conditions— from those who are entirely healthy and simply want an annual checkup to those with major health problems who are recovering from hospitalization to those with chronic conditions who need ongoing monitoring. Outpatient visits to hospitals alone numbered nearly 600 million in 2005 (American Hospital Association, 2007b).

Adult day services (ADS) are particularly relevant to long-term care. ADS represent a daytime program of personal care, therapeutic activities, supervision, socialization, assistance with ADLs, midday meals, and perhaps health-related skilled care. ADS enable frail people who cannot be alone in their own homes to remain in the community. By attending adult day services, people who are functionally disabled due to physical or mental disorders and/or are moderately ill but not in need of round-the-clock nursing care can remain in their homes at night with their families or friends while receiving the care they need during the day. ADS participants may attend on an indefinite basis or just while recovering from an acute episode of illness. They may attend each day, or just 2 or 3 days per week. The goals are to foster the maximum possible health and independence in functioning for each participant and to provide respite and support for each caregiver and family. For many, ADS programs provide an alternative to nursing home care.

ADS programs have grown exponentially since the first formal programs began in the 1970s. Currently, there are about 3,400 ADS programs throughout the nation (Cox, 2006). The average daily census is about 25, but capacity ranges up to 38 or more people, with about three times as many people enrolled as attend on any given day. This means that ADS serve about 85,000 people per day. More than 150,000 people throughout the United States are enrolled in ADS at any given time (National Adult Day Services Association, 2007).

ADS average daily charges were about $56 per day in 2007, but relatively few programs make a profit. Most depend on donations, grants, and other subsidies. Medicare does not pay for ADS; Medicaid pays in selective states, and many individuals pay out-of-pocket.

Licensure varies across states. Some states license ADS as a health service; some license it as a social service. ADS can be accredited by the Commission on Accreditation of Rehabilitation Facilities (CARF). ADS are still gaining recognition by professionals and lay people alike.

A key source of information about adult day services is the National Association for Adult Day Services at http://www.aahsa.org/naads.

Home Health

Home health care is one of the oldest components of the continuum of care. A number of home health agencies across the nation have celebrated their centennials. Home care today consists of several types of services: skilled nursing care and therapies; homemaker/personal care/chore services; high-technology home therapy; durable medical equipment; and hospice. The services may all be provided by one agency, or an agency may specialize in only one. Each service has distinct operating characteristics.

Home health agencies certified by Medicare must serve people who are homebound, have a prognosis of improvement/recovery; have home care ordered by a physician; need skilled nursing, physical therapy, or speech-language therapy; require intermittent care only; and meet conditions of participation specified by the federal Medicare legislation. These home care agencies offer skilled services provided by registered nurses, physical therapists, occupational therapists, speech therapists, social workers, and home health aides. They do not provide personal care or functional support on an indefinite basis. Nearly 3 million people are served by Medicare-certified home care agencies each year (National Association of Home Care, 2007).

Medicare-certified home health agencies numbered about 7,628 in 2004 (National Association for Home Care, 2007). Home health agencies may be freestanding or owned by hospitals, health departments, assisted living complexes, or other community agencies. Nearly one-half are for profit; the others are not-for-profit or government affiliated. The national average payments in 2004 were $129 per visit and $4,050 per patient. Medicare is the largest single payer, although many managed-care and commercial insurers also pay for home care provided by Medicare-certified agencies. Medicare certified home health agencies may be accredited by the Joint Commission or the Community Health

Accreditation Program (CHAP). Detailed information can be found from the National Association for Home Care and Hospice at http://www.nahc.org and from Medicare at http://cms.gov.

Private home care agencies are not certified by Medicare and are thus not restricted by federal regulations. Consequently, they provide a broader spectrum of home services ranging from highly skilled to basic personal support, homemaker, and chore services. Private home care agencies bill by the hour or the service. Many individuals pay privately. In addition, private home care agencies may have contracts with managed-care plans, commercial insurers, Medicaid, or other local government agencies. Statistics on private home care agencies are limited. Private agencies are estimated to number more than 12,000 and to care for more than 5 million people per year. The largest association representing both Medicare-certified and private home care agencies is the National Association for Home Care, which can be accessed at http://www.nahc.org.

High-tech home therapy refers to specialty care provided in the home that requires sophisticated equipment and pharmaceuticals. Examples are chemotherapy, antibiotic therapy, enteral and parenteral nutrition, and home dialysis. High-tech home therapy may be provided by a Medicare-certified or private home care agency or by a company that specializes only in high-tech home care. This service is mentioned separately because it has grown exponentially over the past 30 years and is expected to continue to do so as therapies are moved from inpatient to outpatient venues. Also, high-tech home care requires additional licenses, personnel, and payment mechanisms from those required of standard home care agencies because of the pharmaceuticals and equipment involved, as well as the high level of intensity of illness of the clients.

Hospice

Hospice is a philosophical approach to care rather than a place. Ideally, hospice care occurs in the person's home, including in a nursing home, assisted living complex, or other group residential setting.

Hospice is a concept of comprehensive and palliative care for someone whose death is imminent. The goals are to make the person as comfortable as possible, including using drugs to alleviate pain; achieve emotional acceptance of death by the person and the family; and comfort and assist the family after the person's death. Hospice uses an interdisciplinary team, including pastoral care and bereavement counselors.

The concept of hospice was developed in Great Britain by Dr. Cicely Saunders. The first hospice in the United States opened in 1971. Hospice can be organized independently or from the base of any health care entity, including home health agencies. Medicare has a special hospice provision. This entails detailed regulations for those organizations that seek to be certified Medicare hospice providers, a complex payment system, and certain expectations of and benefits for enrollees. Commercial insurance companies and Medicaid have tended to mirror the Medicare benefit in covering hospice care. For a person to enroll in hospice, he or she must be eligible for Medicare and have a projected life expectancy of 180 days or less. Both the Joint Commission and CHAP accredit hospice programs.

The number of hospices and hospice patients has grown steadily over the past 35 years. In 2007, there were 3,078 hospices certified by Medicare and numerous others that did not seek certification (Hospice Association of America, 2007). The Medicare hospices served more than 890,000 people in 2005, or more than one-third of all those who die during the year. The median length of stay in hospice was less than 21 days in 2006, indicating that many people do not get the benefits of hospice as early as they might.

Detailed information about hospice can be found at http://www.nahc.org, http://www.cms.gov, and http://hhpco.org.

Durable Medical Equipment

Durable medical equipment (DME) is equipment that enables a person to accommodate a disability and maintain independence. DME encompasses a wide range of devices, from simple walkers and canes to sophisticated wheelchairs and beds. DME is paid for by Medicare, Medicaid, and private insurance under conditions specified by each insurer. It may be rented or purchased, depending on the insurer, the person's condition, and whether the need for the equipment is expected to be short-term or indefinite. Companies that provide DME are distinct from other health care agencies, but home health agencies will often assist in arranging for DME that is needed by a person to remain in his or her own home while receiving home care services. DME is an important component of the continuum of care because it enables people with disabilities who might otherwise be dependent on others for assistance to maintain their independence. Detailed information about Medicare's DME provisions can be found at http://cms.gov/center/dme.asp.

Outreach

Outreach programs make health and social services readily available in the community rather than within the formidable walls of a large institution. Health fairs at community events, senior membership programs, emergency response systems, nurse practitioners stationed by health care systems in senior housing complexes, and vans for transportation to medical appointments are all forms of outreach. They are targeted at those who are living in the community for the purpose of keeping them connected with the health care system.

Many outreach programs are provided at no or low charge to the consumer. They may be paid for by a hospital, medical group, managed care company, or other health care organization as a community benefit or a loss leader to market other services. Regardless of the purpose, clients identified through outreach activities should ideally be linked back to the organization's core businesses for purposes of continuity of care.

Wellness

Wellness programs span a wide spectrum from activities provided for those who are basically healthy

and want to stay that way by actively engaging in health promotion to disease management for those with chronic illnesses who want to remain as healthy as possible. Wellness programs include health education classes, exercise programs, health screenings, and disease management regimes offered at health care sites or to be used at home.

Wellness activities may be provided at no or low charge to the client. With a few notable exceptions, wellness activities are not paid for by third-party payers. They tend to be provided free of charge as a public relations tool or because the organization offering the activity appreciates that they will save money on providing care if they can help someone stay healthy.

Disease management (DM) programs have become pervasive and sophisticated in recent years. They are one method for empowering consumers who have diagnosed health problems to control their condition so they do not become severely ill. DM programs may also be structured so that they are a means of facilitating clients with access to the services clients need, when they need them. Health plans and medical groups have been prominent proponents of disease management and often bear the costs.

Housing

Housing is an integral component of the continuum of care, because a person's housing situation affects his or her functional independence and health status, and vice versa. For example, a woman who lives in two-story house in New England with front steps that have no railing might slip on the ice and break her hip. She may not be able to go home from the hospital as soon as possible because she cannot negotiate the front steps or access the bathroom on the second floor. In contrast, a women who lives in a one-story Southern California bungalow with a flat path from the driveway to the house might not slip on the ice in the first place and, if she did break her hip for other reasons, could go home from the hospital more quickly and easily because indoor and outdoor access are all on one level and inclement weather is not likely to inhibit egress mobility.

Housing accommodations for long-term care range from modifying existing independent housing to independent apartments with support services to formal assisted living (with support services incorporated into the building and the pricing) to group homes. Services may be available within a community, such as within continuing care requirement communities (CCRCs) or naturally occurring retirement communities (NORCs); within a facility, such as within independent apartment buildings; or within a person's home, such as board and care homes. Various levels of housing are defined by states, and are typically licensed under housing or social service agencies, not as health care providers. In 2006, the United States had approximately 39,500 assisted living facilities and 2,240 continuing care retirement communities (American Association of Homes and Services for the Aging, 2007).

Payment for housing is usually the responsibility of the individual. In a few states, Medicaid pays for assisted living as a less-expensive alternative to nursing home care, and group homes for the developmentally disabled or mentally ill may be paid for by Medicaid or a state mental health program. Recognizing the frailty of populations served by some types of housing, assisted living facilities may be accredited by either the Joint Commission or CARF.

Despite its close relationship to health status, housing operates for the most part in a different sphere of licensing, regulation, and financing. This separation often poses challenges for those who need integration of housing and health care in order to manage long-term care needs optimally. Two websites pertaining to assisted living are http://www.aahsa.org and http://www.alfa.org.

Characteristics of Major Services

These categories encompass more than 60 distinct services. Each service has its own operating characteristics. Table 9.3 summarizes select operating characteristics of a few of the major services.

The differences pose challenges to organizations and individuals in attempting to manage care in a unified way, as well as to clinicians in attempting to achieve continuity of care across settings and over time for clients. Differences in financing, licensing, regulatory enforcement, and accreditation all pose structural barriers to integration. The integrating mechanisms, described next, are deliberate management actions that can be taken to facilitate clinical integration of the care for the individual client.

INTEGRATING MECHANISMS

From a client's perspective, the many services of the continuum should be seamlessly connected. Multiple services might be used at the same time, and they should be coordinated. Changes in service over time, due to a change in the client's condition, should be accomplished with a smooth transition and a flow of essential information from one provider to the other. Payment should not inhibit access to services.

In reality, at the present time in the U.S. health care delivery system, services are highly fragmented. Access is limited by payment constraints, availability of select services in some geographic areas, capacity of available services, limited health care personnel, and other factors. Moreover, because services have evolved in an individualistic manner, services are not automatically integrated. Thus, to accomplish the seamlessness that is important to a client's care, formal structural integrating mechanisms are essential. The conceptual framework of the continuum of care includes four basic integrating mechanisms, described next.

Inter-Entity Structure and Management

Integrated management of services must be structured both within an organization and across organizations. Client services are not likely to be

Table 9.3. Sample Operating Characteristics of Select Services

Service	Staffing	Top Payers	Licensing	Accreditation*
Skilled nursing facility	1 RN/shift; LVNs, Aides	Medicaid; private	By state department of health	Joint Commission
Home health, Medicare certified	RN, PT, OT, SP, MSW, HHA	Medicare; commercial insurance; other government	By state department of health	Joint Commission CHAP
Home care, private	On-call staff, professional or support persons	Private pay; commercial insurance; government but not Medicare	May be only local business license	Regional
Hospice	Interdisciplinary team of professionals led by MD	Medicare; all insurers	May be separate or part of health organization	Joint Commission CHAP
Adult day services	Activity director, aides, may or may not have skilled professionals	Private pay; Medicaid; Fund-raising	Varies by state; may be only business license, state health department, or state social services	CARF
Assisted living	Personal care staff	Private pay (Medicaid in a few states)	State housing department; varies by state	Joint Commission CARF
CORF	Rehabilitation therapists	Medicare; commercial insurance	By state health department	CARF
Meals on Wheels	Volunteers	Older Americans Act	Not licensed	None

*CARF—Commission on Accreditation of Rehabilitation Facilities.
CHAP—Community Health Accreditation Program.

coordinated unless the units that are providing the services are coordinated administratively, particularly when budgeting and financial issues arise. For example, a person with a hip fracture may be cared for by the emergency department of a hospital, acute care inpatient unit of the same or a different hospital, skilled nursing facility, rehabilitation hospital or unit, home health agency, Medicare-certified home health agency, private home care agency, and durable medical equipment company. Even when all these services are within the same parent organization, the client with fee-for-service insurance will fill out admission papers eight different times, deal with eight different sets of clinicians and

administrators, and receive bills from eight or more distinct provider entities. (A person with managed-care insurance may have a somewhat less complicated experience, but most managed-care plans don't cover long-term care, so fragmentation is the most common model.)

Administrative structures are necessary for a continuum of care to (1) ensure channels of communication and cooperation; (2) establish clear lines of authority, accountability, and responsibility for client services; (3) negotiate budgets and financial trade-offs; (4) address issues of risk management and liability; (5) gather and share data efficiently; and (6) present a cohesive, consistent message in interactions with the patient, external agencies, and the community.

Administrative mechanisms within an organization that promote seamless functioning of a continuum of care include

- a designated senior administrator responsible for decisions that affect several different departments or units.

- an integrated budget that recognizes the contribution of each unit to the performance of the whole, including losses in one unit that produce larger gains in another unit.

- interdepartmental/interentity planning and management teams and committees that cut across services.

- interdisciplinary and interdepartmental task forces focusing on specific short-term issues, including planning new programs or solving operating problems.

- product line management or a matrix structure that spans internal and external service units organized as a continuum of care from the patient perspective.

- contracts articulating transfer agreements.

Management integration is at least in part driven by public policy at the federal, state, and local levels. In efforts to streamline long-term care, several states have enacted programs to reduce the fragmented regulations that often produce lack of access to care and the resulting frustration and poor quality. State efforts have focused on reducing barriers to access caused by removing conflicting eligibility criteria, creating a single entry point or single assessment form, and incorporating funding from several distinct streams into one.

Care Coordination

The clinical care for a person with long-term, multifaceted illness is ideally coordinated over time, across settings, and among various professionals. Quality is enhanced when information is communicated among all the professionals caring for a person, and efficiencies are achieved when duplication of services is avoided. Several techniques have evolved for coordinating clinical care, including case management, interdisciplinary teams, clinical liaisons, single-entry access points, extended care pathways, and some disease management programs.

The most common form of care coordination is case management. Over time this has evolved into a fairly standard process with the following elements (White, 2005):

- case identification

- assessment

- care planning

- service arrangement

- monitoring

- reassessment

The purpose of case management is to have a single individual professional work directly with clients and families over time to assist them in arranging and managing the complex set of resources that the client requires to maintain health and independent functioning. Ideally, the case manager guides the client and family through the maze of services, matches service need with funding authorization and availability, coordinates with clinicians, negotiates with payers, and facilitates changes as the client's needs change over time.

A case manager may be a nurse, social worker, or health care professional trained specifically as a case manager. The range of a case manager's authority varies from the ideal comprehensive role based on the organizational auspice of the case manager and who is paying for this service. Case management is paid for by some third-party payers, by individuals and families, or by a combination. Medicare pays for case management only for highly specialized services. Medicaid and other government sources vary by state and locality but often cover limited case management for those with long-term care needs. Private pay for case management is now so common that associations of private case managers have grown to national presence.

Interdisciplinary teams are another mechanism for coordinating clinical care; these are typical of rehabilitation and hospice programs. As noted earlier, disease management has grown markedly over the past decade and is a structured way of empowering the individual to monitor and coordinate his or her own care with the support of self-help tools backed up by access to professionals.

The cost-effectiveness of care coordination programs has been well documented. Nonetheless, they are often perceived as additional, rather than core services and may not be accessed until the complexity of a person's care overwhelms the individual or family.

Integrated Information Systems

Information systems that compile data over time and across settings are essential for efficient management of the care of individuals with complex and chronic illnesses and the management of organizations. To implement quality assurance and utilization review programs, assess efficiency of operations, track and aggregate client experiences, and calculate the long-term costs of care, comprehensive and integrated data systems and accompanying management reporting systems are imperative. Nonetheless, the United States is only now on the verge of developing and implementing the information systems technology to provide adequate data for long-term care client management. Many health and social service agencies still maintain separate clinical, financial, and management information and reporting systems. Moreover, many small community agencies that are critical providers of long-term care support services do not yet have automated clinical records, let alone ones integrated within the organization, and are far from being able to integrate automated information across organizations.

The financing of long-term care, to be discussed later, cannot evolve until more predictable information is available on the financial costs of care over time and the interaction effect of multiple support services. This type of expansive information over time cannot be achieved until integrated information systems are in place in more organizations and communities. Conceptually, comprehensive information could be maintained by the health care provider, the insurer, or the patient himself.

Computer technology advances that enable storing great quantities of information in small and inexpensive devices and the exponential growth in the availability of the Internet make it possible for providers and consumers alike to maintain computerized health records. Yet, for comprehensive information about the use of services across settings and over time to occur, many providers must be willing to automate their records and use a common format. Privacy concerns and regulations, many implemented by the Health Insurance Privacy and Accountability Act, must be incorporated into a secure means of sharing information. Several forefront activities show great progress toward eventual access to comprehensive, integrated automated health information.

Electronic health records (EHR) are not new but have not yet replaced the prevalence of paper records, despite great advances in computer technology during the past two decades. A movement to speed up adoption of computerized medical records received a national push in 2003 when the president of the United States declared as a federal goal that all citizens should have an electronic health record and then appointed a physician leader as the National Coordinator of Health Information Technology. This attention, along with federal funding, helped bring experts together to determine both content and electronic details for a standardized electronic health record. However, consensus on content has not yet been achieved, and implementation remains the decision and cost of each individual organization.

Regional health information systems (RHIOS) are another advancement that had an earlier life in the form of community health networks. RHIOS, which are collaboratives of private or private and public providers, are being promoted as a way to create the organizational infrastructure needed to bring health organizations within a community together to share health-related information across settings and over time.

Meanwhile, government initiatives by Medicare (adding prescription drug coverage) and Medicaid (continued expansion to managed-care models) may provide unanticipated benefits in enabling access to aggregate and individual data pertaining to the use of health care services by the chronically ill.

Integrated Financing

The financing of long-term care is responsible for the availability of so many services as well as the fragmented way in which the services of the continuum operate. There is no single category of expenditures denoted in federal or state budgets as "long-term care," nor is there a single source of payment. Financial information about long-term care is thus a mosaic of pieces from which to infer the total picture. Table 9.4 shows the expenditures for two types of long-term care, nursing home and home care, as categories of national data on Personal Health Expenditures. As is evident, costs for these two types of services have expanded over time. The magnitude of the costs of long-term care would appear significantly greater if the costs for the full spectrum of continuum services were included and if hospital and physician expenditures were differentiated between acute care and chronic care.

Two perspectives on financing are useful: the service perspective, that is, from whom a provider gets paid, and the payer perspective, that is, what services each source covers.

Who Pays?

Table 9.5 shows just a few of the numerous sources that pay for long-term care, reflecting in part the array of clients described earlier and the public policies driven by advocacy groups that provide resources for specific client populations. Medicaid is the largest single third-party payer of long-term care. Covered services vary by state and even locality but include at minimum nursing home care, home care, durable medical equipment, hospice, and in some states, assisted living and adult day services. Other public programs that provide and/or pay for select long-term care services are Veterans Affairs, Title XX of the Social Security Act, the Aging Network established by the Older Americans Act, state and local mental health services, Ryan White Act (AIDS/HIV), and numerous others. Each public program has specific regulations that cover who is eligible for services and what services can be provided.

In addition to public program support, many individuals pay out-of-pocket for long-term care. For example, nursing home care is the largest single category of long-term care expenditures, and about one-fourth is paid by individuals and their families. Except for a few state Medicaid programs, almost all assisted living is paid for directly by individuals. Other long-term care services that are heavily paid for directly by consumers include private home care, adult day services, and the array of support services engaged by caregivers to help them care for loved ones.

Contrary to what many people believe, Medicare was intended to cover short-term acute episodes of

Table 9.4. Selected National Health Expenditures: United States, 1960–2002 (amount in billions)

Expenditure	1960	1970	1980	1990	2000	2004
Personal health care	$23.3	$62.9	$215.3	$607.5	$1,139.9	$1,560.2
Home health care	0.1	0.2	2.4	12.6	30.6	43.2
Nursing home care	0.9	4.0	19.0	52.6	95.3	115.2

From *National Health Care Expenditures by Type of Expenditure: United States, 1960–2004* (DHHS Pub. No. 2006-1232) (Table 123), retrieved May 19, 2007, from http://cdc.gov/nchs/hus.htm.

Table 9.5. Select Major Federal Government Programs Paying for Various Long-Term Care Services*

Program	Services Covered
Medicare**	Skilled nursing—100 days only
	Home care—skilled only
	Hospice
	LTC hospital
	Rehabilitation
	Mental health
Medicaid	Skilled nursing
	Home care—skilled or support care
	Hospice
	Rehabilitation therapies
	Mental health
	Adult day health care
	Assisted living (some states only)
	Case Management
Veterans Affairs	Skilled nursing
	Home care
	Hospice
	Rehabilitation therapies
	Mental health
	Adult day care
	Respite
Older American Act	Congregate meals
	Meals on Wheels
	Homemaker
	Case management
Title XX	Home care
	Chore service

*Not intended to be complete; illustrative only.
**Assumes short-term prognosis of improvement.

care, and by law, excludes coverage of services for prolonged illness. To be eligible for standard Medicare services, the patient must have a prognosis of improvement or recovery. The majority of people who are eligible for Medicare are either over age 65 or are legally disabled. Medicare is thus faced with creating an artificial distinction of providing acute care for the purposes of "cure" to people with chronic illnesses. In recent years, Medicare has recognized that this distinction is unrealistic and ineffective. The Medicare Prescription Drug and Modernization Act of 2003 (MMA) recognized the need to restructure the legislation to match client needs more appropriately. The MMA now pays for prescription drugs, a particular asset to those with chronic conditions, as well as increased screenings for prevention and health maintenance. When first passed, the MMA also included demonstration projects for disease management and chronic care coordination. Nonetheless, Medicare still has strict limits on its authority to pay for nursing home care, home care, assisted living, adult day services, and most other long-term care services.

Commercial health insurance companies and managed care health plans tend to follow Medicare. They may cover more than Medicare in select program areas, but they tend to be legislatively mandated by state or federal authorities to pay for services associated with acute episodes of care rather than chronic care.

How Do Services Get Paid?

Figure 9.3 shows major payers for select services of the continuum. As is evident, any given service may have several distinct payment sources; furthermore, payers and payment details vary in each geographic locality. This makes management extremely difficult for the individual client, as well as for the provider organizations. Moreover, the fragmented payment system and the detailed regulations that accompany each law inhibit creating a single national policy on long-term care or a single template for long-term care management.

In addition to funding difference services, payment sources affect how a provider operates. All the organizations that participate in the Medicare program must comply with the Conditions of Participations (CoP). Medicare has also implemented specific payment systems that complicate the ability for a provider to combine the costs for a single patient. As a result of the Balanced Budget Act of 1997, Medicare payment mechanisms for providers other than hospitals and physicians were connected

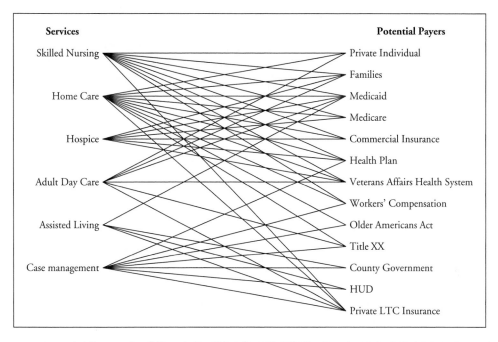

Figure 9.3. Potential Payers for Select Long-Term Care Services

SOURCE: Adapted from "Training Modules for Geriatrics," n.d., U.S. Department of Health and Human Services.

to specific patient assessment tools. These tools serve to limit financing, information sharing, and care across settings, as each service is required to use a different metric to measure client health status and progress. Moreover, Medicare payment systems are continually being revised and refined, making trend data on individuals or groups all the more difficult to track. Table 9.6 shows the name of the payment systems and the accompanying assessment tools as of 2007.

Models of Integrated Financing

Fragmented financing results in fragmented care, particularly when the payment sources have strict eligibility criteria that inhibit clients from accessing the services they need when they need them or payment systems that must be maintained separately. Under the ideal concept of the continuum of care, financial resources would be pooled so that neither the amount nor the restrictions of payment for care

would prevent a person from getting the care they need to manage an illness effectively over time. Despite the barriers to integrating financing from multiple streams, a few examples demonstrate that integrated financing is both possible and cost-effective.

Federal Initiatives. Under Medicare, the federal government established the Social HMOs (S/HMOs), the Program of All-Inclusive Care for the Elderly (PACE), and hospice. Each program targets a different client group but has the legislative authority to blend financing streams or to offer service based on client need rather than regulatory restrictions. All have demonstrated enhanced quality of care and cost-effectiveness compared to care under regular fee-for-service payment systems. PACE and hospice have been incorporated into core Medicare programs; the Social HMO program is being phased out over time.

Table 9.6. Medicare Payment Systems, by Service

Service	Patient Assessment	Classification*	Payment System**
Hospital	Discharge diagnosis data	Diagnostic related groups (DRGs)	IPPS
Inpatient psychiatry	Discharge diagnosis data (only specific conditions qualify)	Diagnostic related groups (DRGs) (1 of 15)	IPF PPS
Rehabilitation	Patient assessment instrument (IRF PAI) (only specific conditions qualify)	Case mix groups	IRF PPS
Long-term care hospital	Discharge diagnosis data	Long-term care hospital diagnostic related groups (LTCH DRGs)	LTCH PPS
Skilled nursing facilities	Minimum data set (MDS)	Resource utilization groups—III (RUGS)	SNF PPS
Home health	Outcome and assessment information set (OASIS)	Home health resource groups (HHRG)	HH PPS

*DRG—Diagnostic related groups. These are a combination of discharge diagnosis, surgery, age, sex, and discharge disposition.

**Prospective payment systems: Inpatient PPS, Inpatient psychiatric facility PPS, Inpatient rehabilitation facility PPS, Long-term care hospital PPS, Skilled nursing facility PPS, Home health PPS.

NOTE: Medicare has yet additional payment systems for various types of ambulatory care services, such as outpatient rehabilitation and outpatient psychiatric services.

Continuing care retirement communities (CCRCs) represent a private model of pooled financing and service. CCRCs provide several levels of housing on the same campus, with a range from entirely independent houses or apartments, to assisted living, to skilled nursing. Home care, chore service, congregate housing with meals, transportation, and other support services may also be available. Physician and hospital care are not typically components of the CCRC service package. Individuals pay a substantial entry fee to buy into the CCRC, with supplemental fees typically charged for additional services and paid directly to the CCRC who is the provider or pays the providers. Long-term care, Medicare supplement, or other health insurance may be required for entry. The CCRC arranges service delivery and coordinates on-site services. CCRCs target the middle- to upper-economic-class clientele. They establish financial ability to pay for services as a requirement for admission and then assist the residents in accessing the services they need when they need them.

LONG-TERM CARE POLICY

The United States has no single public policy on long-term care per se. Rather, a myriad of policies at federal, state, and local levels impact care for specific target populations or select components of the health care delivery system. Table 9.7 is a short list of some of the many federal policies pertaining to long-term care.

Table 9.7. Major Federal Legislation Pertaining to Long-Term Care

Social Security Act, 1935
Veterans Administration, 1963, 1972, 1975, 1980
Mental Health Acts, 1963, 1967, 1971, 1986
Title XVIII (Medicare), Social Security Act, 1965
Title XIX (Medicaid), Social Security Act, 1965
Older Americans Act, 1965, 2001
Housing and Urban Development Act, 1965, 1974
Developmental Disabilities Services and Facilities Act, 1970
Title XVI (Supplemental Security Income), Social Security Act, 1972
Rehabilitation Act, 1973
Title XX, Social Security Act, 1974
Omnibus Budget Reconciliation Act, 1987
Medicare Catastrophic Coverage Act, 1988 (repealed, 1990)
Americans with Disabilities Act, 1990
Patient Self-Determination Act, 1991
Family Medical Leave Act, 1993
Health Insurance Portability and Accountability Act, 1996
Balanced Budget Act, 1997
National Caregiver Support Act, 2000
Ryan White Care Act, 1990, reauthorized 2000
Medicare Prescription Drug, Improvement, and Modernization Act, 2003
Olmstead vs. *L.C.,* 1999 (Supreme Court decision)

SOURCE: From *The Continuum of Long-Term Care,* 3rd Ed., by C. Evashwick (Ed.), 2005, Albany, NY: Delmar Publishers.

Legislation tends to have one (or more) of four major thrusts:

- Direct payment for services (such as Medicare for those age 65 and older).

- Regulations (such as the Balanced Budget Acts of 1997 and 1999).

- Creation of resources (such as the Hill-Burton or Health Manpower Act).

- Direct provision of service (such as the acts creating the hospitals and services provided by Veterans Affairs).

Different advocacy groups have, at different times, lobbied for different types of legislation. The piecemeal approach to public policy to date has produced the fragmented long-term care delivery system that currently exists in the United States. The lack of coordination across services has created the imperative for the four integrating mechanisms that are essential to achieving coordination of care from the perspective of the individual client.

Despite an array of federal laws pertaining to various aspects of long-term care, overall, long-term care is primarily an issue dealt with by state governments. States have recognized the detrimental impact of fragmentation on the quality of care provided to individuals and on the cost to government. Several states have thus implemented systems to streamline their long-term care service delivery. Wisconsin, for example, has long had a single entry point, uniform assessment and case management system that brings together health, social services, and mental health programs. The Robert Wood Johnson Foundation sponsored a nationwide program in the late 1990s that promoted coordination of care at the state level for those with chronic illnesses, particularly for those receiving Medicaid. Efforts to achieve coordination through government programs are likely to continue, but at local, rather than national levels. For the foreseeable future, the individual and family will remain those ultimately responsible for coordinating the long-term care of a person with chronic illness and functional disability.

SUMMARY

The services available to provide assistance to those with long-term disabilities and chronic conditions have grown significantly during the past three decades. However, the population needing long-term care has also grown, and the greatest burst of expansion is anticipated with the aging of the Baby Boom generation. As a nation, the United States is not prepared to provide extensive long-term care that is efficient, effective, and affordable. The challenges to clinicians, administrators, policy makers, and payers demand attention. Nonetheless, they pale in contrast to the challenges faced by families and individuals trying to orchestrate and pay for long-term care on a daily basis.

The following summarizes the current state of long-term care in the United States.

1. Managing a seamless continuum of care is challenging from the perspective of the individual client due to fragmentation of services, different eligibility criteria, and varying payment streams.

2. Managing the continuum of services is difficult for an organization due to the need to coordinate with external organizations and even to coordinate internally.

3. Public policy is not likely to provide any overarching continuity for long-term care in the near future. Meanwhile, federal, state, and local policies are likely to continue to change, requiring constant reorientation of management procedures and policies.

4. The portending swell of people with chronic conditions and multigeneration caregiver needs will add stress to the system.

5. The current and future shortage of health care personnel will add further challenge of long-term care services, which are heavily manpower-intense.

6. LTC services will continue to evolve individually, with emphasis on quality of care, evidence-based performance, and financial viability.

7. Individuals must be engaged in personal planning and policy dialogue in order to forge a better system for the future. Health care executives should thus address their own personal actions and promote personal planning by employees as models and as a basis for knowledge that can be shared with clients.

REVIEW QUESTIONS

1. Describe the continuum of care framework.
2. What is long-term care?
3. Who needs long-term care?
4. Describe and differentiate the roles of hospitals and nursing homes in providing long-term care.
5. Explain the contributions and drawbacks of adult day services.
6. Contrast home health agencies certified by Medicare and private home health agencies.
7. Delineate the components of hospice care and the patients served by hospice.
8. Define the four basic integrating mechanisms and explain why they are essential to achieving a seamless continuum of care.
9. Critique the current state of long-term care policy in the United States.

REFERENCES & ADDITIONAL READINGS

American Association of Homes and Services for the Aging. (2007). *Aging services: The facts*. Retrieved May 17, 2007, from http://www.aahsa.org.

American Health Care Association. http://www.ahca.org.

American Hospital Association. (2007a). *Fast facts*. Retrieved May 16, 2007, from http://www.aha.org.

American Hospital Association. (2007b). *Trendwatch chartbook 2007*. Chart 3.12. Chicago: American Hospital Association.

Assisted Living Facilities of America. http://www.alfa.org.

Centers for Medicare and Medicaid Services. (2007). *The chart series chartbook 2007*. Table 1.11. Retrieved May 14, 2007, from http://www.cms.hhs.gov.

Cox, Nancy. (2006). *Lessons learned: Sustainability of Partners in Caregiving: The Adult Day Services Program*. Princeton, NJ: The Robert Wood Johnson Foundation.

Evashwick, C. (1987). Definition of the continuum of care. In C. Evashwick, & Weiss, L. (Eds.), *Managing the continuum of care.* Gaithersburg, MD: Aspen Publishers.

Evashwick, C. (Ed.) (2005). *The Continuum of Long-Term Care.* Albany, NY: Delmar Publishers.

Hoffman, C., Rice, D. P., & Sung, H. Y. (1996). Persons with chronic conditions: Their prevalence and costs, *Journal of the American Medical Association, 276*(18), 1473–1479.

Hospice Association of America. (2007). *Hospice facts and statistics.* Retrieved May 17, 2007, from http://www.nahc.org/facts.

Katz, S., Ford, A., Moskowitz, R., Jackson, B., & Jaffe, M. (1963). Studies of illness in the aged. *Journal of the American Medical Association, 185,* 914–919.

Lawton, M. P., & Brody, E. M. (1969). Assessment of older people; Self-maintaining and instrumental activities of daily living. *The Gerontologist, 9,* 179–186.

Lu, S., & Green, A. (2000). *Projection of chronic illness and cost inflation.* Santa Monica, CA: Rand.

National Adult Day Services Association. (2007). *Adult day services: The facts.* Retrieved May 27, 2007, from http://www.nadsa.org.

National Association for Home Care. *Home care and Hospice facts.* Retrieved May 17, 2007, from http://www.nahc.org.

National Center for Health Statistics (NCHS). (2005). *Health, United States, 2005.* Table 56. Hyattsville, MD: U.S. Department of Health and Human Services.

National Center for Health Statistics. (2007). *Definitions.* Retrieved May 21, 2007, from http://www.nehs.gov/definitions.

National Hospice and Palliative Care Organization. http://www.nhpco.org.

White, Monika. (2005). Case management. In C. Evashwick (Ed.), *The continuum of long-term care.* Albany, NY: Delmar Publishers.

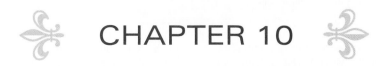

CHAPTER 10

Mental and Behavioral Health Services*

Stephen J. Williams and Paul R. Torrens

CHAPTER TOPICS

- Origins of Mental Health
- The Fundamentals of Mental Health
- Types of Mental Illness
- Epidemiology of Mental Illness
- Organization and Financing of Mental Health Services
- Mental Health Financing
- The Future of Mental Health Services

LEARNING OBJECTIVES

Upon completing this chapter, the reader should be able to

1. Understand the basis for defining mental health services.
2. Appreciate the history of mental health.
3. Assess the epidemiology of mental health.
4. Understand the various settings and arrangements for delivering mental health services.
5. Appreciate the financing issues in mental health.
6. Assess present and future challenges in mental health.

*Chapter adapted from *Mental Health: A Report of the Surgeon General—Executive Summary,* Rockville, MD: U.S. Department of Health and Human Services, 1999, and websites of Substance Abuse and Mental Health Services Administration, Center for Mental Health Services, National Institutes of Health, and National Institute of Mental Health.

The nation's contemporary mental health enterprise, like the broader field of health, is rooted in a population-based public health model. The public health model is characterized by concern for the health of a population in its entirety and by awareness of the linkage between health and the physical and psychosocial environment. This chapter describes mental health services and systems in the United States. Definitions and historical perspectives on mental health, delivery systems, and many complex issues are discussed. Examples of various mental and behavioral illnesses are described to illustrate the complex and evolving nature of these conditions.

Many ingredients of mental health may be identifiable, but mental health is not easy to define. What it means to be mentally healthy is subject to many different interpretations that are rooted in value judgments that may vary across cultures.

Mental illness is the term that refers collectively to all diagnosable mental disorders. Mental disorders are health conditions that are characterized by alterations in thinking, mood, or behavior (or some combination thereof) associated with distress and/or impaired functioning. Alzheimer's disease exemplifies a mental disorder largely marked by alterations in thinking (especially forgetting). Depression exemplifies a mental disorder largely marked by alterations in mood. Attention-deficit/hyperactivity disorder exemplifies a mental disorder largely marked by alterations in behavior (over activity) and/or thinking (inability to concentrate).

Considering health and illness as points along a continuum helps one appreciate that neither state exists in pure isolation from the other. In another, but related, context, everyday language tends to encourage a misperception that "mental health" or "mental illness" is unrelated to "physical health" or "physical illness." In fact, the two are inseparable.

Seventeenth-century philosopher René Descartes conceptualized the distinction between the mind and the body. He viewed the "mind" as completely separable from the "body" (or "matter" in general). The mind (and spirit) was seen as the concern of organized religion, whereas the body was seen as the concern of physicians.

Instead of dividing physical from mental health, the more appropriate and neutral distinction is between "mental" and "somatic" health. Somatic is a medical term that derives from the Greek word *soma* for "body." Mental health refers to the successful performance of mental functions in terms of thought, mood, and behavior. Mental disorders are those health conditions in which alterations in mental functions are paramount. Somatic conditions are those in which alterations in nonmental functions predominate. While the brain carries out all mental functions, it also carries out some somatic functions, such as movement, touch, and balance. That is why not all brain diseases are mental disorders. For example, a stroke causes a lesion in the brain that may produce disturbances of movement, such as paralysis of limbs. When such symptoms predominate in a patient, the stroke is considered a somatic condition. But when a stroke mainly produces alterations of thought, mood, or behavior, it is considered a mental condition (e.g., dementia). The point is that a brain disease can be seen as a mental disorder or a somatic disorder depending on the functions it perturbs.

ORIGINS OF MENTAL HEALTH

Stigmatization of people with mental disorders has persisted throughout history. It is manifested by bias, distrust, stereotyping, fear, embarrassment, anger, and/or avoidance. Stigma leads others to avoid living, socializing, or working with, renting to, or employing people with mental disorders. It reduces patients' access to resources and opportunities (e.g., housing, jobs) and leads to low self-esteem, isolation, and hopelessness. It deters the public from seeking, and wanting to pay for, care. Explanations for stigma stem, in part, from the misguided split between mind and body first proposed by Descartes. Another source of stigma lies in the nineteenth century separation of the mental health treatment system in the United States from the mainstream of health.

In colonial times in the United States, people with mental illness were described as "lunatics" and were largely cared for by families. There was no concerted effort to treat mental illness until urbanization in the early nineteenth century created a societal problem that had previously been relegated to families scattered among small rural communities. Social policy assumed the form of isolated asylums where persons with mental illness were administered the reigning treatments of the era. Throughout the history of institutionalization in asylums (later renamed mental hospitals), reformers strove to improve treatment and curtail abuse. Several waves of reform culminated in the deinstitutionalization movement that began in the 1950s with the goal of shifting patients and care to the community.

In the 1950s, the public viewed mental illness as a stigmatized condition and displayed an unscientific understanding of mental illness. The public was not particularly skilled at distinguishing mental illness from ordinary unhappiness and worry and tended to see only extreme forms of behavior—namely psychosis—as mental illness. Mental illness carried great social stigma, especially linked with fear of unpredictable and violent behavior.

By the mid-1990s Americans had achieved greater scientific understanding of mental illness. But the increases in knowledge did not defuse social stigma. The public learned to define mental illness and to distinguish it from ordinary worry and unhappiness. It expanded its definition of mental illness to encompass anxiety, depression, and other mental disorders. The public attributed mental illness to a mix of biological abnormalities and vulnerabilities to social and psychological stress.

There is likely no simple or single panacea to eliminate the stigma associated with mental illness. Overall approaches to stigma reduction involve programs of advocacy, public education, and contact with persons with mental illness through schools and other societal institutions. Another way to eliminate stigma is to find causes and effective treatments for mental disorders. History suggests this to be true. When pellagra was traced to a nutrient deficiency, and nutritional supplementation with niacin was introduced, the condition was eventually eradicated in the developed world. Pellagra's victims with delirium had been placed in mental hospitals early in the twentieth century before its etiology was clarified.

Ironically, the mental health field was adversely affected when causes and treatments were identified. As advances were achieved, each condition was transferred from mental health to another medical specialty. For instance, dominion over syphilis was moved to dermatology, internal medicine, and neurology upon advances in etiology and treatment. Dominion over hormone-related mental disorders was moved to endocrinology under similar circumstances. The mental health field became the repository for mental disorders whose etiology was unknown. Yet the stigma surrounding *other* mental disorders not only persists but may also be inadvertently reinforced by leaving to mental health care only those behavioral conditions without known causes or cures.

When people understand that mental disorders are not the result of moral failings or limited will power but are legitimate illnesses that are responsive to specific treatments, much of the negative stereotyping may dissipate. As stigma abates, a transformation in public attitudes should occur. People should become eager to seek care. They should become more willing to absorb its cost. And, most importantly, they should become far more receptive to the messages that mental health and mental illness are part of the mainstream of health, and they are a concern for all.

THE FUNDAMENTALS OF MENTAL HEALTH

The past 25 years have been marked by several discrete, defining trends in the mental health field. These have included the extraordinary pace and productivity of scientific research on the brain and behavior; the introduction of a range of effective treatments for most mental disorders; a dramatic transformation of our society's approaches to the organization and financing of mental health care; and the emergence of powerful consumer and family movements.

The brain has emerged as the central focus for studies of mental health and mental illness. New scientific disciplines, technologies, and insights have begun to weave a seamless picture of the way in which the brain mediates the influence of biological, psychological, and social factors on human thought, behavior, and emotion in health and in illness. Molecular and cellular biology and molecular genetics, which are complemented by sophisticated cognitive and behavioral sciences, are preeminent research disciplines in the contemporary neuroscience of mental health.

These disciplines are affording unprecedented opportunities for "bottom-up" studies of the brain. This term refers to research that is examining the workings of the brain at the most fundamental levels. Studies focus, for example, on the complex neurochemical activity that occurs within individual nerve cells, or neurons, to process information; on the properties and roles of proteins that are expressed, or produced, by a person's genes; and on the interaction of genes with diverse environmental influences. All these activities are now understood, with increasing clarity, to underlie learning, memory, the experience of emotion, and, when these processes go awry, the occurrence of mental illness or a mental health problem.

Equally important to the mental health field is "top-down" research; here, as the term suggests, the aim is to understand the broader behavioral context of the brain's cellular and molecular activity and to learn how individual neurons work together in well-delineated neural circuits to perform mental functions.

As information accumulates about the basic workings of the brain, it is the task of translational research to transfer new knowledge into clinically relevant questions and targets of research opportunity—

to discover, for example, what specific properties of a neural circuit might make it receptive to safer, more effective medications. To elaborate on this example, theories derived from knowledge about basic brain mechanisms are being wedded more closely to brain imaging tools such as functional magnetic resonance imaging (MRI) that can observe actual brain activity. Such a collaboration would permit investigators to monitor the specific protein molecules intended as the "targets" of a new medication to treat a mental illness or, indeed, to determine how to optimize the effect on the brain of the learning achieved through psychotherapy.

In its entirety, the new "integrative neuroscience" of mental health offers a way to circumvent the antiquated split between the mind and the body that has historically hampered mental health research. It also makes it possible to examine scientifically many of the important psychological and behavioral theories regarding normal development and mental illness that have been developed in years past. The unswerving goal of mental health research is to develop and refine clinical treatments as well as preventive interventions that are based on an understanding of specific mechanisms that can contribute to, or lead to, illness but can also protect and enhance mental health.

Mental health clinical research encompasses studies that involve human participants, conducted, for example, to test the efficacy of a new treatment. A noteworthy feature of contemporary clinical research is the new emphasis being placed on studying the effectiveness of interventions in actual practice settings. Information obtained from such studies increasingly provides the foundation for services research concerned with the cost, cost-effectiveness, and "deliverability" of interventions and the design— including economic considerations—of service delivery systems.

The multifaceted complexity of the brain is fully consistent with the fact that it supports all behavior and mental life. Proceeding from an acknowledgment that all psychological experiences are recorded ultimately in the brain and that all psychological phenomena reflect biological processes, the modern neuroscience of mental health offers an enriched understanding of the inseparability of human experience, brain, and mind. Mental functions, which are disturbed in mental disorders, are mediated by the brain. In the process of transforming human experience into physical events, the brain undergoes changes in its cellular structure and function. Few lesions or physiologic abnormalities define the mental disorders, and for the most part their causes remain unknown. Mental disorders, instead, are defined by signs, symptoms, and functional impairments. Diagnoses of mental disorders made using specific criteria are as reliable as those for general medical disorders.

TYPES OF MENTAL ILLNESS

Mental disorders are common in the United States and internationally. An estimated 22.1 percent of Americans ages 18 and older suffer from a diagnosable mental disorder in a given year. The more prominent of these illnesses are described in this section and some are listed in Table 10.1.

Depressive Disorders

Depressive disorders encompass major depressive disorder, dysthymic disorder, and bipolar disorder. Bipolar disorder is included because people with this illness have depressive episodes as well as manic episodes. Approximately 18.8 million American adults, or about 9.5 percent of the U.S. population age 18 and older in a given year, have a depressive disorder. Nearly twice as many women as men are affected by a depressive disorder each year. Depressive disorders often co-occur with anxiety disorders and substance abuse. Major depressive disorder is the leading cause of disability in the United States and established market economies worldwide. Symptoms of dysthymic disorder (chronic, mild depression) must persist for at least 2 years in adults (1 year in children) to meet criteria for the diagnosis. About 40 percent of adults with dysthymic disorder also meet criteria for major depressive disorder or bipolar disorder in a given year. Dysthymic disorder often begins in childhood, adolescence, or early adulthood.

The economic cost for a depressive illness is high, but the cost in human suffering cannot be estimated. Depressive illnesses often interfere with normal functioning and cause pain and suffering not only to those who have a disorder, but also to those who care about them. Serious depression can destroy family life as well as the life of the ill person. But much of this suffering is unnecessary. Most people with a depressive illness do not seek treatment, although the great majority—even those whose depression is extremely severe—can be helped. There are now medications and psychosocial therapies such as cognitive/behavioral, "talk" or interpersonal that ease the pain of depression.

Types of Depression

Major depression is manifested by a combination of symptoms that interfere with the ability to work, study, sleep, eat, and enjoy once pleasurable activities. Such a disabling episode of depression may occur only once, but more commonly occurs several times in a lifetime. A less severe type of depression, *dysthymia,* involves long-term, chronic symptoms that do not disable but keep one from functioning well or from feeling good. Many people with dysthymia also experience major depressive episodes at some time in their lives. Another type of depression is *bipolar disorder,* also called manic-depressive illness. Not nearly as prevalent as other forms of depressive disorders, bipolar disorder is characterized by cycling mood changes: severe highs (mania) and lows (depression). Sometimes the mood switches are dramatic and rapid, but most often they are gradual. When in the depressed cycle, an individual can have any or all of the symptoms of a depressive disorder. When in the manic cycle, the individual may be overactive, over-talkative, and have a great deal of energy. Mania often affects thinking, judgment, and social behavior in ways that cause serious problems and embarrassment. Bipolar disorder affects approximately 2.3 million American adults, or about 1.2 percent of the U.S. population age 18 and older in a given

Table 10.1. Prevalence Rates (Percent of Group) for Selected Mental Disorders among Adults, Past 12 Months, *National Health Interview Survey,* **1999**

Demographic Characteristic	Selected Mental Disorder		
	Major Depression	Generalized Anxiety	Panic Attack
Total	6.3	2.8	2.7
Age			
18–24 years	6.5	2.7	2.9
25–44 years	6.6	3.1	3.2
45–64 years	7.2	3.1	2.9
65+ years	3.7	1.5	0.9
Sex			
Male	4.5	1.9	1.7
Female	8.0	3.6	3.6
Race/Ethnicity			
White	6.6	2.8	2.8
Black	6.2	2.6	2.9
Hispanic	4.8	2.9	2.0
Family Income			
$20,000 or more	5.6	2.2	2.4
Less than $20,000	9.5	5.1	3.9
Education			
Less than high school	7.0	3.8	2.9
High school or some college	6.9	2.9	3.1
College graduate	4.1	1.5	1.7
Marital Status			
Married	4.7	2.2	2.1
Divorced/Separated/Widowed	10.2	4.4	3.7
Unmarried/Single	7.3	3.1	3.4

SOURCE: From *Mental Health, United States, 2002* [DHHS Pub. No. (SMA) 3938], by R. W. Manderscheid and M. J. Henderson, eds., 2004, Rockville, MD: Substance Abuse and Mental Health Services Administration.

year. The average age at onset for a first manic episode is the early twenties.

Some types of depression run in families, suggesting that a biological vulnerability can be inherited. This seems to be the case with bipolar disorder. In some families, major depression also seems to occur generation after generation. However, it can also occur in people with no family history of depression. People who low self-esteem, who consistently view themselves and the world with pessimism, or who are readily overwhelmed by stress, are prone to depression. In recent years, researchers have shown that physical changes in the body can be accompanied by mental changes as well. Medical illnesses such as stroke, a heart attack, cancer, Parkinson's diseases, and hormonal disorders can cause depressive illness, making the sick person apathetic and unwilling to care for his or her physical needs, thus prolonging the recovery period. Also, a serious loss, difficult relationship, financial problem, or any stressful (unwelcome or even desired) change in life patterns can trigger a depressive episode. Very often, a combination of genetic, psychological, and environmental factors is involved in the onset of a depressive disorder.

In 2003, 31,484 people died by suicide in the United States. More than 90 percent of people who kill themselves have a diagnosable mental disorder, commonly a depressive disorder or a substance abuse disorder. Four times as many men as women die by suicide; however, women attempt suicide two to three times as often as men.

Women with Depression. Women experience depression about twice as often as men. Many hormonal factors may contribute to the increased rate of depression in women—particularly such factors as menstrual cycle changes, pregnancy, miscarriage, postpartum period, premenopause, and menopause. Many women also face additional stresses such as responsibilities both at work and home, single parenthood, and caring for children and for aging parents.

Men with Depression. Although men are less likely to suffer from depression than women, 3 to 4 million men in the United States are affected by the illness. Men are less likely to admit to depression, and doctors are less likely to suspect it. Men's depression is often masked by alcohol or drugs, or by the socially acceptable habit of working excessively long hours. Depression typically shows up in men not as feeling hopeless and helpless, but as being irritable, angry, and discouraged.

Depression in the Elderly. Depression in the elderly, undiagnosed and untreated, causes needless suffering for the family and for the individual who could otherwise live a fruitful life. When he or she does go to the doctor, the symptoms described are usually physical, for the older person is often reluctant to discuss feelings of hopelessness, sadness, loss of interest in normally pleasurable activities, or extremely prolonged grief after a loss.

Children with Depression. Only in the past two decades has depression in children been taken very seriously. The depressed child may pretend to be sick, refuse to go to school, cling to a parent, or worry that the parent may die. Older children may sulk, get into trouble at school, be negative, be grouchy, and feel misunderstood. Because normal behaviors vary from one childhood stage to another, it can be difficult to tell whether a child is just going through a temporary "phase" or is suffering from depression.

Treatment

The first step to getting appropriate treatment for depression is a physical examination by a physician. Treatment choice will depend on the outcome of the evaluation. There are a variety of antidepressant medications and psychotherapies that can be used to treat depressive disorders. Some people with milder forms may do well with psychotherapy alone. People with moderate to severe depression most often benefit from antidepressants. Most do best with combined treatment: medication to gain relatively quick symptom relief and psychotherapy to learn more effective ways to deal with life's problems, including depression. Electroconvulsive therapy (ECT) is useful, particularly for individuals whose depression is severe or life threatening or who cannot take antidepressant medication. In recent years, ECT has been much improved. A muscle relaxant is given before treatment, which is done under brief anesthesia.

There are several types of antidepressant medications used to treat depressive disorders. These include newer medications—chiefly the selective serotonin reuptake inhibitors (SSRIs)—the tricyclics, and the monoamine oxidase inhibitors (MAOIs). The SSRIs—and other newer medications that affect neurotransmitters such as dopamine or norepinephrine—generally have fewer side effects than tricyclics. Lithium has for many years been the treatment of choice for bipolar disorder, as it can be effective in smoothing out the mood swings common to this disorder. Other mood-stabilizing drugs are anticonvulsants, carbamazepine, and valproate.

In the past few years, much interest has risen in the use of herbs in the treatment of both depression and anxiety. St. John's wort (*Hypericum perforatum*) is an herb used extensively in the treatment of mild to moderate depression in Europe.

Many forms of psychotherapy, including some short-term (10–20 week) therapies, can help depressed individuals gain insight into and resolve their problems through verbal exchange with the therapist. "Behavioral" therapists help patients learn how to obtain more satisfaction and rewards through their own actions and how to unlearn the behavioral patterns that contribute to or result from their depression. Two of the short-term psychotherapies that research has shown helpful for some forms of depression are interpersonal and cognitive/ behavioral therapies. Interpersonal therapists focus on the patient's disturbed personal relationships that both cause and exacerbate (or increase) the depression. Cognitive/behavioral therapists help patients change the negative styles of thinking and behaving often associated with depression. Psychodynamic therapies, which are sometimes used to treat depressed persons, focus on resolving the patient's conflicted feelings. These therapies are often reserved until the depressive symptoms are significantly improved.

Schizophrenia

Approximately 2.2 million American adults, or about 1.1 percent of the population age 18 and older in a given year, have schizophrenia. Schizophrenia is a chronic, severe, and disabling brain disease. Approximately 1 percent of the population develops schizophrenia during their lifetime. Schizophrenia affects men and woman with equal frequency but often appears earlier in men. People with schizophrenia often suffer terrifying symptoms such as hearing internal voices not heard by others, or believing that other people are reading their minds, controlling their thoughts, or plotting to harm them. These symptoms may leave them fearful and withdrawn. Their speech and behavior can be so disorganized that they may be incomprehensible or frightening to others. Most people with schizophrenia continue to suffer some

symptoms throughout their lives; it has been estimated that no more than one in five individuals recovers completely. Research is gradually leading to new and safer medications and unraveling the complex causes of the disease. Schizophrenia is found all over the world. The severity of the symptoms and long-lasting, chronic pattern of schizophrenia often cause a high degree of disability. Medications and other treatments for schizophrenia, when used regularly and as prescribed, can help reduce and control the distressing symptoms of the illness.

The sudden onset of severe psychotic symptoms is referred to as an "acute" phase of schizophrenia. "Psychosis," a common condition in schizophrenia, is a state of mental impairment marked by hallucinations, which are disturbances of sensory perception, and/or delusions, which are false yet strongly held personal beliefs that result from an inability to separate real from unreal experiences. Less obvious symptoms, such as social isolation or withdrawal, or unusual speech, thinking, or behavior, may precede, be seen along with, or follow the psychotic symptoms.

Causes of Schizophrenia

There is no known single cause of schizophrenia. Many diseases, such as heart disease, result from an interplay of genetic, environmental, and behavioral factors, and this may be the case for schizophrenia as well. It has long been known that schizophrenia runs in families. People who have a close relative with schizophrenia are more likely to develop the disorder than are people who have no relatives with the illness. It appears likely that multiple genes are involved in creating a predisposition to develop the disorder. In addition, factors such as prenatal difficulties like intrauterine starvation or viral infections, perinatal complications, and various nonspecific stressors, seem to influence the development of schizophrenia. Several regions of human genome are being investigated to identify genes that may confer susceptibility for schizophrenia. Some evidence has suggested that chromosomes 6, 8, and 13 may be involved. Identification of specific genes involved in the development of schizophrenia will provide important clues into what goes wrong in the brain to produce and sustain the illness and will guide the development of new and better treatments.

Treatment

Because schizophrenia may not be a single condition and its causes are not yet known, current treatment methods are based on both clinical research and experience. These approaches are chosen on the basis of their ability to reduce the symptoms of schizophrenia and to lessen the chances that symptoms will return. Antipsychotic medications have been available since the mid-1950s. They have greatly improved the outlook for individual patients. These medications reduce the psychotic symptoms of schizophrenia and usually allow the patient to function more effectively and appropriately. Antipsychotic drugs are the best treatment now available, but they do not "cure" schizophrenia or ensure that there will be no further psychotic episodes.

A number of new antipsychotic drugs (the so-called "atypical antipsychotics") have been introduced since 1990. The first of these, clozapine, has been shown to be more effective than other antipsychotics, although the possibility of severe side effects—in particular, a condition called agranulocytosis (loss of the white blood cells that fight infection)—requires that patients be monitored with blood tests every 1 or 2 weeks. Even newer antipsychotic drugs, such as risperidone and olazapine, are safer than the older drugs or clozapine, and they may also be better tolerated. Antipsychotic drugs are often very effective in treating certain symptoms of schizophrenia, particularly hallucinations and delusions; unfortunately, the drugs may not be as helpful with other symptoms, such as reduced motivation and emotional expressiveness. It is with these psychological, social, and occupational problems that psychosocial treatments may help most. While psychosocial approaches have limited value for acutely psychotic patients, they may be useful for patients with less severe symptoms or for patients whose psychotic symptoms are under control.

Very often, patients with schizophrenia are discharged from the hospital into the care of their family, so it is important that family members learn all they can about schizophrenia and understand the difficulties and problems associated with the illness. Self-help groups for people and families dealing with schizophrenia are becoming increasingly common. Although not led by a professional therapist, these groups may be therapeutic because members provide continuing mutual support as well as comfort in knowing that they are not alone in the problems they face.

Anxiety Disorders

Anxiety disorders include panic disorder, obsessive-compulsive disorder (OCD), posttraumatic stress disorder (PTSD), generalized anxiety disorder, and phobias (social phobia, agoraphobia, and specific phobia). Approximately 19.1 million American adults ages 18 to 54, or about 13.3 percent of people in this age group in a given year, have an anxiety disorder. Anxiety disorders frequently co-occur with depressive disorders, eating disorders, or substance abuse. Many people have more than one anxiety disorder. Women are more likely than men to have an anxiety disorder. Approximately twice as many women as men suffer from panic disorder, posttraumatic stress disorder, generalized anxiety disorder, agoraphobia, and specific phobia, although about equal numbers of women and men have obsessive-compulsive disorder and social phobia.

Approximately 2.4 million American adults ages 18 to 54, or about 1.7 percent of people in this age group in a given year, have panic disorder. Approximately 3.3 million American adults ages 18 to 54, or about 2.3 percent of people in this age group in a given year, have OCD. The first symptoms of OCD often begin during childhood or adolescence. Approximately 5.2 million American adults ages 18 to 54, or about 3.6 percent of people in this age group in a given year, have PTSD. About 30 percent of Vietnam veterans experienced PTSD at some point after the war. The disorder also frequently occurs after violent personal assaults such as rape, mugging, or domestic violence; terrorism; natural or human-caused disasters; and accidents.

Approximately 5.3 million American adults ages 18 to 54, or about 3.7 percent of people in this age group in a given year, have social phobia which typically begins in childhood or adolescence. Agoraphobia involves intense fear and avoidance of any place or situation where escape might be difficult or help unavailable in the event of developing sudden paniclike symptoms. Specific phobia involves marked and persistent fear and avoidance of a specific object or situation. Approximately 6.3 million American adults ages 18 to 54, or about 4.4 percent of people in this age group in a given year, have some type of specific phobia.

Eating Disorders

The three main types of eating disorders are anorexia nervosa, bulimia nervosa, and binge-eating disorder. Females are much more likely than males to develop an eating disorder. Only an estimated 5 to 15 percent of people with anorexia or bulimia and an estimated 35 percent of those with binge-eating disorder are male.

Attention-Deficit/ Hyperactivity Disorder

Attention-deficit/hyperactivity disorder (ADHD), one of the most common mental disorders in children and adolescents, affects an estimated 4.1 percent of youths ages 9 to 17 in a 6-month period. About two to three times more boys than girls are affected. ADHD usually becomes evident in preschool or early elementary years. The disorder frequently persists into adolescence and occasionally into adulthood.

Autism

Autism affects an estimated 1 to 2 per 1,000 people. Autism and related disorders (also called autism spectrum disorders or pervasive developmental disorders) develop in childhood and are generally apparent by age 3. Autism is about four times more common in boys than girls. Girls with the disorder, however, tend to have more severe symptoms and greater cognitive impairment.

Alzheimer's Disease

Alzheimer's disease, the most common cause of dementia among people age 65 and older, affects an estimated 4 million Americans. As more and more Americans live longer, the number affected by Alzheimer's disease will continue to grow unless a cure or effective prevention is discovered. The duration of illness, from onset of symptoms to death, averages 8 to 10 years.

EPIDEMIOLOGY OF MENTAL ILLNESS

About one in five Americans experiences a mental disorder in the course of a year. Approximately 15 percent of all adults who have a mental disorder in one year also experience a co-occurring substance (alcohol or other drug) use disorder, which complicates treatment. Range of treatments of well-documented efficacy exists for most mental disorders. Two broad types of intervention include psychosocial treatments—for example, psychotherapy or counseling—and psychopharmacologic treatments; these are often most effective when combined. In the mental health field, progress in developing preventive interventions has been slow because, for most major mental disorders, there is insufficient understanding about etiology (or causes of illness) and/or there is an inability to alter the *known* etiology of a particular disorder. Still, some successful strategies have emerged in the absence of a full understanding of etiology.

About 10 percent of the U.S. adult population use mental health services in the health sector in any year, with another 5 percent seeking such services from social service agencies, schools, or religious or self-help groups. Yet critical gaps exist between those who need service and those who receive service. Gaps also exist between optimally effective treatment and what many individuals receive in actual practice settings. Mental illness and less severe mental health problems must be understood in a social and cultural context, and mental health services must be designed and delivered in a manner that is sensitive to the perspectives and needs of racial and ethnic minorities.

The consumer movement has increased the involvement of individuals with mental disorders and their families in mutual support services, consumer-run services, and advocacy. They are powerful agents for changes in service programs and policy. The notion of recovery reflects renewed optimism about the outcomes of mental illness, including that achieved through an individual's own self-care efforts, and the opportunities open to persons with mental illness to participate to the full extent of their interests in the community of their choice.

Persons with mental illness and, often their families, welcome a proliferating array of support services—such as self-help programs, family self-help, crisis services, and advocacy—that help them cope with the isolation, family disruption, and possible loss of employment and housing that may accompany mental disorders. Support services can help dissipate stigma and to guide patients into formal care as well.

Mental health and mental illness are dynamic, ever-changing phenomena. At any given moment, a person's mental status reflects the sum total of that individual's genetic inheritance and life experiences. The brain interacts with and responds—both in its function and in its very structure—to multiple influences continuously, across every stage of life. At different stages, variability in expression of mental health and mental illness can be very subtle or very pronounced. As an example, the symptoms of separation anxiety are normal in early childhood but are signs of distress in later childhood and beyond. It is all too common for people to appreciate the impact of developmental processes in children yet not to extend that conceptual understanding to older people. In fact, people continue to develop

and change throughout life. Different stages of life are associated with vulnerability to distinct forms of mental and behavioral disorders and also with distinctive capacities for mental health.

Even more than is true for adults, children must be seen in the context of their social environments, that is, family and peer group, as well as that of their larger physical and cultural surroundings. Childhood mental health is expressed in this context, as children proceed along the arc of development. A great deal of contemporary research focuses on developmental processes, with the aim of understanding and predicting the forces that will keep children and adolescents mentally healthy and maintain them on course to become mentally healthy adults. Research also focuses on identifying what factors place some at risk for mental illness and, yet again, what protects some children but not others despite exposure to the *same* risk factors. In addition to studies of normal development and of risk factors, much research focuses on mental disorders in childhood and adolescence and what can be done to prevent or treat these conditions and on the design and operation of service settings best suited to the needs experienced by children.

For about one in five Americans, adulthood—a time for achieving productive vocations and for sustaining close relationships at home and in the community—is interrupted by mental illness. In years past, the onset, or occurrence, of mental illness in the adult years was attributed principally to observable phenomena—for example, the burden of stresses associated with career or family, or the inheritance of a disease viewed to run in a particular family. Such explanations may now appear naive at best. Contemporary studies of the brain and behavior are racing to fill in the picture by elucidating specific neurobiological and genetic mechanisms that are the platform upon which a person's life experiences can either strengthen mental health or lead to mental illness.

It now is recognized that factors that influence brain development prenatally may set the stage for a vulnerability to illness that may lie dormant throughout childhood and adolescence. Similarly, no single gene has been found to be responsible for any specific mental disorder; rather, variations in multiple genes contribute to a disruption in healthy brain function that, under certain environmental conditions, results in a mental illness. Moreover, it is now recognized that socioeconomic factors affect individuals' vulnerability to mental illness and mental health problems. Certain demographic and economic groups are more likely than others to experience mental health problems and some mental disorders. Vulnerability alone may not be sufficient to cause a mental disorder; rather, the causes of most mental disorders lie in some combination of genetic and environmental factors, which may be biological or psychosocial.

The fact that many, if not most, people have experienced mental health problems that mimic or even match some of the symptoms of a diagnosable mental disorder tends, ironically, to prompt many people to underestimate the painful, disabling nature of severe mental illness. In fact, schizophrenia, mood disorders such as major depression and bipolar illness, and anxiety often are devastating conditions. Yet relatively few mental illnesses have an unremitting course marked by the most acute manifestations of illness; rather, for reasons that are not yet understood, the symptoms associated with mental illness tend to wax and wane. These patterns pose special challenges to the implementation of treatment plans and the design of service systems that are optimally responsive to an individual's needs during every phase of illness. Enormous strides are being made in diagnosis, treatment, and service delivery, placing the productive and creative possibilities of adulthood within the reach of persons who are encumbered by mental disorders.

Late adulthood is when changes in health status may become more noticeable and the ability to compensate for decrements may become limited. As the brain ages, a person's capacity for certain mental tasks tends to diminish, even as changes in other mental activities prove to be positive and rewarding. Well into late life, the ability to solve novel problems can be enhanced through training in cognitive skills and problem-solving strategies.

The promise of research on mental health promotion notwithstanding, a substantial minority of older people are disabled, often severely, by mental disorders including Alzheimer's disease, major depression, substance abuse, anxiety, and other conditions. In the United States today, the highest rate of suicide—an all-too-common consequence of unrecognized or inappropriately treated depression—is found in older males. This fact underscores the urgency of ensuring that health care provider training properly emphasize skills required to differentiate accurately the causes of cognitive, emotional, and behavioral symptoms that may, in some instances, rise to the level of mental disorders, and in other instances be expressions of unmet general medical needs.

As the life expectancy of Americans continues to extend, the sheer number—although not necessarily the proportion—of persons experiencing mental disorders of late life will expand, confronting our society with unprecedented challenges in organizing, financing, and delivering effective mental health services for this population. An essential part of the needed societal response will include recognizing and devising innovative ways of supporting the increasingly more prominent role that families are assuming in caring for older, mentally impaired and mentally ill family members.

ORGANIZATION AND FINANCING OF MENTAL HEALTH SERVICES

A broad array of services and treatments exists to help people with mental illnesses—as well as those at particular risk of developing them—to suffer less emotional pain and disability and live healthier, longer, and more productive lives. Mental disorders and mental health problems are treated by a variety of caregivers who work in diverse, relatively independent, and loosely coordinated facilities and services—both public and private.

About 15 percent of all adults and 21 percent of U.S. children and adolescents use services in the system each year. The system is usually described as having four major components or sectors. The *specialty mental health* sector consists of mental health professionals such as psychiatrists, psychologists, psychiatric nurses, and psychiatric social workers who are trained specifically to treat people with mental disorders (Table 10.2).

The great bulk of specialty treatment is now provided in outpatient settings such as private office-based practices or in private or public clinics. Most acute hospital care is now provided in special psychiatric units of general hospitals or beds scattered throughout general hospitals (Table 10.3). Private psychiatric hospitals and residential treatment centers for children and adolescents provide additional intensive care in the private sector. Public sector facilities include state/county mental hospitals and multiservice mental health facilities, which often coordinate a wide range of outpatient, intensive case management, partial hospitalization, and inpatient services. Altogether, slightly less than 6 percent of the adult population and about 8 percent of children and adolescents (ages 9 to 17) use specialty mental health services in a year.

The *general medical/primary care* sector consists of health care professionals such as general internists, pediatricians, and nurse practitioners in office-based practice, clinics, acute medical/surgical hospitals, and nursing homes. More than 6 percent of the adult U.S. population use the general medical sector for mental health care, with an average of about 4 visits per year—far lower than the average of 14 visits per year found in the specialty mental health sector. The general medical sector has long been identified as the initial point of contact for many adults with mental disorders; for some, these providers may be their only source of mental health services. However, only about 3 percent of children and adolescents contact general medical physicians for mental health services; the human services sector (discussed later) plays a much larger role in their care.

The *human services* sector consists of social services, school-based counseling services, residential rehabilitation services, vocational rehabilitation, criminal justice/prison-based services, and religious professional counselors. For children, school mental health services are a major source of care, as are services in the child welfare and juvenile justice systems. The *voluntary support network* sector, which consists of self-help groups, such as 12-step programs and peer counselors, is a rapidly growing component of the mental and addictive disorder treatment system.

Public and Private Sectors

The de facto mental health service system is divided into public and private sectors. The term "public sector" refers both to services directly operated by government agencies (e.g., state and county mental hospitals) and to services financed with government resources (e.g., Medicaid, a federal-state program for financing health care services for people who are poor and disabled, and Medicare, a federal health insurance program primarily for older Americans and people who retire early due to disability). Publicly financed services may be provided by private organizations. The term "private sector" refers both to services directly operated by private agencies and to services financed with private resources (e.g., employer-provided insurance).

State and local governments have been the major payers for public mental health services historically and remain so today. Since the mid-1960s, however, the role of the federal government has increased. In addition to Medicare and Medicaid, the federal government funds special programs for adults with serious mental illness and children with serious emotional disability. Although small in relation to state and local funding, these federal programs provide additional resources. They include the Community Mental Health Block Grant, Community Support programs, the PATH program for people with mental illness who are homeless, the Knowledge Development and Application Program, and the Comprehensive Community Mental Health Services for Children and Their Families Program.

Table 10.2. Estimated Number of Selected Clinically Active or Trained Mental Health Personnel and Rate per 100,000 Civilian Population, by Discipline: United States, various years

Region	Psychiatry (2001)		Psychology (2002)		Social Work (2002)		Psychiatric Nursing (2000)		Marriage and Family Therapy (2002)	
	Number Persons	Rate per 100,000	Number Persons	Rate per 100,000	Number Persons	Rate per 100,000	Number Persons	Rate per 100,000	Number Persons	Rate per 100,000
United States	38,436	13.7	88,491	31.1	99,341	35.3	18,269	6.5	47,111	16.7
New England	3,749	26.9	7,425	53.0	11,233	80.7	3,043	21.8	1,763	12.7
Middle Atlantic	8,759	22.1	19,770	49.7	24,327	61.3	3,632	9.1	2,104	5.3
East North Central	4,842	10.7	14,727	32.5	16,793	37.2	3,150	6.9	3,356	7.4
West North Central	1,833	9.5	6,879	35.6	4,924	25.6	930	4.8	1,627	8.4
South Atlantic	6,690	12.9	12,878	24.4	15,348	29.6	3,310	6.3	4,469	8.6
East South Central	1,403	8.2	2,681	15.6	3,080	18.1	1,367	8.0	1,248	7.3
West South Central	2,684	8.5	4,600	14.4	6,445	20.5	573	1.8	3,973	11.3
Mountain	1,843	10.1	5,263	28.2	5,393	29.7	760	4.1	2,061	11.3
Pacific	6,633	14.7	14,268	31.1	11,798	26.2	1,503	3.3	26,512	58.3

SOURCE: From *Mental Health, United States, 2002* [DHSS Pub. No. (SMA) 3938], by R. W. Manderscheid and M. J. Henderson, eds., Rockville, MD: Substance Abuse and Mental Health Services Administration.

Table 10.3. Mental Health Organizations and Beds for 24-Hour Hospital and Residential Treatment: United States, 1986 and 1998

Type of Organization	1986	1998
	Number of mental health organizations	
State and county mental hospitals	285	229
Private psychiatric hospitals	314	348
Nonfederal general hospital psychiatric services	1,351	1,707
Department of Veterans Affairs medical centers	139	145
Residential treatment centers for emotionally disturbed children	437	461
All other organizations*	2,221	2,832
	Number of beds	
State and county mental hospitals	119,033	63,769
Private psychiatric hospitals	30,201	34,154
Nonfederal general hospital psychiatric services	45,808	55,145
Department of Veterans Affairs medical centers	26,874	13,742
Residential treatment centers for emotionally disturbed children	24,547	33,997
All other organizations*	21,150	65,922

*Includes freestanding psychiatric outpatient clinics, partial care organizations, and multiservice mental health organizations.

These federally funded public sector programs buttress the traditional responsibility of state and local mental health systems and serve as the mental health service "safety net" and "catastrophic insurer" for those citizens with the most severe problems and the fewest resources in the United States. The public sector serves particularly those individuals with no health insurance, those who have insurance but no mental health coverage, and those who exhaust limited mental health benefits in their health insurance.

Each sector of the de facto mental health service system has different patterns and types of care and different patterns of funding. Within the specialty mental health sector, state- and county-funded mental health services have long served as a safety net for people unable to obtain or retain access to privately funded mental health services. The general medical sector receives a relatively greater proportion of federal Medicaid funds, while the voluntary support network sector, staffed principally by people with mental illness and their families, is largely funded by private donations of time and money to emotionally supportive and educational groups.

Effective functioning of the mental health service system requires connections and coordination among many sectors (public–private, specialty–general health, health–social welfare, housing, criminal justice, and education). Without coordination, it can readily become organizationally fragmented, creating barriers to access. Adding to the system's complexity is its dependence on many streams of funding, with their sometimes competing incentives.

Patterns of Use

Americans use the mental health service system in complex ways, or patterns. A total of about 15 percent of the U.S. adult population use mental health services in any given year. About 6 percent of the adult population use specialty mental health care; 5 percent of the population receive their mental health services from general medical and/or human services providers, and 3 to 4 percent of the population receive their mental health services from other human service professionals or self-help groups. Nineteen percent of the adult U.S. population have a mental disorder alone (in one year); 3 percent have both mental and addictive disorders; and 6 percent have addictive disorders alone. A substantial *majority* of those with specific mental disorders do not receive treatment.

Although 9 percent of the entire child/adolescent sample received some mental health services in the health sector (i.e., the general medical sector and specialty mental health sector), the largest provider of mental health services to this population was the school system. Many children served by schools do not have diagnosable mental health conditions; some may have other diagnoses such as adjustment reactions or acute stress reactions. One percent of children and adolescents received their mental health services from human service professionals, such as those in child welfare and juvenile justice.

The mental health treatment system is a dynamic array of services accessed by patients with different levels of disorder and severity, as well as different social and medical service needs and levels and types of insurance financing. Disparities in access are due to sociocultural factors. In a system in which substantial numbers of those with even the most severe mental illness do not receive any mental health care, the match between service use and service need is far from perfect. But not everyone with a diagnosable mental disorder perceives a need for treatment, and not all who desire treatment have a currently diagnosable disorder. Providing access to appropriate mental health services is a fundamental concern for mental health policy makers in both the public and private arenas.

The Costs of Mental Illness

Mental disorders impose an enormous emotional and financial burden on ill individuals and their families. They are also costly for our nation in reduced or lost productivity (indirect costs) and in medical resources used for care, treatment, and rehabilitation (direct costs).

The *indirect costs* of all mental illness reflects morbidity costs—the loss of productivity in usual activities because of illness. But indirect costs also include mortality costs (lost productivity due to premature death), and productivity losses for incarcerated individuals and for the time of individuals providing family care. Indirect cost estimates are conservative because they do not capture some measure of the pain, suffering, disruption, and reduced productivity that are not reflected in earnings.

The fact that morbidity costs comprise about 80 percent of the indirect costs of all mental illness indicates an important characteristic of mental disorders: Mortality is relatively low, onset is often at a younger age, and most of the indirect costs are derived from lost or reduced productivity at the workplace, school, and home.

Disability adjusted life years (DALYs) are now being used as a common metric for describing the burden of disability and premature death resulting from the full range of mental and physical disorders throughout the world. Mental disorders account for more than 15 percent of the burden of disease in established market economies; unipolar major depression, bipolar disorder, schizophrenia, and obsessive-compulsive disorder are identified as among the top 10 leading causes of disability worldwide.

Mental health expenditures for treatment and rehabilitation are an important part of overall health care spending but differ in important ways from other types of health care spending. Many mental health services are provided by separate specialty providers—such as psychiatrists, psychologists, social workers, and nurses in office practice—or by facilities such as hospitals, multiservice mental health organizations, or residential treatment centers for children. Insurance coverage of mental health services is typically less generous than that for general health, and government plays a larger role in financing mental health services compared to overall health care.

A majority of private health insurance plans have a benefit that combines coverage of mental illness and substance abuse. However, most of the treatment services for mental illness and for substance abuse are separate (and use different types of providers), as are virtually all the public funds for these services. This separation causes problems for treating the substantial proportion of individuals with comorbid mental illness and substance abuse disorders, who benefit from being treated for both disorders together.

Alzheimer's disease and other dementias have historically been considered as both mental and somatic disorders. However, efforts to destigmatize dementias and improve care have removed some insurance coverage limitations. Once mostly the province of the public sector, Alzheimer's disease now enjoys more comprehensive coverage, and care is better integrated into the private health care system.

MENTAL HEALTH FINANCING

Funding for the mental health service system comes from both public and private sources. Approximately 53 percent of the funding for mental health treatment comes from public payers. Of the 47 percent of expenditures from private sources, more than half are from private insurance. Most of the remainder is out-of-pocket payments. These out-of-pocket payments include copayments from individuals with private insurance, copayments and prescription costs not covered by Medicare, and payment for direct treatment from the uninsured or insured who choose not to use their insurance coverage for mental health care.

Among the fastest-rising expenses for mental health services are outpatient prescription drugs. Although these medications are prescribed in both specialty and general medical sectors, they are increasingly being covered under general medical rather than mental health private insurance benefits. The higher than average growth rate of spending for prescription drugs reflects, in part, the increasing availability and application of medications of demonstrable efficacy in treating mental disorders. Only one-third of psychotropic medications are prescribed by psychiatrists, with two-thirds prescribed by primary care physicians and other medical specialists.

During the past two decades there have been important shifts in what parties have final responsibility for paying for mental health care. The role of direct state funding of mental health care has been reduced, whereas Medicaid funding of mental health care has grown in relative importance. This is in part due to substantial funding offered to the states by the federal government. One consequence of this shift is that Medicaid program design has become very influential in shaping the delivery of mental health care. State mental health authorities, however, continue to be an important force in making public mental health services policy, working together with state Medicaid programs.

Health Insurance

Private insurance coverage has played a somewhat more limited role in mental health financing in the past decade. Various cost-containment efforts have been pursued aggressively in the private sector through the introduction of managed care. Private insurance coverage for prescription drugs has expanded dramatically over the past 15 years. Insurance coverage for mental health treatments is on par with coverage for other illnesses. Accompanying this pattern of private insurance coverage are the availability of innovative new prescription drugs aimed at treating major mental illnesses and a shift in mental health spending in private insurance toward pharmaceutical agents.

Private health insurance is generally more restrictive in coverage of mental illness than in coverage for somatic illness. This is motivated by several concerns. Insurers fear that coverage of mental health services could result in high costs associated with long-term and intensive psychotherapy and extended hospital stays. They are also reluctant to pay for long-term, often custodial, hospital stays that are guaranteed by the public mental health system, the provider of "catastrophic care." These factors have encouraged private insurers to limit coverage for mental health services.

Some private insurers refuse to cover mental illness treatment; others simply limit payment to acute care services. Those who do offer coverage choose to impose various financial restrictions, such as separate and lower annual and lifetime limits on care (per person and per episode of care), as well as separate (and higher) deductibles and co-payments. As a result, individuals pay out-of-pocket for a higher proportion of mental health services than general health services and face catastrophic financial losses (and/or transfer to the public sector) when the costs of their care exceed the limits.

Federal public financing mechanisms, such as Medicare and Medicaid, also impose limitations on coverage, particularly for long-term care, of "nervous and mental disease" to avoid a complete shift in financial responsibility from state and local governments to the federal government. Existence of the public sector as a guarantor of "catastrophic care" for the uninsured and underinsured allows the private sector to avoid financial risk and focus on acute care of less-impaired individuals, most of whom receive health insurance benefits through their employer.

The purpose of health insurance is to protect individuals from catastrophic financial loss. While the majority of individuals who use mental health services incur comparatively small expenses, some who have severe illness face financial ruin without the protection afforded by insurance. For people with health insurance, the range of covered benefits and the limits imposed on them ultimately determine where they will get service, which, in turn, affects their ability to access necessary and effective treatment services. Adequate mental health treatment resources for large population groups require a wide range of services in a variety of settings, with sufficient flexibility to permit movement to the appropriate level of care.

Health insurance, whether funded through private or public sources, is one of the most important factors influencing access to mental health services. Most Americans have some sort of insurance coverage—primarily private insurance obtained through the workplace. However, adequacy for mental health care is extremely variable across types of plans and sponsors.

Low-income individuals on public support receive Medicaid coverage. The average cost of this coverage is 2.5 times higher than that in the private sector. An explanation for this higher average cost is the severity of illness of this population and greater intensity of services needed to meet their needs. Finally, funds from state/local government and from other federal government block grants and Veterans Affairs cover mental health services for the uninsured. Most of the uninsured are members of employed families who cannot afford to purchase insurance coverage. Individuals with severe and persistent mental illness who are uninsured have the highest annual costs, leaving few resources for treatment for those with less severe disorders.

From the time they were introduced in 1929 until the 1990s, fee-for-service (indemnity) plans, such as Blue Cross/Blue Shield, were the most common form of health insurance. Insurance plans would identify the range of services they considered effective for the treatment of all health conditions and then reimburse physicians, hospitals, and other health care providers for the usual and customary fees charged by independent practitioners. To prevent the overuse of services, insurance companies would often require patients to pay for some portion of the costs out-of-pocket (i.e., co-insurance) and would use annual deductibles, much as auto insurance companies do, to minimize the administrative costs of processing small claims.

For most health insurance plans covering somatic illness, to protect the *insured*, costs above a certain "catastrophic limit" are borne entirely by the insurance company. To protect the *insurer* against potentially unlimited claims, however, "annual" or "lifetime limits" are imposed for most medical or surgical conditions. It is expected that any expenses beyond that limit are the responsibility of the patient's family.

In contrast, in the case of coverage for mental health services, insurance companies often set lower annual or lifetime limits to protect themselves against costly claims leaving patients and their families exposed to much greater personal financial risks. The legacy of the public mental health system safety net as the provider of catastrophic coverage encourages such practices. Further, when federal financing mechanisms such as Medicare and Medicaid were introduced, they also limited coverage of long-term care of "nervous and mental disease" to avoid shifting financial responsibility from state and local government to the federal government.

For potential insurers of mental health care or general health care, two financial concerns are key: *moral hazard* and *adverse selection*. Moral hazard reflects a concern that if people with insurance no longer have to pay the full costs of their own care, they will use more services—services that they do not value at their full cost. To control moral hazard, insurers incorporate cost sharing and care management into their policies. Adverse selection reflects a concern that, in a market with voluntary insurance or multiple insurers, plans that provide the most generous coverage will attract individuals with the greatest need for care, leading to elevated service use and costs for those insurers independent of their efficiency in services provision. To control adverse selection, insurers try to restrict mental health coverage to avoid enrolling people with higher mental health service needs.

While these economic forces are important, insurer responses to them may have been exaggerated. In the fee-for-service insurance system, for example, some insurers have addressed their concerns about moral hazard by assigning higher cost sharing to mental health services. Coverage limitations, imposed to control costs, have been applied unevenly, however, and without full consideration of their consequences. In particular, higher cost sharing, such as placing a 50 percent copayment on outpatient psychotherapy, may reduce moral hazard and inappropriate use, but it may also reduce

appropriate use. Limits on coverage may reduce adverse selection but leave people to bear catastrophic costs themselves.

Managed Care and Mental Health

Managed care represents a confluence of several forces shaping the organization and financing of health care. These include the drive to deliver more highly individualized, cost-effective care; a more health-promoting and preventive orientation (often found in health maintenance organizations); and a concern with cost containment to address the problem of moral hazard. Managed care implies a range of financing and payment strategies that depart in important ways from traditional fee-for-service indemnity insurance.

Health maintenance organizations (HMO) initially treated only those mental disorders that were responsive to short-term treatment, but they reduced copayments and deductibles for any brief therapy. There was an implicit reliance on the public mental health system for treatment of any chronic or severe mental disorder—especially those for whom catastrophic coverage was needed.

In carve-out managed behavioral health care, segments of insurance risk—defined by service or disease—are isolated from overall insurance risk and covered in a separate contract between the payer (insurer or employer) and the carve-out vendor. Even with highly restrictive admission criteria, many HMOs have recently found it cost effective to carve out mental health care for administration by a managed behavioral health company, rather than relying on in-house staff. This arrangement permits a larger range of services than can be provided by existing staff without increasing salaried staff and management overhead costs. Carve-outs generally have separate budgets, provider networks, and financial incentive arrangements. Covered services, utilization management techniques, financial risk, and other features vary depending on the particular carve-out contract. The employee as a plan member may be unaware of any such arrangement. These separate contracts delegate management of mental health care to specialized vendors known as *managed behavioral health care organizations (MBHOs)*.

There are two general forms of carve-outs: *payer carve-outs* and *health plan subcontracts*. In payer carve-outs, an enrollee chooses a health plan for coverage of health care with the exception of mental health and must enroll with a separate carve-out vendor for mental health care. In health plan subcontracts, administrators of the general medical plan arrange to have mental health care managed by a carve-out vendor or MBHO; the plan member does not have to take steps to select mental health coverage.

Managed-care arrangements (HMO, PPO, or POS plans), which fundamentally alter the way in which health care resources are allocated, now cover the majority of Americans. Managed care has also made significant inroads into publicly funded health care. In Medicaid, growth is primarily focused on the population receiving Temporary Aid to Needy Families (TANF) support as opposed to the population with severe and chronic mental illness, eligible for Medicaid because of Supplemental Security Income.

The administrative mechanisms have changed the incentive structure for mental health professionals, with "supply-side" controls (e.g., provider incentives) replacing "demand-side" controls (e.g., benefit limits) on service use and cost. In addition, the privatization of service delivery is increasing in the public sector. As a result of these changes, access to specific types of mental health services is increasingly under the purview of managed behavioral-care companies and employers.

As the states have adopted Medicaid managed care for mental health, at least two distinct models have emerged. States that entered managed care early have tended to issue contracts to private sector organizations to perform both administrative (payments, network development) and management (utilization review) functions. States that entered managed care more recently have tended to contract administrative functions with administrative services organizations (ASOs), while retaining control of management functions.

In a managed-care system, the moral hazard of unnecessary utilization need not be addressed through benefit design. Utilization is typically controlled at the level of the provider of care, through a series of financial incentives and through direct management of the care. For example, managed care reduces cost in part by shifting treatment from inpatient to outpatient settings, negotiating discounted hospital and professional fees, and using utilization management techniques to limit unnecessary services. In this fashion, at least theoretically, unnecessary utilization, the moral hazard, is eliminated at the source, on a case-by-case basis.

Adverse selection may be addressed through regulations, such as mandates in coverage that require all insurers in a market to offer the same level of services. In this way, no one insurer runs the risk that offering superior coverage will necessarily attract people who are higher utilizers of care. Efforts to regulate adverse selection may not produce the intended effect, however, when insurers that offer the same services use management techniques to control costs by restricting care to those who use services most intensely—effectively denying care to those who need it most. In such instances, patients with the greatest needs might become concentrated in plans with the most generous management of care. This may lead to financial losses for such plans or encourage them to cut back on services for those who need care most or to divert resources from other beneficiaries.

The range of management controls currently applied to enrollees in covered plans extends from simple utilization review of hospitalizations on an administrative services only (ASO) contract to prepaid, at-risk contracts with extensive employee assistance plan (EAP) screening and networks of eligible mental health specialists and hospitals providing services for discounted fees.

Managed care demonstrably reduces the cost of mental health services. That was one of its goals—to remove the excesses of overutilization, such as unnecessary hospitalization, and to increase the number of individuals treated by using more cost-effective care. This was to be accomplished through case-by-case "management" of care. The risk of cost containment, however, is that it can lead to under-treatment. Excessively restrictive cost-containment strategies and financial incentives to providers and facilities to reduce specialty referrals, hospital admissions, or length or amount of treatment may ultimately contribute to lowered access and quality of care. These restrictions pose particular risk to people on either end of the severity spectrum: Individuals with mental health problems may be denied services entirely, while the most severely and persistently ill patients may be undertreated.

The term "access to mental health services" refers generally to the ability to obtain treatment with appropriate professionals for mental disorders. Having health insurance—and the nature of its coverage and administration—are critical determinants of such access. But so are factors such as the person's clinical status and personal and socio-cultural factors affecting desire for care; knowledge about mental health services and the effectiveness of current treatments; the level of insurance copayments, deductibles, and limits; ability to obtain adequate time off from work and other responsibilities to obtain treatment; and the availability of providers in close proximity, as well as the availability of transportation and child care. In addition, because the stigma associated with mental disorders is still a barrier to seeking care, the availability of services organized in ways that reduce stigma—such as employee assistance programs—can provide important gateways to further treatment when necessary.

Current incentives both within and outside managed care do not generally encourage an emphasis on quality of care. Nonetheless, some managed mental health systems recognize the potential uses of quality assessment of their services. These include monitoring and ensuring quality of care to public and private oversight organizations; developing programs to improve services or outcomes

from systematic empirical evaluation; and permitting reward on the basis of quality and performance, not simply cost. Clinical outcome data systems, although more expensive and complicated than administrative data systems, have potential for evaluating how programs and practices actually affect patient outcomes.

Another way to measure quality takes into account outcomes outside the mental health specialty sector. When management and financial incentives limit access to mental health care or encourage a shift to general health care services for mental health care, disability may increase and work performance decline. These losses to employers may well offset management-based savings in mental health specialty costs.

Many of the administrative techniques used in managed care (such as case management, utilization review, and implementation of standardized criteria) have the potential to improve the quality of care by enhancing adherence to professional consensus treatment guidelines and possibly improving patient outcomes. However, little is known about what happens when management is introduced into service systems in combination with high cost sharing.

Parity in Mental Health

"Parity" refers to the effort to treat mental health financing on the same basis as financing for general health services. The fundamental motivation behind parity legislation is the desire to cover mental illness on the same basis as somatic illness. A parity mandate requires all insurers in a market to offer the same coverage, equivalent to the coverage for all other disorders. The potential ability of managed care to control costs (through utilization management of moral hazard) without limiting benefits makes a parity mandate more affordable than under a fee-for-service system.

Managed care coupled with parity laws offers opportunities for focused cost control by eliminating moral hazard without unfairly restricting coverage through arbitrary limits or cost sharing and by controlling adverse selection. However, continued use of unnecessary limits or overly aggressive management may lead to undertreatment or to restricted access to services and plans.

Despite both the cost-controlling impact of managed care and advocacy to expand benefits, inequitable limits continue to be applied to mental health services. Parity legislation in the states and federal government has attempted to redress this inequity.

Federal legislative efforts to achieve parity in mental health insurance coverage date from the 1970s and have continued through to the present time. The drive for mental health parity culminated in passage of the Mental Health Parity Act in 1996. Implemented in 1998, this legislation focused on only one aspect of the inequities in mental health insurance coverage: "catastrophic" benefits. It prohibited the use of lifetime and annual limits on coverage that were different for mental and somatic illnesses. As federal legislation, it included within its mandate some of the nation's largest companies that are self-insured and otherwise exempted from state parity laws because of the Employment Retirement Income Security Act.

Although it was seen as an important first substantive step and rhetorical victory for mental health advocacy, the Parity Act was limited in a number of important ways. Companies with fewer than 50 employees or that offered no mental health benefit were exempt from provisions of the law. The parity provisions did not apply to other forms of benefit limits, such as per episode limits on length of stay or visit limits, or copayments or deductibles, and they did not include substance abuse treatment. In addition, insurers who experienced more than a 1 percent rise in premium as a result of implementing parity could apply for an exemption.

State efforts at parity legislation paralleled those at the federal level. A growing number of states have implemented parity. Some target their parity legislation narrowly to include only people with severe mental disorders; others use a broader defi-

nition of mental illness for parity coverage and include, in some cases, substance abuse. Some states focus on a broad range of insured populations; others focus on only a single population.

Evidence of the effects of parity laws shows that their costs are minimal. Introducing or increasing the level of managed care can significantly limit or even reduce the costs of implementing such laws. Within carve-out forms of managed care, parity results in less than a 1 percent increase in total health care costs. In plans that have not previously used managed care, introducing parity simultaneously with managed care can result in an actual reduction in such costs.

THE FUTURE OF MENTAL HEALTH SERVICES

Mental health is fundamental to health and human functioning. Mental illnesses are real health conditions that are characterized by alterations in thinking, mood, or behavior—all mental, behavioral, and psychological symptoms mediated by the brain. Mental illnesses exact a staggering toll on millions of individuals, as well as on their families and communities and our nation as a whole. Appropriate treatment can alleviate, if not cure, the symptoms and associated disability of mental illness. With proper treatment, the majority of people with mental illness can return to productive and engaging lives. There is no "one size fits all" treatment; rather, people can choose the type of treatment that best suits them from the diverse forms of treatment that exist.

Even as we approach the end of the decade, the majority of those who need mental health treatment do not seek it. The reluctance of Americans to seek care for mental illness is all too understandable, given the many barriers that stand in their way.

The nation has realized immense dividends from five decades of investment in research focused on mental illness and mental health. Yet to realize further advances in treatment and, ultimately, prevention, the nation must continue to invest in research at all levels. Today, integrative neuroscience and molecular genetics present some of the most exciting basic research opportunities in medical science. Molecular and genetic tools are being used to identify genes and proteins that might be involved in the origins of mental illness and that clearly are altered by drug treatment and by the environment. Genes and gene products promise to provide novel targets for new medications and psychosocial interventions. The opportunities available underscore the need for the mental health research community to strengthen partnerships with both the biotechnology and the pharmaceutical industries. A plethora of new pharmacologic agents and psychotherapies for mental disorders affords new treatment opportunities but also challenges the scientific community to develop new approaches to clinical and health services interventions research.

Responding to the calls of managed mental and behavioral health care systems for evidence-based interventions will have a much needed and discernible impact on practice. Research is a potent weapon against stigma, one that forces skeptics to let go of misconceptions and stereotypes concerning mental illness and the burdens experienced by persons who have these disorders.

Special effort is required to address pronounced gaps in the mental health knowledge base. Key among these is the urgent need for research evidence that supports strategies for mental health promotion and illness prevention.

Americans are often unaware of the choices they have for effective mental health treatments. There exists a constellation of treatments for most mental disorders. Treatments fall mainly under several broad categories—counseling, psychotherapy, medication therapy, rehabilitation—yet within each category are many more choices.

All human services professionals, not just health professionals, have an obligation to be better informed about mental health treatment resources in their communities. Managed-care companies and other health insurers need to publish clear information about their mental health benefits (usually called "behavioral health benefits"). At present, many beneficiaries appear not to know *if* they have mental health coverage, much less where to seek help for problems.

The service system as a whole, as opposed to treatment services considered in isolation, dictates the outcome of treatment. The fundamental components of effective service delivery include integrated community-based services, continuity of providers and treatments, family support services (including psychoeducation), and culturally sensitive services. Effective service delivery for individuals with the most severe conditions also requires supported housing and supported employment. For adults and children with less severe conditions, primary health care, the schools, and other human services must be prepared to assess and, at times, to treat individuals who come seeking help. All services for those with a mental disorder should be consumer oriented and focused on promoting recovery. That is, the goal of services must not be limited to symptom reduction but should strive for restoration of a meaningful and productive life.

The supply of well-trained mental health professionals is also inadequate in many areas of the country, especially in rural areas. Particularly keen shortages are found in the numbers of mental health professionals serving children and adolescents with serious mental disorders and older people. More mental health professionals also need to be trained in cognitive-behavioral therapy and interpersonal therapy, two forms of psychotherapy shown by rigorous research to be effective for many types of mental disorders.

To be effective, the diagnosis and treatment of mental illness must be tailored to individual circumstances, while taking into account, age, gender, race, culture, and other characteristics that shape a person's image and identity. Services that take these demographic factors into consideration have the greatest chance of engaging people in treatment, keeping them in treatment, and helping them to recover thereafter. The successful experiences of individual patients will positively influence attitudes toward mental health services and service providers, thus encouraging others who may share similar concerns or interests to seek help.

While women and men experience mental disorders at almost equal rates, some mental disorders such as depression, panic disorder, and eating disorders affect women disproportionately. The mental health service system should be tailored to focus on women's unique needs.

Members of racial and ethnic minority groups account for an increasing proportion of the nation's population. Mental illness is at least as prevalent among racial and ethnic minorities as in the majority white population. Yet many racial and ethnic minority group members find the organized mental health system to be uninformed about cultural context and, thus, unresponsive and/or irrelevant.

The mental health service system is highly fragmented. Many who seek treatment are bewildered by the maze of paths into treatment; others in need of care are stymied by a lack of information about where to seek effective and affordable services. In recent years, some progress has been made in coordinating services for those with severe mental illness, but more can be accomplished. Public and private agencies have an obligation to facilitate entry into treatment. There are multiple "portals of entry" to mental health care and treatment, including a range of community and faith-based organizations. Primary health care could be an important portal of entry for children and adults of all ages with mental disorders. The schools and child welfare system are the initial points of contact for most children and adolescents and can be useful sources of first-line assessment and referral, provided that expertise is available. The juvenile justice system represents another pathway, although many overburdened facilities tend to lack the staff required to deal with the magnitude of the mental health problems encountered. Of equal concern are the adult criminal jus-

tice and corrections systems, which encounter substantial numbers of detainees with mental illness. Individuals with mental disorders are often neglected or victimized in these institutions.

It is essential for first-line contacts in the community to recognize mental illness and mental health problems, to respond sensitively, to know what resources exist, and to make proper referrals and/or to address problems effectively themselves. For the general public, primary care represents a prime opportunity to obtain mental health treatment or an appropriate referral. Yet primary health care providers vary in their capacity to recognize and manage mental health problems. Many highly committed primary care providers do not know referral sources or do not have the time to help their patients find services.

Some people do not seek treatment because they are fearful of being forced to accept treatments not of their choice or of being treated involuntarily for prolonged periods. For most, these fears are unwarranted: Coercion, or involuntary treatment, is restricted by law only to those who pose a direct threat of danger to themselves or others or, in some instances, who demonstrate a grave disability. Coercion takes the form of involuntary commitment to a hospital; in about 40 states and territories, it includes certain outpatient treatment requirements. Advocates for people with mental illness hold divergent views regarding coercion. Some advocates crusade for more stringent controls and treatment mandates, whereas others adamantly oppose coercion on any grounds. One point is clear: The *need* for coercion should be reduced significantly when adequate services are readily accessible to individuals with severe mental disorders who pose a threat of danger to themselves or others.

Financial obstacles discourage people from seeking treatment and from staying in treatment. Repeated surveys have shown that concerns about the cost of care are among the foremost reasons why people do not seek care. Mental health coverage is often arbitrarily restricted. Individuals and families are consequently forced to draw on relatively—and substantially—more of their own resources to pay for mental health treatment than they pay for other types of health care. This inequity is a deterrent to treatment and needs to be redressed.

SUMMARY

Mental health celebrates scientific advances in a field once shrouded in mystery. These advances have yielded unparalleled understanding of mental illness and the services needed for prevention, treatment, and rehabilitation. The journey ahead must firmly establish mental health as a cornerstone of health; place mental illness treatment in the mainstream of health care services; and ensure consumers of mental health services access to respectful, evidenced-based, and reimbursable care.

REVIEW QUESTIONS

1. What have been the fundamental changes in our understanding of mental health services over the past 50 years?
2. Describe the structure of the U.S. mental and behavioral health system.
3. Describe the patterns of mental health service use in the United States.
4. How do we pay for mental health services?
5. Describe the concepts of moral hazard and adverse selection.
6. What does parity refer to in mental health, and how has it influenced legislation in the United States?
7. What are the major challenges facing mental health services for the future?

REFERENCES & ADDITIONAL READINGS

Brown, R. S., Snyder, D. M., & Peterson, D. W. (2000). *Textbook for mental health: A narrative approach.* Boston: Pearson Cuystom Publishers.

Drake, R. E. (2005). *Evidence based mental health practice: A textbook.* New York: W.W. Norton.

Grob, G. (1994). *The mad among us: A history of the care of America's mentally ill.* New York: Free Press.

Grob, G. N. (1997). Deinstitutionalization: The illusion of policy. *Journal of Policy History, 19*(1), 48–73.

Grob, G. (1998). Psychiatry's holy grail: The search for the mechanisms of mental diseases. *Bulletin of the History of Medicine, 72*(2), 189–219.

Kornstein, S. G., & Clayton, A. H. (Eds.). (2002). *Women's mental health.* New York: Guilford Press.

Manderscheid, R. W., & Henderson, M. J. (Eds.). (2004). *Mental health, United States, 2002.* [DHHS Pub. No. (SMA) 3938]. Rockville, MD: Substance Abuse and Mental Health Services Administration.

Mechanic, D. (1999). *Mental health and social policy: The emergence of managed care* (4th ed.). Boston: Allyn and Bacon.

President's Commission on Mental Health. *Report to the President from the President's Commission on Mental Health* (4 vols.). (1978). Washington, DC: U.S. Government Printing Office.

Tsuang, M. T., & Tohen, M. (Eds.). (2002). *Textbook in psychiatric epidemiology.* New York: Wiley-Liss.

U.S. Department of Health and Human Services. *Health people 2010: Understanding and improving health* (2nd ed.). (2000). Washington, DC: U.S. Government Printing Office.

Welfel, E. R., & Ingersoll, R. E. (Eds.). (2001). *The mental health desk reference.* New York: Wiley.

FOUR

Nonfinancial Resources for Health Care

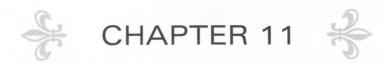

CHAPTER 11

The Pharmaceutical Industry*

CHAPTER TOPICS

- Regulatory and Legal Issues
- From Idea to Treatment: The Long, Uncertain Research and Development Process
- Access, Pricing, and Patent Issues
- The Value of Medicines

LEARNING OBJECTIVES

Upon completing this chapter, the reader should be able to

1. Understand the nature of the pharmaceutical industry.
2. Understand the drug discovery process.
3. Appreciate the role of pharmaceuticals in promoting health.
4. Appreciate the complex legal and regulatory issues facing the industry.
5. Understand the role of government and public policy with regard to pharmaceuticals.

*This chapter is adapted from *Pharmaceutical Industry Profile 2007*, Pharmaceutical Research and Manufacturers of America (PhRMA), 2007, Washington, DC: PhRMA. Copyright © 2007 by the Pharmaceutical Research and Manufacturers of America.

Breakthrough medicines and vaccines have played a central role in this century's unprecedented progress in the treatment of fatal diseases. New medicines generated 40 percent of the 2-year gain in life expectancy achieved in 52 countries between 1986 and 2000. Leading causes of death have been eliminated, and people of all ages enjoy vastly increased life expectancy and improved health. Antibiotics and vaccines figured importantly in the near eradication of syphilis, diphtheria, whooping cough, polio, and measles. Likewise, cardiovascular drugs, ulcer therapies, and anti-inflammatories have had a major impact on heart disease, ulcers, emphysema, and asthma. Advances in biomedical science and revolutionary new research techniques are helping to develop novel approaches to attack infectious, chronic, and genetic diseases. By unraveling the underlying causes of disease, today's research holds the promise that tomorrow's medicines will move beyond the treatment of the symptoms of disease to the prevention or cure of the disease itself. While much progress has been made, many challenges remain. The role of the pharmaceutical industry in addressing the challenges of disease and illness is the subject of this chapter.

Improvements in life expectancy are due in large part to historic discoveries of anti-infective therapies. Introduction of the first sulfa drug in 1935 stimulated interest in pharmaceutical research and set the stage for the successful development of penicillin. The 15 years between 1938 and 1953 became known as "The Age of Antibiotics" as the result of the introduction of an unprecedented number of new anti-infective agents. Antibiotics and vaccines played a major role in the near-eradication of many major diseases of the 1920s, including syphilis, diphtheria, whooping cough, measles, and polio. Since 1920, the combined death rate from influenza and pneumonia has been reduced by 85 percent. Despite a recent resurgence of tuberculosis (TB) among the homeless and immunosuppressed populations, antibiotics have reduced the number of TB deaths to one-tenth the levels experienced in the 1960s. Before antibiotics, the typical TB patient was forced to spend 3 to 4 years in a sanitarium and faced a 30 to 50 percent chance of death. Today, most patients can recover in 6 to 12 months with a full and proper course of antibiotics. Lack of compliance among the homeless and the subsequent emergence of drug-resistant strains of TB remain a challenge to public health officials.

Pharmaceutical discoveries since the 1950s have helped to cut death rates for chronic as well as acute conditions. Cardiovascular drugs such as beta-blockers and ACE inhibitors have contributed to a 74 percent reduction in the death rate for atherosclerosis. Similarly, H2 blockers, proton pump inhibitors, and combination therapies have cut the death rate for ulcers by 72 percent. Anti-inflammatory therapies and bronchodilators have helped reduce the death rate from emphysema by 57 percent and provided relief for those with asthma. Similarly, since 1960, vaccines have greatly reduced the incidence of childhood diseases—many of which once killed or disabled thousands of American children. A vaccine has helped to cut the incidence of hepatitis B, a leading cause of liver cancer in the United States.

The twenty-first century beckons as the Biotechnology Century. Rapid scientific advances—in biochemistry, molecular biology, cell biology, immunology, genetics, and information technology—are transforming drug discovery and development, paving the way for unprecedented progress in developing new medicines to conquer disease.

In the 1980s, scientists identified the gene causing cystic fibrosis; this discovery took 9 years. Scientists located the gene that causes Parkinson's disease—in only 9 days! Gene chips will offer a road map for the prevention of illnesses throughout a lifetime.

Biotechnology offers new approaches to the discovery, design, and production of drugs, vaccines, and diagnostics. The new technology will make it possible to prevent, treat, and cure more diseases than is possible with conventional therapies; to develop more precise and effective new medicines with fewer side effects; to anticipate and prevent disease rather than just react to disease symptoms; to replace human proteins on a large scale that would not otherwise be available in sufficient quantities, such as insulin for diabetics and erythropoietin for cancer patients; and to eliminate the contamination risks of infectious pathogens by avoiding the use of human and animal sources for raw materials, as with the use of recombinant Factor III for the treatment of hemophilia and human growth hormone for growth-deficient children. Through modern biological science, particularly genomics—the study of genes and their function—we better understand the underlying cause of disease, the ways in which drugs operate, and how to create new therapies.

REGULATORY AND LEGAL ISSUES

The drug discovery and development process is time consuming, complex, and highly risky. At the same time, to ensure safety, the research-based pharmaceutical industry is one of the most heavily regulated in the country. The historic Food and Drug Administration (FDA) Modernization Act of 1997 has enabled the agency to further reduce regulatory approval times. Manufacturers are able to make new cures and treatments available to patients about a year earlier than would otherwise have been possible.

Drug Discovery and Testing

The process of discovering and developing a new drug is long and complex. In the discovery phase, pharmaceutical companies employ thousands of scientists to search for compounds capable of affecting disease. While this was once a process of trial and error and serendipitous discovery, it has become more rational and systematic through the use of more sophisticated technology.

From discovery through postmarketing surveillance, drug sponsors and the FDA share an overriding focus to ensure that medicines are safe and effective. The drug development and approval process takes so long in large part because the companies

and the FDA proceed extremely carefully and methodically to ensure that drug benefits outweigh any risks. More clinical trials are being conducted than ever before. More patients are participating in the trials than ever before. As a result, more information on benefits and risks is being developed than ever before. The companies and FDA cannot, however, guarantee that a drug will be risk-free. Drugs are chemical substances that have benefits and potential risks. The FDA does not approve a drug unless it determines that its overall health benefits for the vast majority of patients outweigh its potential risks. But there will always be some risks to some patients.

The FDA and the pharmaceutical industry follow elaborate scientific procedures to ensure safety in four distinct stages:

1. Preclinical safety assessment
2. Preapproval safety assessment in humans
3. Safety assessment during FDA regulatory review
4. Postmarketing safety surveillance

The relative safety of newly synthesized compounds is initially evaluated in both in vitro and in vivo tests. If a compound appears to have important biological activity and may be useful as a drug, special tests are conduced to evaluate safety in the major organ systems (e.g., central nervous, cardiovascular, and respiratory systems). Other organ systems are evaluated when potential problems appear. These pharmacology studies are conduced in animals to ensure that a drug is safe enough to be tested in humans. An important goal of these preclinical animal studies is to characterize any relationship between increased doses of the drug and toxic effects in the animals. Development of a drug is usually halted when tests suggest that it possesses a significant risk for humans, especially organ damage, genetic defects, birth defects, or cancer.

A drug sponsor may begin clinical studies in humans once the FDA is satisfied that the preclinical animal data do not show an unacceptable safety risk to humans. The time ranges from a few to many years for a clinical development program to gather sufficient data to prepare a new drug application (NDA) seeking FDA regulatory review to market a new drug. Every clinical study evaluates safety, regardless of whether safety is a stated objective. During all studies, including quality-of-life and pharmacoeconomic studies, patients are observed for adverse events. These are reported to the FDA and, when appropriate, the information is incorporated in a drug's package labeling. The average NDA for a novel prescription drug is based on almost 70 clinical trials involving more than 4,000 patients—more than twice the number of trials and patients for the NDAs submitted in the early 1980s.

Clinical studies are conduced in three stages:

- *Phase I:* Most drugs are evaluated for safety in health volunteers in small initial trials. A trial is conducted with a single dose of the drug, beginning with small doses. If the drug is shown to be safe, multiple doses of the product are evaluated for safety in other clinical trials.

- *Phase II:* The efficacy of the drug is the primary focus of these second-stage trials, but safety is also studied. These trials are conducted with patients instead of healthy volunteers; data are collected to determine whether the drug is safe for the patient population intended to be treated.

- *Phase III:* These large trials evaluate safety and efficacy in groups of patients with the disease to be treated, including the elderly, patients with multiple diseases, those who take other drugs, and/or patients whose organs are impaired.

Investigators must promptly report all unanticipated risks to human subjects. Investigators are also required to report all adverse events that occur during a trial. A sponsor must report an adverse event that is unexpected, serious, and possibly drug-related to the FDA within 15 days. Every individual adverse event that is fatal or life threatening must be reported within 7 days.

A sponsor submits an NDA to the FDA for approval to manufacture, distribute, and market a drug in the United States based on the safety and efficacy data obtained during the clinical trials. In addition to written reports of each individual study included in the NDA, an application must contain an integrated summary of all available information received from any source concerning the safety and efficacy of the drug.

The FDA usually completes its review of a "standard" drug in 10 to 12 months. One hundred and twenty days prior to a drug's anticipated approval, a sponsor must provide the agency with a summary of all safety information in the NDA, along with any additional safety information obtained during the review period. While the FDA is approving drugs more expeditiously, the addition of 600 new reviewers has been made possible by user fees. Over the years, the percentage of applications approved and rejected by the FDA has remained stable. Two decades ago, 10 to 15 percent of NDAs were rejected—the same as today.

Postapproval Safety and Marketing

Monitoring and evaluating a drug's safety becomes more complex after it is approved and marketed. Once on the market, a drug will be taken by many more patients than in the clinical trials, and physicians are free to use it in different doses, different dosing regimens, different patient populations, and in other ways that they believe will benefit patients. This wider use expands the safety information about a drug. Adverse reactions that occur in fewer than 3,000–5,000 patients are unlikely to be detected in Phase I–III investigational clinical trials and may be unknown at the time a drug is approved. These adverse reactions are more likely to be detected when large numbers of patients are exposed to a drug after it have been approved.

Safety monitoring continues for the life of a drug. Postmarketing surveillance is a highly regulated and labor-intensive global activity. Even before a drug is approved, multinational pharmaceutical companies establish large global systems to track, investigate, evaluate, and report adverse drug reactions (ADRs) for that product on a continuing basis to regulatory authorities around the world. As a condition of approval, the FDA may require a company to conduct a postmarketing study, or a company may decide on its own to undertake such a study to gather more safety information. A company may also undertake a study if it believes that the report of ADRs it has received requires such action. These studies may consist of new clinical trials or they may be evaluations of existing databases. The FDA collects reports of ADRs from companies (which submit more than 90 percent of the reports), physicians, and other health care professionals. The agency evaluates the reports for trends and implications and may require a company to provide more data, undertake a new clinical trial, revise a drug's labeling, notify health care professionals, or even remove a product from the market.

In addition to meeting regulatory requirements necessary to prove drug safety and efficacy, manufacturers must also comply with FDA regulations to ensure the quality of pharmaceutical manufacturing. These "good manufacturing practice" (GMP) requirements govern quality management and control for all aspects of drug manufacturing. To enforce GMP requirements, the FDA conducts field inspections where training investigators periodically visit manufacturing sites to ensure that a facility is in compliance with the regulations.

The FDA also regulates all aspects of pharmaceutical marketing. These regulations are to ensure that health care professionals and the public are provided with adequate, balanced, and truthful information and that all promotional claims are based on scientifically proven clinical evidence. Key aspects of marketing regulations include labeling, advertisements, promotional claims, investigational new drugs, and advertising in the form of Internet, television, and direct-to-consumer marketing.

Labeling

Labels and other written, printed, or graphic matter on a drug or its packaging (including all other promotional material such as brochures, slides, video tapes, and other sales aids) must not be false or misleading in any way. The labeling must include adequate directions for use of a product, warnings when needed against use in children and people with certain conditions, dosage information, and methods and duration of use. Labeling must include a brief summary of a drug's side effects, contraindications, and effectiveness. Any deviation from labeling regulations is considered "misbranding," a serious violation of federal law.

Advertising and Promotional Claims

All advertising is subject to the same requirements that apply to drug labeling. An ad must include a brief summary that gives a balanced presentation of side effects, contraindications, and effectiveness. It also must include information on all indications for which a drug is approved but may not include any information on unapproved or "off-label" uses. All promotional claims must be in agreement with the most current information and scientific knowledge available. The FDA may cite an ad as false, misleading, or lacking in fair balance based on its emphasis or manner of presentation.

Claims of safety relate to the nature and degree of side effects and adverse reactions associated with a drug or the overall risk benefit ratio of the drug. Claims of effectiveness relate to the ability of a drug to achieve its indicated therapeutic effect. Any product claims relating to safety and effectiveness must be supported by adequate and well-controlled studies. The FDA Modernization Act allows promotion of economic claims to HMOs based on "competent and reliable scientific evidence."

Investigational New Drugs

Unapproved drugs under clinical development or approved drugs under investigation for a new indication can be discussed in scientific literature and at medical conferences but cannot be promoted as safe or effective. The FDA may authorize distribution of the unapproved treatment investigational new drug to seriously ill patients who are not participating in clinical studies.

FROM IDEA TO TREATMENT: THE LONG, UNCERTAIN RESEARCH AND DEVELOPMENT PROCESS

According to the National Science Foundation, pharmaceutical product development comprises one of the most research-intensive sectors in the United States. The industry is one of the largest employers of scientists in the United States—and its success or failure relies heavily on their ability to make breakthroughs.

On average it takes 10 to 15 years and costs more than $800 million (and up to $1.2 billion for a biologic) to advance a potential new medicine from a research idea to a treatment approved by the FDA. That means that for more than a decade, scientists, engineers, and physicians strive every day in laboratories and hospitals searching for a new discovery and a way to deliver those new medicines to patients. It may entail trying to understand how to turn a key gene on or off. Researchers may test thousands of chemicals for biochemical activity in the body. It might involve attempting to create a completely new chemical compound, one so unique that the U.S. government grants its inventor a patent.

The research doesn't end with the understanding of how a gene works or the creation of a new molecule—scientists must then transform those discoveries into medicines. The chemicals and biologics must be safe and work as they should when ingested. They must be engineered so that the body absorbs them in the proper quantities and transports them to their sites of action.

Even after a medicine is discovered, teams of engineers, biologists, chemists, and physicists must spend long hours figuring out how to mass-produce the results achieved by an individual scientist at his or her lab bench. Often promising experiments are not replicable on a large scale. The research may fail because it is not possible to manufacture the drug safely or to the proper specifications.

Teams of physicians must study the effects of a new medicine on patients to discover whether it really works in a population and works without causing unacceptable side effects. Clinical trials may take years and involve thousands of patients and procedures. On average each new trial requires many procedures and increasingly larger numbers of patients.

After a decade or more of the scientists', engineers', and physicians' efforts, still only one out of five medicines that enter clinical trials is approved for patient use by the FDA. The process is long, risky, fraught with failure, and ultimately expensive. Failure at the clinical trial stage could completely nullify 15 years of work.

The United States is the world leader in pharmaceutical research. During the 1990s, the United States surpassed Europe as the leading site for pharmaceutical research and development (R&D). The increased concentration of research efforts in the United States is reflected by the fact that 8 of the top 10 medicines by sales originate from the United States, compared to 2 from Europe.

Americans are also conducting more pharmaceutical-related research in universities and public institutions as compared to their European counterparts (Figure 11.1). However, academic scientists

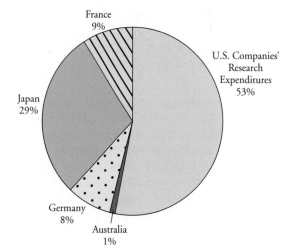

Figure 11.1. Worldwide Pharmaceutical Research

SOURCE: *Pharmaceutical Industry Profile 2004*, 2004, Washington, DC: Pharmaceutical Research and Manufacturers of America (PhRMA).

might use National Institutes of Health (NIH) dollars to discover how two genes interact to cause a disease, but a scientist in a pharmaceutical research company lab will discover how to create a medicine to regulate those genes, thus inventing the treatment or cure for a disease.

Last year pharmaceutical research companies spent $33 billion on research to develop new and better medicines, a 7 percent increase from the previous year. Over time, this investment will yield new medicines that will make progress in better treating a range of diseases that impose large direct and indirect costs on patients and society.

The innovation taking place in pharmaceutical research leads to new and better treatments for disease (Exhibit 11.1). The products of this innovation will allow millions of patients to live longer, better, and more productive lives. New medicines also help curb overall health care costs by often reducing the need for hospitalization and more invasive procedures, such as surgery, or by delaying nursing home admission. The combination of innovation in new medicines and a shift to prescription medications as preferred medical intervention means that spending on prescription drugs has increased.

Since 1990, pharmaceutical research company scientists have invented and developed more than 300 completely new medicines, vaccines, and biologics approved by the FDA to treat more than 150 conditions, ranging from infectious diseases to chronic diseases—and from diseases affecting millions of patients to those afflicting less than 200,000 people. Recent pharmaceutical research company advances are helping to meet the emerging diabetes epidemic, save the lives of cancer patients, and forestall the burden of Alzheimer's disease. The progress made in reducing death rates from heart disease and stroke, for example, is saving the lives of more than 1 million Americans each year. In addition, pharmaceutical research has created new medicines for a number of serious, but rare, conditions such as Fabry's disease, cystic

EXHIBIT 11.1 A Decade of Innovation

Today, patients who would have faced death or disability a few years ago have treatments options available to help them live healthier, more productive lives. A sampling of these innovations are as follows.

- Patients suffering from Alzheimer's disease (AD), a neurological condition that leads to cognitive decline among older people, had few treatment options until the past decade, when the FDA approved new medicines to treat AD and slow impairment. A new class of drugs is the first approved treatment for moderate to severe AD. New medicines are still greatly needed to stem the enormous costs of AD because the number of cases continues to rise.

- High blood pressure can lead to stroke, blindness, heart problems, and kidney damage. Since 1995, scientists have developed two new classes of blood pressure medications, angiotensin-II antagonists and selective aldosterone receptor antagonists. These new medicines improve blood pressure control with individualized treatment plans and have fewer side effects.

- Schizophrenia is an incapacitating mental illness that impairs the patient's sense of reality, reduces the ability to relate to people, and, in many cases, causes hallucinations.

- New atypical antipsychotic medicines treat schizophrenia with fewer problematic side effects than older drugs, which makes them easier for patients to tolerate and continue taking. As a result, many people with schizophrenia can now lead more normal, independent lives.

fibrosis, sickle cell anemia, and a number of rare cancers.

Medical literature today includes countless studies demonstrating medicines' ability to help patients avoid hospitalization and invasive surgery, or delay the need for long-term nursing home care. In addition to improving patient quality of life and giving physicians more options to tailor treatment to the needs of individual patients, the use of new medicines also reduces overall health care costs. For example, by preventing complications, side effects, and symptoms, new medicines drastically reduce the need for hospitalization.

Examples of Pharmaceutical Invention

Scientists have developed new medicines to treat a number of gastrointestinal disorders over the past two decades. Since these medicines have become available to patients, the need for surgical procedures to correct ulcers has slowed, and today ulcer surgery is a relic of the past.

A new Alzheimer's drug slows the progression of cognitive decline, allowing patients to maintain their independence longer and delay entering a nursing home by an average of 30 months. Nursing home care is more costly than in-home care, so this delay can significantly reduce health care expenditures—and the economic and emotional burden on both patient and caregiver.

The health of AIDS patients is not only improved by new medicines, but those medicines also reduce the need for costly hospital care. After the introduction of highly active antiretroviral therapy (HAART) for the treatment of AIDS, pharmaceutical expenditures increased by about 33 percent, while hospital expenditures decreased by about 43 percent. Overall, total health care expenditures decreased by 16 percent (between 1996 and 1998).

New medicines to reduce the incidence of breast cancer can help women avoid later chemotherapy and surgery. Because of the high-technology science needed to develop these new prescription drugs,

the medication costs as much as $1,050 a year. However, surgery, chemotherapy, or other invasive treatments for women suffering from breast cancer may cost as much as $14,000 a year.

Medicines have played a significant role in the life expectancy gains made in the United States and around the world. New medicines are estimated to have generated 40 percent of the 2-year gain in life expectancy achieved in 52 countries between 1986 and 2000.

In many cases new medicines and vaccines help prevent disease, in addition to those that may cure or alleviate previously fatal or debilitating conditions. For example, new medicines contributed to the decline in U.S. HIV/AIDS death rates.

Some cancers have become a "chronic disease much like asthma, diabetes, and, more recently, AIDS" as a result of new diagnostic techniques and innovative medicines. Today there are 3 million more cancer survivors than there were a decade ago. The chance of surviving for five years after diagnosis has risen by 10 percentage points over the past two decades to 62 percent today.

New and better medicines are not only extending more people's lives but also giving them higher quality, more productive years. Risks for chronic disabilities such as stroke and dementia have declined sharply.

As patients and health care professionals have turned increasingly to medications as cost-effective alternatives to invasive surgery and hospitalization, spending on prescription medicines has naturally increased. Although prescription medicines are often portrayed as the main driver of rising health care costs, prescription drugs accounted for 16 percent of total health care spending increases in a recent year.

In addition to more than 70,000 scientists, the pharmaceutical research industry directly employs more than 315,000 Americans. New medicines also benefit the economy by increasing worker productivity and reducing absenteeism. Many types of medicines—including those for depression, migraines, diabetes, and allergies—help boost worker productivity.

ACCESS, PRICING, AND PATENT ISSUES

Ultimately, innovative medicines make a difference only when patients have access to them and use them. Underutilization of effective new medicines is a serious concern that limits the potential public health impact of pharmaceutical discoveries (Exhibit 11.2). Strategies to contain pharmaceutical costs have led to less access to needed medicines for patients. However, some important programs that broaden access to innovative medicines illustrate the positive impact of this approach.

In recent years, many Medicaid programs have instituted preferred drug lists (PDLs), which specify the reimbursable medicines physicians can freely prescribe. Drugs not on the PDL are reimbursed only if a patient's doctor first obtains special permission from the insurer to prescribe the drug (known as "prior authorization"). Although the intent of this mechanism is to control costs, the result has been less access to needed medicines for patients. Prior authorization and restrictive PDLs limit a physician's ability to choose the most appropriate medicine(s) for the patient. Yet one size does not fit all when it comes to medicines because individual differences in drug response are common.

Access restrictions are particularly onerous for low-income patients, who lack the resources to pay

---

EXHIBIT 11.2   Underutilization of Drugs

Use of medicines is increasing as more patients take medicines for a broader range of conditions. This is indicative of new medicines offering new treatment options (e.g., Alzheimer's disease and chemotherapy-induced anemia) and changing standards of medical care that call for earlier use of medicines to prevent the progression of disease, use of combination therapy rather than a single medicine, and improved therapies. Nonetheless, increasing use of medicines is often cited in policy debates as indicating widespread overuse of medicines.

In fact, while only limited research indicates overuse of prescription drugs, there is much evidence that large numbers of patients underuse needed medical care, including prescription medicines, for many serious health conditions. Such underuse is not limited to patients without health insurance or prescription drug coverage—it clearly afflicts patients who have health insurance with prescription drug coverage.

A RAND study found that nearly half of all adults in the United States fail to receive recommended health care. Only 45 percent of patients with diabetes received the care they needed; only 68 percent of patients with coronary artery disease received recommended care; only 45 percent of heart attack patients received medications that could reduce their risk of death; only 54 percent of patients with colorectal cancer received recommended care; and less than 65 percent of patients with high blood pressure received recommended care. According to the RAND researchers, "the deficiencies in care . . . pose serious threats to the health of the American public that could contribute to thousands of preventable deaths in the United States each year" (McGlynn et al., 2003).

In assessing underuse and overuse of health care services, the study included an examination of nine health conditions that require treatment with prescription medicines. There was underuse of prescription medications in seven of the nine conditions. Those seven conditions were asthma, cerebrovascular disease, congestive heart failure, diabetes, hip fracture, hyperlipidemia, and hypertension.

for innovative medicines out of pocket. If the most appropriate medicines for them are not on the PDL, they face fighting their way through the bureaucracy of prior authorizations and/or lengthy appeals processes—or doing without.

Yet experience shows that denial of the most appropriate drug therapy ultimately lowers quality of care and increases use of more expensive services, such as hospitalization. For example, clinicians treating patients in Michigan's Medicaid program reported that the prior authorization process was overly burdensome and time consuming for them and their patients. The process also harmed vulnerable Medicaid beneficiaries, such as an HIV/AIDS patient who had to be hospitalized due to a delay in obtaining prior authorization for a necessary medication.

While Medicaid PDLs seek to restrict access to medicines, alternative approaches seek to improve quality of care and achieve overall health cost savings by promoting the correct use of medicines, thereby avoiding the later need for more costly interventions. Increases in expenditures for prescription medicines often help patients lead healthier lives while avoiding expensive hospitalizations, emergency room visits, and long-term care. Disease management programs work to increase patient access to innovative medicines to improve health and reduce overall health care costs.

Patient-focused disease management programs promote appropriate use of pharmaceuticals and medical resource utilization. In these programs, patients receive more intensive education, assistance, and monitoring in following a treatment plan tailored to their needs. Managed-care organizations and large employers make up the majority of disease management clients, although some state Medicaid programs also offer them. Disease management programs rely heavily on giving patients access to innovative medicines to reduce health care costs and improve outcomes.

For example, disease management programs, which target patient populations with specific high-cost, high-risk chronic conditions, have shown that increased spending on medicines that manage disease helps reduce surgeries, hospitalizations, and emergency room visits. Patient-focused disease management programs promote appropriate use of pharmaceuticals and medical resource utilization.

Direct-to-consumer advertising (DTCA) brings Food and Drug Administration approved information about prescription medicines to patients and families. Through print and broadcast channels, many people learn about new medications for symptoms they are experiencing.

The ability of patients without insurance coverage to access medicines is essential to maintaining health. Pharmaceutical research companies employ a number of programs—discount cards, supporting clinics, donated medicines—to help patients gain access to the medicines they need. Through these programs, companies provide prescription drugs free of charge to patients who might otherwise not have access to necessary medicines, such as those who do not have prescription drug insurance coverage or who are underinsured with either private and/or government health plans. Companies also allow physicians, hospitals, community pharmacies, home health companies, and others to obtain drugs for patients in need. In 2003, an estimated 6.2 million patients received prescription medicines through these programs.

In the United States today, a vigorously competitive pharmaceutical market provides incentives for scientists to be the first to bring a new product to market and potentially earn rewards after more than a decade of costly research. Pricing through a competitive market also allows innovators to earn returns on successful inventions, thus providing the substantial funds necessary to continue other research projects.

However, in parts of the world where the government controls prescription drug prices, both innovation and patient access to innovation suffer. In many European countries where governments impose prescription drug price controls, patients must wait as long as 2 years for new medicines to get to market while bureaucrats decide on price levels.

Some national health care systems restrict access to a new medicine even after setting its price. In the

United Kingdom (UK), a governmental board, the National Institute for Clinical Excellence (NICE), issues recommendations based on a number of factors (including cost effectiveness) as to whether the National Health Service (NHS) should make medicines available to patients covered by the government-run health care system. European price controls often restrict patient access to medicines that American doctors cite as essential for proper patient care. There are huge differences in the access to medicines among the various European countries. The shift of research and development (R&D) investment and the physical relocation of pharmaceutical research laboratories from Europe to the United States especially with consolidation underline the significance of free-market policies for producing innovation.

Patents and Drugs

Another policy important to innovation is governments' granting of patents as an incentive for research and for inventors to share their discoveries with the public. In the United States, patents are granted according to strict standards by trained examiners at the U.S. Patent and Trademark Office (USPTO). They are granted only to inventions proved as new, useful, and nonobvious and provide only a limited period of exclusivity to the inventor (20 years in the United States), after which anyone can replicate or use the invention.

Patent incentives encourage the development of new medicines by attempting to provide a level of certainty to inventors. If granted a patent, scientists and the companies they work for know that they have a protected period of time in which they may prevent others from selling their invention. The exclusive right to exclude others from selling the new invention during this time gives them the opportunity to potentially recoup the hundreds of millions of dollars invested in researching and developing a new medicine.

Under current law, generic drug manufacturers can infringe unexpired patents in order to prepare their copies for Food and Drug Administration approval and the market, and can—in an increasing number of instances—enter the market with their copies years before patents expire. In fact, a growing number of generics seek to enter the market as quickly as 5 years after an innovator medicine is approved. Yet pharmaceuticals already have fewer effective years of patent protection than other U.S. products.

Continuing Innovation

Over the past several decades, scientists have invented and discovered a steady stream of new and better medicines, advanced our scientific and technological capabilities, and improved our knowledge of disease. The work of these scientists is far from over.

In some labs geneticists are striving to unlock the secrets of the human genome and to develop new scientific techniques for regulating the genes that cause disease. In other labs chemists are developing new and more efficient ways to combine chemical compounds to produce new treatments for patients. Engineers and computer scientists are designing robots to screen new compounds for biochemical activity and design new and faster computers and applications to analyze data on potential drug targets. Biologists are trying to understand and replicate the complex structure of proteins and are looking for new tools to combat antibiotic-resistant bacteria and bioterrorism agents.

Prescription drugs save lives, alleviate suffering, and improve the quality of life. They also often reduce the need for other more invasive and expensive treatments. A narrow focus on the cost of drugs, without regard to their value and their role in the health system as a whole, would discourage innovation and harm the prospects for health advances.

Better quality patient care is often more efficient care. For example, large percentages of patients with conditions such as diabetes, depression, hypertension, and high cholesterol are not receiving needed care, yielding worse health outcomes and higher overall costs. Focusing on promoting solutions that improve quality will lead to better results for patients and more affordable medical care.

Instead of focusing on reducing the prescription drug line item, some health plans are emphasizing disease management programs, which recognize the value of medicines in both improving patient care and offsetting other health care expenditures. Furthermore, a competitive market provides greater opportunity for access to medicines.

THE VALUE OF MEDICINES

Medicines save lives, relieve pain and cure and prevent disease. Medicines help keep families together longer and improve the quality of life for patients and caregivers. Medicines keep employees on the job and productive in the community. They also help people—and the health care system—avoid disability, surgery, hospitalization and nursing home care, often decreasing the total cost of caring for an illness.

Ulcer treatment provides a good example of the ability of pharmaceutical innovation to reduce costs, both for individuals and for the health care system. Before 1977, the year in which stomach-acid-blocking H2 antagonist drugs were introduced, 97,000 ulcer surgeries were performed each year. By 1987, the number of surgeries per year had dropped to fewer than 19,000. In the early 1990s, the annual cost of drug therapy per person was about $900, compared to about $28,000 for surgery. The discovery that the *H. pylori* bacterium is the principal cause of ulcers led to the use of antibiotics in combination with H2 antagonists to treat duodenal ulcers.

Every 5 years since 1965, roughly one additional year has been added to life expectancy at birth. These longer life spans are due, in large part, to the conquest of diseases by pharmaceuticals: Vaccines have virtually wiped out such diseases as diphtheria, whooping cough, measles and polio in the United States. The influenza epidemic of 1918

killed more Americans than all the battles fought during the World War I. Since that time, medicines have helped reduce the combined U.S. death rate from influenza and pneumonia by 85 percent; in large part to new medicines, deaths from heart disease have been cut by more than half since 1950. And this steady decline is continuing; deaths from all cancers combined as well as for the top 10 cancer sites declined in the United States between 1990 and 1997, due to better treatments and early detection; and since 1965, drugs have helped cut emphysema deaths by 57 percent and ulcer deaths by 72 percent.

Medicines are helping more children grow into healthy adults. In 1949, more than one in every hundred babies died of respiratory distress syndrome due to immature lungs. Today, thanks in large part to new medicines that accelerate lung maturity in premature babies, infant mortality rates have sunk to record lows. Polio, which killed nearly 2,000 American children in 1950, is now virtually unknown, thanks to vaccines. Before routine measles vaccination began in the 1960s, more than 3 million cases of this childhood disease and 500 deaths from measles were reported each year. Cases of bacterial meningitis among young children dropped nearly 80 percent over 11 years after the introduction of a vaccine.

Treating cystic fibrosis patients with a breakthrough medicine reduces hospitalization and related medical costs. This medicine, when used in conjunction with standard treatments, was proven in clinical trials to reduce the risk of respiratory tract infections requiring intravenous antibiotic therapy by 27 percent. For asthma patients, increased drug spending kept patients out of the hospital. Total health care costs declined nearly 25 percent and hospitalization rates dropped by 50 percent for asthma patients using new inhaled corticosteroid therapy.

New medicines have helped reduce the toll of cancer, and ongoing pharmaceutical research promises to continue and accelerate the impressive progress made against cancer in the past decade (Exhibit 11.3). Researchers are using new knowledge

EXHIBIT 11.3   New Chemotherapy: Nineteen Years from Idea to Approval

In 2000 the FDA approved a new chemotherapy treatment, Mylotarg®, for patients with relapsed acute myelogenous leukemia. The approval came 19 years after scientists at Lederle Labs, now Wyeth, first discovered a microorganism in a soil sample that produced a powerful anticancer substance called calicheamicin.

Scientists learned that calicheamicin destroys cell DNA, which results in the cell's death. Thus, in theory, targeting it to cancerous cells could eliminate them. In developing any cancer treatment, a key challenge is finding a way to kill cancer cells while minimizing or avoiding damage to the body's other healthy cells. However, calicheamicin's exceptionally high toxicity (between 1,000 and 10,000 times more toxic than traditional anticancer medicines) meant that scientists had to find a novel way to deliver the drug only to cancer cells.

Before concentrating on making the medicine safe for patient use, the pharmaceutical researchers first had to figure out how to make large quantities of calicheamicin for experimentation. During the next 5 years, they worked to understand its structure and how to stabilize it.

The team spent the next 3 years trying to develop a "linker" molecule that would bind tightly to the calicheamicin to deliver it directly to cancer cells without releasing it in the bloodstream. Although they found linkers that worked in animals, they had problems converting them to a form usable in humans. Working virtually around the clock, only stopping for a break on Christmas day, the pharmaceutical research company scientists tested 35 linkers before finding one that worked. Finally, in 1995, 14 years after discovering calicheamicin, the new medicine Mylotarg® entered human clinical trials. After nearly 5 years of successful clinical trials, the FDA approved the medicine for widespread patient use.

and innovative techniques to hone in on cancer cells without damaging healthy cells.

Pharmaceutical companies have developed a number of drugs that improve the quality of life for cancer patients and, in some cases, lower the cost of cancer treatment. Drugs that prevent nausea during chemotherapy are making treatment easier to bear for many patients, as are medicines that help restore the energy that chemotherapy can take away. Another medicine, called a colony stimulating factor, helps patients whose immune systems are weakened by high-dose chemotherapy. A shift from intravenous to newer forms of oral chemotherapy is also yielding savings both in quality of life and in cost reductions.

Prescription medicines can reduce disability and absenteeism and increase productivity—while improving the quality of life for employees. Migraine headaches not only cause pain to those who suffer from them—they also take a huge toll in absenteeism and lost productivity. Thanks to a breakthrough drug, however, the human and economic costs of migraine headaches are dropping. Total costs of treating patients for migraine headaches declined 41 percent as the result of the new drug treatment. The drug saved employers $435 per month per treated employee due to a reduction in lost productivity costs, while the monthly cost of the drug per employee was only $43.78.

Depression affects nearly 18 million Americans. Its annual toll on U.S. businesses amounts to about $70 billion in medical expenditures, lost productivity, and other costs. Innovative prescription medicines are reducing employers' costs and absenteeism drops when depressed workers are treated with prescription medicines. Savings from improved productivity and the reduction in work loss and medical costs far outweighed the cost of the drug.

Hay fever, or seasonal allergic rhinitis, affects an estimated 13 million working adults and has been shown to cause absenteeism and diminished work productivity. But new nonsedating antihistamines actually increase worker productivity.

Women live an average of 7 years longer than men. The bad news is they are more susceptible to a number of diseases and more likely to experience illness or disability. Pharmaceutical companies are targeting diseases that disproportionately afflict women. Over 300 medicines are in development for such diseases as rheumatoid arthritis, multiple sclerosis, lupus, osteoporosis, breast cancer, ovarian cancer, diabetes, and depression.

Breast cancer is the second leading cause of cancer death among U.S. women, exceeded only by lung cancer. Breast cancer afflicts 8 million American women and takes 40,000 lives each year. Breast cancer deaths have declined due to early detection and better treatments, including new medicines. Some of the latest medicines developed for breast cancer are a genetically engineered version of one of the body's own weapons for killing invaders; an oral anticancer drug to shrink hard-to-treat tumors; and a drug that can reduce the incidence of breast cancer in high-risk women.

Multiple sclerosis, or MS, is a chronic, often progressive disease of the central nervous system in which scattered patches of the covering of nerve fibers in the brain and spinal cord are destroyed. MS is most often diagnosed in people in their twenties and thirties, and women develop the disease at a rate almost double that of men. An estimated 350,000 Americans have this disease. The average annual cost of MS exceeds $34,000 per person, while the lifetime cost is more than $2.2 million per person.

Treatment with a breakthrough medicine slows the cognitive impairment often suffered by people with relapsing MS. The medicine has also been shown to reduce relapses and slow the progression of the disease. A combination of two powerful drugs may help patients who continue to suffer flare-ups on one-drug treatment.

One of every two women will have an osteoporosis-related fracture at some point in her life. In osteoporosis, a reduction in bone mass leads to fractures, particularly of the vertebrae, hips, and wrist. Bone-density screening for early detection, strengthening exercises, and innovative medicines can help people avoid osteoporosis. Several types of medicines are available to help prevent osteoporosis and to reduce the human and economic toll of this disease. Because fractures due to osteoporosis often lead to disability and nursing home admission, new medicines for osteoporosis are the best hope of cutting the cost of this disease.

Heart disease is America's number-one killer, and stroke is third, following cancer. Heart disease and stroke claim almost a million lives and cost $300 billion each year. New treatments, including innovative medicines, have helped cut deaths from heart disease and stroke in half in the past 30 years and are also reducing the economic toll of these diseases. The widespread use of blood pressure drugs over the past half century appears to have sharply reduced dangerous hypertension and potentially lethal enlargement of the heart's main pumping chamber. A blood thinning drug reduces the risk of new heart attacks, strokes, and death by 20 percent a year in people being treated for mild heart attacks and bad chest pain. ACE inhibitor drugs for patients with congestive heart failure helped avoid $9,000 per person in hospitalization costs and reduce deaths. The use of a beta-blocker medicine to treat high blood pressure and congestive heart failure sharply reduces hospital admissions. Combining two common medicines can significantly reduce the risk of death for patients with mild heart failure: Using beta-blockers and ACE inhibitors in combination can reduce the risk of death from heart failure by 30 percent. A study sponsored by the National Institutes of Health (NIH) found that treating stroke patients promptly with a clot-busting medicine reduces the need for hospitalization, rehabilitation, and nursing home care.

Some historians have called the era from the 1940s through the 1990s "the Golden Age of

Medicine." But many scientists predict that even those accomplishments will be dwarfed by the achievements of the twenty-first century. Stunning advances in the knowledge about disease, increases in targets available for drug discovery, and our growing ability to design effective medicines open the door to exciting possibilities. No one can predict the future with great accuracy, but here are some of the developments scientists believe are possible in this next "Platinum Age" of medicine: Medicines can already stop the AIDS virus from reproducing. The next breakthrough may be medicines that can stop the virus from entering the cell in the first place; drugs that will slow the progression of Alzheimer's disease; "cocktails" of treatments, including vaccines, monoclonal antibodies, immune system boosters, and drugs that cut off a tumor's blood supply in an all-out attack against cancer; medicines that will prompt the heart to grow new blood vessels, reducing the need for bypass surgery; and treatments that may regenerate nerves damaged by brain disease or spinal cord injury.

Arthritis

Rheumatoid arthritis (RA) is a chronic inflammatory autoimmune disease that primarily affects the joints. In this disease, the body's immune system attacks the cells of a fluid that surrounds the joints. This fluid normally lubricates and nourishes the bones and cartilage within a joint, but with RA, the inflammatory process causes this fluid to become thicker and begin to destroy the cartilage and bone. This leads to RA's characteristic effects on the joints: pain, swelling, loss of function. RA can also lead to bone loss that causes osteoporosis, as well as the development of anemia, neck pain, dry eyes and mouth, bumps under the skin, and very rarely, inflammation of the blood vessels, the lining of the lungs, or the sac enclosing the heart.

Medicines seek to relieve the symptoms of RA in three main ways: reducing pain, decreasing inflammation, and slowing damage to the joints. Before 1998, treatment of rheumatoid arthritis depended largely on nonsteroidal anti-inflammatory drugs (NSAIDs) like aspirin. However, since 1998, patients suffering from rheumatoid arthritis have benefited from a surge in the approval of new treatments for their often painful condition. In 1998, the FDA approved the first new disease modifying anti-rheumatic drug (DMARD) specifically developed for the treatment of rheumatoid arthritis in more than a decade. This class has the potential to reduce or prevent joint damage, preserve joint integrity and function, and ultimately, reduce the total costs of health care and maintain economic productivity of the patient with RA. That same year, the FDA also approved the first in a new category of biologic products known as biological response modifiers. Medical products in this category reduce inflammation by blocking the protein in the immune system that causes excessive inflammation in those with RA.

Advances in drug treatment continued in 1998 with the FDA's approval of a medicine in a third new class of drugs known as COX-2 (cyclo-oxygenase-2) inhibitors. Like NSAIDs, these drugs block COX-2, an enzyme that causes inflammation. However, unlike NSAIDs, they do not block COX-1, an enzyme that protects the lining of the stomach, thus reducing risk of the gastrointestinal ulcers and bleeding that can occur with NSAIDs. In 2004, these drugs faced a challenge due to concerns about elevated cardiovascular risks in clinical use.

Although RA still has no cure, drug treatments are helping patients live more comfortable, productive lives. New drugs in development focus on the early stages of the immune response to block only those specific immune system cells involved in autoimmune disease; so-called "next generation biologics," including co-stimulatory blockers that prevent the initial signaling and chain of chemical reactions that turn on the immune system; and therapies that inhibit the migration of inflammatory cells into the joint tissues, thus preventing cartilage and bone destruction. Trials of gene therapy products that affect factors regulating the immune system have also shown promising results.

HIV/AIDS

Like other viruses, the human immunodeficiency virus (HIV) that causes acquired immune deficiency syndrome (AIDS) replicates by entering a healthy cell and taking over its machinery. Most medicines available to treat HIV infection have gained FDA approval in the past decade, including four new classes of medicines that target three different stages of the HIV virus's life cycle. Two new classes of medicines, along with one class approved in the late 1980s, use different mechanisms to interfere with the reverse transcriptase enzyme, thereby interrupting an early stage of the HIV life cycle. Medicines in the earliest class of drugs, nucleoside analogues, provide faulty DNA building blocks, halting the DNA chain that the virus uses to make copies of itself.

A second drug class, introduced in 1996 and called nonnucleoside reverse transcriptase inhibitors, binds to the enzyme so it cannot copy itself. The third class, nucleotide analogue reverse transcriptase inhibitors, was first introduced in 2001. These drugs block the reverse transcriptase to prevent replication of the HIV virus. A second enzyme, protease, is a critical player in a later stage of the HIV life cycle. The first drug in a class of protease inhibitors to combat this enzyme was approved in 1995. Health care providers combine protease inhibitors with the other classes of antiviral medicines in a strategy known as combination therapy (using more than one type of medicine to treat a condition). This strategy has been used to treat both early-stage and advanced-stage HIV disease and is an important factor behind the significant decline in AIDS deaths in the United States in recent years.

In 2003, the FDA approved the first in another new class of drugs that prevents the HIV virus from attaching to healthy cells. This class, known as fusion inhibitors, blocks the virus's ability to infect certain components of the immune system. Recent clinical trials showed that when added to combination therapy regimens, fusion inhibitors can decrease the amount of virus in the bloodstream to undetectable levels. Because these drugs attack the HIV virus in a totally different way, they can be of particular benefit to individuals who have developed resistance to previously available medicines.

Beyond the entirely new classes of drugs, important innovations within existing drug classes have made the treatment of people living with HIV/AIDS more effective as well as more tolerable. For example, the first treatments had to be taken multiple times a day, but many new drugs are available in twice-daily or even once-daily dosage forms.

Medicines under development for AIDS and AIDS-related conditions include, among others, an antisense gene therapy medicine that uses two novel technologies to boost immune responsiveness against HIV; a new medicine that blocks a third enzyme, known as integrase, that the HIV virus uses to copy itself; and a number of HIV/AIDS vaccines that may prevent the spread of the virus.

Although a cure has not yet been found for HIV/AIDS, new medicines that are the product of research have dramatically affected the length and quality of life for those infected with the HIV virus. Because people receiving pharmaceutical therapy for HIV/AIDS are better able to maintain their health, they use fewer health care services and use them less often.

Neurology and Mental Health

Parkinson's disease is a condition that results from the breakdown of neurons in the part of the brain that controls movement. This breakdown causes a shortage of a chemical called dopamine. Dopamine is responsible for relaying the brain's instructions for movement, and a lack of it causes the tremors, rigidity, and slower-than-normal movement that many Parkinson's patients experience. Until recently, patients suffering from Parkinson's disease were usually first treated with levodopa, a chemical that is converted to dopamine once it enters the brain. Unfortunately, levodopa is often broken down in the bloodstream before it reaches its target in the brain, causing decreased effectiveness.

In 1997, researchers made a major advance in treating Parkinson's disease by introducing a second generation of medicines called dopamine agonists. These medicines mimic the effect of dopamine and stimulate neurons to act as though sufficient dopamine were present in the brain. A new class of drugs introduced in 1998, known as COMT (catechol O-methyltransferase) inhibitors, blocks the enzymes that break down levodopa as it moves through the bloodstream, allowing it to get to the brain and be converted to dopamine. Consistent exposure to dopamine allows patients to function more independently and for longer periods of time between doses with fewer of the burdensome symptoms of Parkinson's disease.

Alzheimer's disease (AD) is a progressive neurological disease that affects memory, personality, and behavior. The pathological processes involved in AD disrupt the three key functions of nerve cells in the brain—communication, metabolism, and repair. When these processes are disturbed, brain cells stop working, lose connections with each other, and eventually die. Over a period of years, those with AD gradually lose their ability to remember things and think clearly.

All four of the prescription medicines, belonging to two therapeutic classes, approved by the FDA to treat Alzheimer's disease have been developed in the past decade. The first class, acetylcholinesterase inhibitors, prevents the breakdown of a neurotransmitter in the brain called acetylcholine. This chemical is thought to carry messages between nerve cells. The breakdown of acetylcholine can lead to disruptions in thinking and memory. These medicines were first introduced in 1993. The second class, cholinesterase inhibitors, also prevents the breakdown of acetylcholine as well as another similar chemical, butyrylcholine. This class was first approved for use in 2000.

By preventing the breakdown of these chemicals, these new medicines ensure that more acetylcholine is available for memory-related and cognitive functioning. They also help with some behavioral problems commonly experienced by those with AD, including delusions and agitation.

Although these drugs do not stop or reverse AD, they allow people with the disease to maintain their independence for longer periods of time. These AD treatment innovations are the current standard of care among neurologists for those with mild to moderate AD.

Another medicine in recent clinical trials is the first in a new class of drugs known as NMDA (N-methyl D-aspartate) receptor antagonists. The medicine works by modulating the levels of glutamate, a nerve signaling agent in the brain. Too much glutamate can lead to the death of nerve cells. As the Baby Boom generation reaches its older years, the number of Americans suffering from Alzheimer's disease is likely to increase dramatically, and this will have major financial and social consequences. As a result, the search for new AD treatment strategies is a high priority.

Schizophrenia is a condition that causes those who suffer from it to lose their sense of reality, become delusional, suffer from hallucinations, become emotionally unstable, and find it difficult to make decisions and relate to people. Little is known about the causes of schizophrenia and it has no cure, but medications are now available to treat many of the symptoms. The first medicines to treat schizophrenia were introduced in the 1950s, but these drugs often caused side effects such as muscle stiffness, tremor, and abnormal movements.

The past decade witnessed the introduction of new atypical antipsychotic medicines. These atypical antipsychotic medicines work by blocking receptors of the neurotransmitters dopamine and serotonin. Serotonin controls mood, emotion, sleep, and appetite and is thus implicated in the control of numerous behavioral and physiological functions, while dopamine acts on the cardiovascular, renal, hormonal, and central nervous systems. These drugs appear to change the chemical balance of serotonin and dopamine in the brain. The new medications are able to control the so-called "positive" symptoms of schizophrenia—symptoms and behavior that should not be there—as well as the "negative" symptoms—lack of characteristics that should be present—thereby allowing patients to lead more normal, independent lives.

Diabetes and Heart Disease

Diabetes is a metabolic disorder in which the body is unable to make enough of and/or properly use the hormone insulin to control blood glucose levels. Glucose provides the basic fuel for all cells in the body, and insulin transports glucose from the blood into the cells for storage. When glucose builds up in the blood instead of going into cells, it can cause two problems. Immediately, cells may be starved for energy, and over time, serious problems develop for many body systems. During the past decade, research breakthroughs have led to the approval of new insulin products to treat Type 1 and advanced Type 2 diabetes. One closely mimics the action of human insulin by providing a slow release over a 24-hour period, with no pronounced peak. Another medicine works quickly and for a short period of time, allowing patients to take the medication right before they eat a meal, instead of the 30 minutes before eating that insulin doses have traditionally required. Beginning in 1995, a string of additional treatment advances have allowed people with Type 2 diabetes to more effectively manage their condition.

Until 1995, only one category of oral medicines was available in the United States to treat patients with Type 2 diabetes. This category of drugs, the sulfonylureas (SU), was a major advance in treatment for Type 2 diabetes because it was the first oral medicine that could be used to treat the disease. Available in the United States since 1954, SU drugs stimulate the pancreas of a patient with Type 2 diabetes to produce more insulin and remain an important part of diabetes treatment today. New SU drugs with fewer side effects have been developed and are used as "monotherapy" or as part of combination therapy with other types of diabetes pills or insulin.

In 1995, one class of medicines known as biguanides was introduced in the United States after having been available in Europe for a number of years. This class lowers blood sugar levels by preventing the liver from making too much glucose and by improving the sensitivity of the muscle to the body's own insulin.

Since 1995, four totally new classes of medicines have been introduced in the United States, allowing doctors to better customize treatment regimens to fit their patients' needs. Alpha-glucosidase inhibitors, controls blood sugar by slowing down the digestion of carbohydrates in the small intestine after meals. By blocking the enzyme that digests carbohydrates, the medicine keeps blood sugar levels from rising too dramatically after a diabetic eats a meal. Thiazolidinediones are designed to reduce insulin resistance. These medicines were first introduced in 1997. By making cells more sensitive to insulin, thiazolidinediones allow insulin to move sugar from the blood into cells more effectively. The third class of Type 2 diabetes medications, meglitinides, was also introduced in 1997. The drugs stimulate insulin secretion from the pancreas, which lowers blood sugar levels. The first drug in the most recent class of new medicines for Type 2 diabetes was approved by the FDA in 2000. The class, D-phenylalanine derivatives, stimulates rapid, short-acting insulin secretion from the pancreas, effectively lowering overall blood sugar levels and blunting the increases in these levels that most people with Type 2 diabetes experience after meals.

Because these medications have different mechanisms of action and different side effects, combination therapy can prevent patients from becoming hypoglycemic or experiencing serious complications such as kidney problems. Experimental pharmaceutical treatments in development include a protein to promote increased insulin secretion when blood glucose levels are high, but not when they are normal; inhaled forms of insulin that do not require injections; dual-acting sensitizers that increase muscle cell uptake of blood sugar and inhibit the liver's production of blood sugar, as well as reduce blood lipid levels; and drugs that are designed to lessen diabetic nerve disease and complications involving small blood vessels, such as those in the eye or kidney.

Approximately one in every four adults has high blood pressure, a condition in which the force of blood against the walls of the arteries remains too high for an extended period of time. High blood pressure is a symptomless condition, and nearly one-third of people with it do not know they have it. Fewer than 3 out of 10 people with high blood pressure have it adequately controlled by medication. High blood pressure can lead to stroke, blurred vision or blindness, congestive heart failure, heart attack, kidney damage, and hardening of the arteries.

Major advances continue to be made in treating this condition. As researchers have learned more about existing drug classes—such as calcium channel blockers, ACE inhibitors, alpha-blockers, beta-blockers, and diuretics—they have been able to develop new medicines with easier dosing schedules (such as once-daily dosing) and better side effect profiles. Researchers also have learned that combining multiple types of high blood pressure medications can help patients.

Over the past decade, two new therapeutic classes for treating high blood pressure have been developed. The first class, introduced in 1995 and known as angiotensin-II antagonists, blocks the hormone angiotensin-II. This hormone normally causes blood vessels to narrow, but angiotensin-II antagonists cause blood vessels to dilate, resulting in decreased blood pressure. The formulation of these medicines allows patients to take them once daily and provides smooth, gradual, 24-hour blood pressure reduction.

In 2002, the FDA approved a second new class of medicines to treat high blood pressure—selective aldosterone receptor antagonists. These medicines work to block aldosterone, a hormone that helps the kidneys absorb sodium and water. If too much absorption takes place in the kidneys, blood pressure can increase. By blocking the hormone, selective aldosterone receptor antagonists can prevent that increase in blood pressure. High blood cholesterol is a primary risk factor for coronary artery disease, the nation's number-one killer. Nearly 100 million Americans now meet the definition of having high blood cholesterol.

Researchers have continued to develop the class of breakthrough cholesterol-lowering drugs known as statins (HMG-CoA reductase inhibitors). First introduced in the late 1980s, statins act by preventing the body from manufacturing cholesterol, reducing absorption of dietary cholesterol, or removing cholesterol from the bloodstream. Some statins work by slowing down the liver's production of cholesterol and increasing that organ's ability to remove low-density lipoprotein (LDL) cholesterol already in the blood. Some statins also modestly increase high-density lipoprotein (HDL), which carries cholesterol to the liver, where it can be broken down and removed from the body, and reduce other fats in the blood.

In 2002, a new class of medicines was approved by the FDA. These medicines, called cholesterol absorption inhibitors, act in the small intestine, keeping cholesterol from ever entering the liver. This means that less cholesterol is stored in the liver, and more is removed through the blood. Because this class works differently than statins, it can be used in combination with statins, resulting in improved cholesterol levels.

New drugs are discovered, tested, and approved for marketing for numerous conditions. Often new applications of existing products are identified. Recently, for example, in the area of cardiovascular health clopidogrel bisulfate was found to be beneficial for certain heart attack victims in emergency rooms without the capability to perform angioplasty procedures. Sometimes drugs reach the market, but use in large numbers of individuals uncovers serious adverse side effects such as happened for certain nonsteriodal anti-inflammatory agents. Unfortunately, the United States does not have in place an ongoing comprehensive surveillance program for population drug use.

SUMMARY

The pharmaceutical industry has contributed to improvements in the nation's health. Yet many complex issues remain unresolved including pricing, testing, approval procedures and standards, distribution and access issues, international equity, and legal and regulatory concerns. The industry will continue to be a key part of the national health care system, but its nature and operations will likely adapt to changes in technology, demands for accountability, public policy issues, and many other complex factors.

REVIEW QUESTIONS

1. What is the role of the pharmaceutical industry in the health care system?
2. What are the regulatory and legal issues related to drug and pharmaceutical development and sale?
3. What is the role of the pharmaceutical and biotechnology industry in making products available to the poor in the United States?
4. How are drugs priced in the United States, and how does it differ from drug pricing in other countries?
5. What economic benefits are derived from the use of prescription drugs and other interventions?
6. What does the pharmaceutical industry need to do to thrive in the future?

REFERENCES & ADDITIONAL READINGS

Altman, S. H., & Parks-Thomas, C. (2002). Controlling spending for prescription drugs. *New England Journal of Medicine, 346*(11), 855–856.

McGlynn, E. A., et al. (2003). The quality of health care delivered to adults in the United States. *New England Journal of Medicine, 348*(26), 2635–2645.

Rosenthal, M. B., Berndt, E. R., Donohue, J. M., Frank, R. G., & Epstein, A. M. (2002). Promotion of prescription drugs to consumers. *New England Journal of Medicine, 346*, 498–505.

Scherer, F. M. (2004). The pharmaceutical industry—prices and progress. *New England Journal of Medicine, 351*(9), 927–932.

Schweitzer, S. O. (1997). *Pharmaceutical economics and policy*. New York: Oxford University Press.

Topol, E. J. (2004). Failing the public health—Rofecoxib, Merck, and the FDA. *New England Journal of Medicine, 351*(17), 1707–1709.

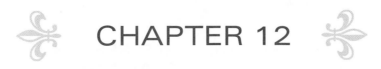

CHAPTER 12

Health Care Professionals

Stephen S. Mick and Kenneth R. White

CHAPTER TOPICS

LEARNING OBJECTIVES

Upon completing this chapter, the reader should be able to

1. Appreciate the growth and changes in the composition of the health profession workforce during the twentieth century and into the twenty-first century.

2. Understand the key role of physicians and osteopaths in the workforce, and account for the growth in physician supply.

3. Account for the various trends and changes in dentistry, public health, nursing, and pharmacy and the forces affecting these health professionals.

4. Comprehend the importance and potential of physician assistants and nurse practitioners in the health care system.

5. Understand the various major transitions occurring in the health care workforce, with particular emphasis on current and impending shortages.

Health care professionals play a key role in the provision of health services to meet the needs and demands of the population. This chapter highlights health care professional trends and discusses issues of provider supply, education and training, distribution, specialization, and the impact of recent market and regulatory changes on the health professions workforce.

EMPLOYMENT TRENDS IN THE HEALTH CARE SECTOR

At the dawn of the twenty-first century, observers now look back at the latter part of the twentieth century and are struck by the dramatic growth in the number and types of personnel employed in the health care sector. Table 12.1 shows the large gains in health sector employment in the United States over the period 1970 to 2003, starting with a pool of about 4.246 million employed persons and growing to 13.615 million. These figures include people who work in hospitals and all other health services organizations and include professional clinicians as well as those without professional training such as clerical staff, artisans, laborers, and others who have supporting roles in the delivery of health services. Although these nonclinical workers

are not discussed in this chapter, they are important because they evidence the role the health care sector has played for new employment opportunities in the service-oriented economy that now characterizes the United States.

The health care sector has maintained a steadily increasing proportion of all persons employed, and it currently includes almost 1 in 10 persons (9.9 percent) working in the U.S. labor force. Thus, growth in employment in the health care sector between 1970 and 2003 (221 percent increase) has outpaced growth in overall employment in the economy (79 percent increase) as well as total population growth (43 percent increase). The health sector is clearly a major engine of economic growth in the U.S. economy. This assertion is underscored by the 124 percent increase in the rate of health care personnel per 100,000 population, from 2,090 in 1970 to 4,682 in 2003 (Table 12.1). In a 33-year span, the number of people involved in health care has increased by about 2,592 workers per 100,000 population, an extraordinary reflection of the central place health and health care have in the lives of Americans.

At least as extraordinary as the increased supply of health care personnel has been the emergence of a wide variety of new categories of personnel, including physicians' assistants (PAs), nurse practitioners (NPs), dental hygienists, laboratory technicians, nursing aids, orderlies, attendants, home

Table 12.1. The Health Sector as a Proportion of All Employed Persons, 1970, 1980, 1990, 2000, 2003

	1970	1980	1990	2000	2003
Employment in health sector (thousands)	4,246	7,339	9,447	11,597	13,615
Total number of persons employed (thousands)	76,805	99,303	117,914	136,891	137,736
Health sector as a proportion of all occupations	5.5%	7.4%	8.0%	8.5%	9.9%
Total resident U.S. population (millions)	203.2	226.5	248.7	281.4	290.8
Number of health personnel per 100,000 population	2,090	3,240	3,799	4,121	4,682

SOURCE: From *Health, United States, 2004, with Chartbook on Trends in the Health of Americans,* National Center for Health Statistics, 2004, Hyattsville, MD: U.S. Government Printing Office.

health aids, occupational and physical therapists, medical records technicians, X-ray technicians, dietitians and nutritionists, social workers, and the like. The Department of Labor recognizes about 400 different job titles in the health sector. Some of the most rapid growth in the supply of health care personnel has occurred in these recently developed categories.

The traditional health care occupations of physician, dentist, and pharmacist have generally experienced declines, some dramatic, in their relative proportion of all health care personnel. For example, physicians (including osteopaths) constituted 30 percent of all persons in health occupations as the decade of the 1920s began, but had declined to 8.0 percent by 2000. Over the same period, dentists declined from 8 to 1.9 percent, and pharmacists 11 to 2.3 percent. Registered nurses have fluctuated up, then down, during this 80-year period: about 20 percent in 1920 to a high of 36 percent in 1940, then a steady decline to 23.4 percent in 2000. The group of health care workers that has gained the largest share of the overall number includes allied health technicians, technologists, aides, and assistants: They composed a mere 1 to 2 percent in 1920, but in 2000, they made up over 54 percent. These figures should not mask the fact that *all* groups of health care personnel have increased in absolute number from year to year as inspection of any of the tables of this chapter will show. What the data emphasize is the higher rate of growth of nontraditional allied health and support personnel, who now constitute the majority of all personnel employed in the health care sector.

The primary reasons for the increased supply and wide variety of health care personnel into the twenty-first century are the interrelated forces of technological growth, specialization, health insurance coverage, the aging of the population, the emergence of the hospital and hospital systems and their associated ambulatory clinics as the central institution of the health care system, and the large array of posthospitalization treatment venues that include nursing homes, rehabilitation facilities, hospices, and home health organizations. The hospital

has become the setting where new technology can be used and where medical, nursing, and other health professional students can be educated. The technological revolution has led to diagnostic and treatment procedures that, in turn, have led to an increased use of hospitals, with a corresponding concentration of health personnel. The rise of private health insurance in the 1940s, plus enactment of the publicly funded insurance systems in the mid-1960s (Medicare and Medicaid), fueled hospital growth because reliable payment mechanisms provided hospitals with assured revenues. These funding sources, intersecting with the ineluctable aging of the population, have given rise to an extensive network of care options for the elderly, all leading to increasing demand for such personnel as home health aides and inhalation or respiratory therapists as well as nursing personnel.

Technological innovation has also led to increased specialization of health care personnel, primarily during the last 40 years. This specialization has resulted in new categories of health care providers within the traditional professions [e.g., pediatric nephrologists and gastroenterologists in medicine, periodontists in dentistry, intensive care unit (ICU) specialists in nursing]. Notable among new medical specialists are hospitalists—physicians who work solely or mostly in hospitals—and intensivists—physicians who work solely or mostly in hospital intensive care units. In 2005, hospitalists numbered about 15,000, and their roles were focused on improving patient quality and safety, increasing patient flow, and affording convenience and support for community physicians (Society of Hospital Medicine, 2005). There has also been the advent of new types of allied health professions (e.g., occupational and radiological technicians and speech pathologists).

Health care personnel will be discussed in greater detail by focusing on five of the more traditional groups of professions—physicians and osteopaths, dentists, public health professionals, nurses, pharmacists—and two of the more recently developed categories of personnel—PAs and NPs.

THE SUPPLY OF PHYSICIANS

From a Surplus to a Shortage?

The number of physicians in the United States has increased rapidly in the last four decades, with an estimated 845,684 active nonfederal physicians, including osteopaths (described more fully in a later section), practicing in 2005 (Figure 12.1). Between 1965 and 2005, there was a 218 percent increase in the supply of active physicians, resulting in an average of approximately 285 physicians per 100,000 population. Over the same period, the physician to 100,000 population ratio increased by 105 percent. In 1980, the Graduate Medical Education National Advisory Committee (GMENAC) reported to the Secretary of the U.S. Department of Health and Human Services that there would be a surplus of physicians of 70,000 in 1990, and roughly 140,000 in 2000, underscoring the belief that the nation could substantially reduce its subsidization of medical education (Graduate Medical Education National Advisory Committee, 1980). In 1999, the Council on Graduate Medical Education (COGME), an advisory group to the federal government, noted that despite the warning of a surplus made 20 years previously, only limited progress had been made in reducing the growth of the U.S. physician supply (Council on Graduate Medical Education, 1999).

But, by the early 2000s, some observers were raising the spectre of a physician shortage, especially among some specialty groups (Cooper et al., 2002). Figure 12.1 shows that for the first time since at least 1965, between 2000 and 2005, there was a slight decrease in the ratio of physicians per 100,000 civilian population (288 to 285), which draws attention to this new concern. How could the fears of a surplus change so quickly into fears of a shortage? The answer to this question is complex. Although part of the response lies in the way that differing methodologies and assumptions yield varying physician requirement and supply projections, the more pertinent answer lies in the crosscutting forces that have affected the U.S. health care system in the last several decades.

First, although managed care remains a formidable force in the organization and delivery of

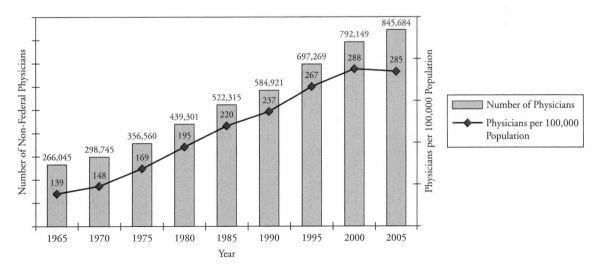

Figure 12.1. Total Number of Nonfederal Physicians and Number of Physicians per 100,000 Civilian Population, 1965–2005

health care, its more restrictive elements have been blunted due to widespread physician and patient dissatisfaction, particularly with limits on choice. Medicine's distaste of tightly controlled reimbursement and of nonphysicians' attempts to control their work fueled much of this backlash (Lesser, Ginsburg, & Devers, 2003). The outcome of this has been a movement away from capitated insurance arrangements back to coverage that more closely resembles fee-for-service plans, especially preferred provider organizations (Mick, 2004). The move away from more efficient forms of organized medical practice commonly means that more physicians will be necessary to deliver the same level of care (Weiner, 2004). Physicians and patients seem to prefer choice to efficiency, which will add pressure for more physicians and is the first of several possible factors fueling fears of a new shortage.

Second, in the early 2000s, a historic first was reached in U.S. medical schools. The proportion of first-year students who were women basically reached parity with men: The entering class of medical students in 2004–2005 was 49.5 percent female; the proportion of all medical students who were women was 48.6 percent. Aside from the social and economic features of this remarkable change (two decades before in 1983–1984, the total proportion of women enrolled was just 30.7 percent), the impact on physician supply is generally thought to be one that will require somewhat more physicians to do the same work previously done predominately by men (Dedobbeleer, Contandriopoulous, & Desjardins, 1995; Carr et al., 1998; Pearse, Haffner, & Primack, 2001). The reasons for this are clear: Women still do a majority of the tasks surrounding the raising of children and maintaining a home, leaving less time available for practice. Taken together this important demographic shift within the workforce may produce more pressure for more rather than fewer physicians.

Third, physician preferences now favor a more "controllable lifestyle." This factor stems in part from the increasing number of women in the workforce, but it affects men as well. Generally, younger physicians seek a different lifestyle that allows for weekends off, limits on the number of hours worked per week, and other amenities that allow for activities outside the workplace. Taken together, these preferences have had and will probably continue to have the effect of reducing the amount of time available for patient care (Dorsey, Jarjoura, & Rutecki, 2003).

Fourth, on the demand side, there has been unusual growth of the U.S. population fueled in large measure by immigration. Since the mid-twentieth century, immigration has dramatically increased so that almost one-third of U.S. population growth in the decade 1990–1999 was due to net legal migration (Philip & Midgley, 2006). The present population of the United States of roughly 297 million is expected to increase to slightly over 400 million by 2050. In the presence of this population pressure, the need for more physicians will inevitably increase.

Fifth, within the general increase in the U.S. population, there exists the ever-increasing lifespan of Americans, with their attendant levels of chronic conditions. In 2000, 12.4 percent of the U.S. population was 65 years of age or older; in 2050, the figure is projected to be 20.6 percent (U.S. Census Bureau, 2007). This change will produce a steadily increasing demand for physician services and a consequent increase in the need for physicians.

On the other hand, there are those who argue that before any effort is made to increase the supply of physicians, consideration should be given to several key problems with the way medical care has been and currently is delivered. The first argument in favor of caution derives from the apparent abandonment of efforts to extract more efficiency from the physicians we already have through innovative delivery arrangements and combinations of different levels of providers. This is the obverse of the point already made about the decline of managed care.

A second factor revolves around the use of physician substitutes or "extenders" in health care delivery. If, for example, nurse practitioners and physician assistants, among others, were increasingly used to provide primary care, there would be less pressure to increase physician supply. The rate of increase of these so-called "midlevel" practitioners has been very high since the 1990s, and their ability to deliver a large proportion of primary care services is no longer argued (Cooper, Laud, & Dietrich, 1998; Cooper, 2001). The extent to which these clinicians continue to grow in number, and are more widely used, will have a restraining influence on how many more physicians need to be trained.

The third argument stems from decades of analysis—called Small Area Variation Analysis—that has documented wide variation in the use of physician services without any obvious connection to levels of health of patients and populations (Wennberg, 2004). These findings raise the question of why there should be more physicians if areas with high levels of physicians—particularly specialists—have health outcomes that are no better than those in areas with low levels of physicians (Goodman, 2005). This lack of evidence about whether present levels of physician supply are optimal leads to the worry about how projections of future supply based on current patterns can be justified. Thus, without a clear demonstration that increasing physician supply will have a positive impact on health outcomes, this position is skeptical of calls to add 3,000 more physicians in residency training programs and to increase medical school enrollment by 15 percent over the next decade (Council on Graduate Medical Education, 2005).

A fourth, and related, point is the relatively new movement by payers and insurers toward a "pay for performance" reimbursement approach, particularly for office-based practice. The essence of these payment schemes is to reduce unnecessary diagnostic and procedural work, to tie clinical processes to outcomes, and to emphasize evidence-based medicine. Much of the variation in physician work is skewed toward more rather than less work, and thus, any reduction in variation will probably reduce work. If this is true, the aggregate amount of work necessary for a given population of patients will experience a dampening effect, which, in turn, could add pressure for fewer rather than for more physicians.

It is difficult to determine what the net effect of forces favoring and disfavoring growth in the physi-

cian supply will be. However, the focus of debate has now shifted from a putative surplus to a possible shortage. Advocates and analysts on either side of the question are pressing hard for policy responses, and over the next several years, a clearer picture will emerge about the issue.

International Medical Graduates

The issue of an appropriate supply of physicians is complicated because of the fact that there exist two distinct avenues to becoming a practicing physician in the United States. The first is the domestic track consisting of persons who are U.S. citizens and who are trained in U.S. medical schools. The second track consists of persons who are foreign-trained physicians known as international medical graduates (IMGs).

As for U.S. medical graduates, Table 12.2 shows the substantial increase in both the number of medical schools and the number of medical students (first year and total enrolled) between the period 1965 and the early 1980s. By 1980–1981, the yearly number of graduates had more than doubled the 1965–1966 number. This increase can be directly attributed to massive federal outlays for training, research, and construction in the 1960s and 1970s. By the early 1970s, 40 to 50 percent of medical school support came from federal sources.

However, the retreat of the federal government from an active role in the financial support of medical education was initiated in the early 1980s as a result of pressures to reduce federal spending, of the perception that there was an adequate supply of physicians in the United States, and of a conservative administrative ideology regarding federal intervention in medical education. The effect of this is seen in Table 12.2: From the early 1980s to the present time, the number of first-year medical students, total medical students, medical school graduates, and medical schools has been constant. By the early 1990s, the federal government provided about 20 to 25 percent of medical school financial support through direct subsidies and research, down from about 44 percent in 1970. The extraordinary

Table 12.2. Number of Allopathic Medical Schools, Applicants, Students, Graduates, and Ratio of First-Year Students to Applicants: Selected Academic Years 1965–1966 through 2004–2005

| Academic Year | Number of Schools | Number of Applicants | Number of Students | | Number of Graduates | Ratio of First-Year Students to Applicants |
			Total	First Year		
1965–1966	88	18,703	32,835	8,759	7,574	1:2.4
1970–1971	103	24,987	40,487	11,348	8,974	1:2.2
1975–1976	114	42,303	56,244	15,351	13,561	1:2.8
1980–1981	126	36,100	65,497	17,204	15,667	1:2.0
1985–1986	127	32,893	66,604	16,929	16,125	1:1.9
1990–1991	126	29,243	64,986	16,803	15,481	1:1.7
1995–1996	125	46,591	66,906	17,024	16,029	1:2.7
1999–2000	125	38,529	66,550	16,856	15,830	1:2.3
2004–2005	125	35,735	67,296	17,109	16,066	1:2.1

SOURCES: Adapted from the following: "Undergraduate Medical Education," 1980, *Journal of the American Medical Association 243*, pp. 849–866; "Educational Programs in U.S. Medical Schools," by H. Jonas, S. Etzel, & B. Barzansky, 1991, *Journal of the American Medical Association, 226*, pp. 913–923; "Educational Programs in U.S. Medical Schools, 1995–1996," by B. Barzansky, H. Jonas, & S. Etzel, 1996, *Journal of the American Medical Association, 276*, pp. 714–719; "Educational Programs in U.S. Medical Schools, 1999–2000," by B. Barzansky, H. Jonas, & S. Etzel, 2000, *Journal of the American Medical Association, 284*, pp. 1114–1120; "Educational Programs in U.S. Medical Schools, 2004–2005," by B. Barzansky, & S. Etzel, 2005, *Journal of the American Medical Association, 294*, pp. 1068–1074.

leveling off of U.S. medical school production is an important ingredient in the current debate about a possible impending shortage.

The second important factor in the supply of physicians has been the influx of IMGs into the United States. In 2005, 204,369, or 24 percent, of the total active nonfederal physician population of 845,684 physicians were IMGs. The inflow of IMGs began after World War II when the U.S. Congress passed legislation that made it relatively easy for professionals from foreign countries to come to this country to obtain advanced graduate training. This effort was in response to the need for skilled personnel in many developing countries and of other countries' rebuilding after the war's destruction to educate a new cadre of professional personnel. It was also an attempt to inculcate the values of democracy into a new generation of young professionals who were also offered advanced education in the then communist Bloc counties where they were exposed to communist ideological positions.

By the mid-1960s, favorable immigration policies for physicians had encouraged this movement; there was, in addition, an unceasing demand for interns and residents in U.S. hospitals as measured by the existence each year of unfilled house officer positions. By the early 1970s, IMGs accounted for more than 40 percent of new physician licentiates, 30 percent of filled residency positions, and 20 percent of the active physicians in the United States. One-third of the growth in physician supply in the 1970s was due to increases in the number of physicians trained outside the United States.

After a period of decline in the number of IMGs filling residency positions during the 1980s, their numbers steadily increased in the 1990s, hitting the mid-20,000s by 1995 and remaining at that level until the present time; in 2005, there were 26,720 IMGs in residency positions of all types.

The question is, How can it be that so many IMGs entered U.S. medicine when there was a supposed "surplus" of physicians as announced by the Graduate Medical Education National Advisory Committee (GMENAC) in 1980 and reaffirmed by the important federal advisory group, the Council on Graduate Medical Education (COGME), in its various reports from the late 1980s to the late 1990s (Council on Graduate Medical Education, 1999)? Although there is no clear and proven answer to this question, there are a number of probable reasons. First, although the United States may have had a surplus of physicians, that is, more physicians than there were requirements for their services, they have continued to be distributed too often in nonprimary care specialties; in urban and suburban locations and insufficiently in rural and inner city locations; in practice settings that are desirable, for example, group practices, well-established HMOs, and the like, and not in less desirable settings, for example, public hospitals, state mental hospitals, prison health services. Thus, IMGs who have entered the U.S. health care system "fill gaps" to some extent, frequently practicing in specialties, geographic locations, and employment settings avoided by U.S. medical graduates (Mick, Lee, & Wodchis, 2000). This rationale remains true today.

A second reason for the large IMG presence in the United States has been that teaching hospitals, that is, those in which physicians, nurses, and most other health professionals are trained, have enjoyed relatively generous funding via the Medicare program to underwrite the costs of graduate medical education (Council on Graduate Medical Education, 1995a). The result has been that many more residency positions exist than there are U.S. medical graduates to fill them. This acts as a sort of "suction" or "pull" factor to bring IMGs to the United States. Often, these hospitals serve large numbers of persons who are poor or without health insurance, or both, as well as those on Medicaid. Estimates of the number of hospitals that are "dependent" on IMG residents *and* that serve the poor vary between 77 and 276, many concentrated in New York, Texas, New Jersey, Michigan, and Illinois (Whitcomb &

Miller, 1995). However, the number of hospitals falling into this category is probably greater than these figures because the authors used conservative criteria to determine "IMG dependence."

A third reason for the IMG presence has been brought on by the increased market penetration of managed-care plans in urban areas. Notwithstanding the decline in the power of managed-care plans in the late 1990s and early 2000s, it remains true that these plans are generally not linked to teaching hospitals and therefore do not train residents or any other health professionals. Nor do they incur the costs of research, as do the teaching hospitals. Managed-care plans can therefore charge lower premiums and offer lower cost services to employers and other groups anxious to cut their rising health care costs. Teaching hospitals, in order to compete, have searched for lower cost substitutes, and residents—often IMGs— may actually provide a lower cost substitute than skilled nurse, NP, or PA services because the latter work fixed hours per week and are generally paid higher overtime rates. A resident works longer hours, is paid a fixed salary, and is a physician. Thus, as managed care has spread in urban markets where IMG residents are traditionally located, there has been more pressure on teaching hospitals to increase the residency complement.

Other factors have undoubtedly played a role in the increase of IMGs. Because of the concern of many in the medical community and groups such as the Institute of Medicine (1996) and others such as the Pew Health Professions Commission (2005), there have been calls for limits on IMG immigration. But, no such action was ever taken, and in view of the arguments of some that there may be a new shortage of physicians, enacting policies to restrict the inflow of IMGs is not likely to happen. Still, the IMG "issue" continues to generate controversy.

The United States has never had a coordinated physician personnel policy as has, for example, France or Canada; in particular, undergraduate and graduate medical education systems have operated largely independently of each other. Thus, past and future policies of increasing the number of U.S. medical schools and U.S. medical graduates have

Table 12.3. Number of Active Physicians (MDs) and Percentage Distribution by Specialty Groups: Selected Years, 1980, 1990, 2000, 2002

Specialty	1980 Number	1980 Percent	1990 Number	1990 Percent	2000 Number	2000 Percent	2002 Number	2002 Percent	Percent Change 1980–2002
All specialties	435,264	100.0	559,988	100.0	737,504	100.0	768,498	100.0	76.6
Primary care specialties[a]	170,705	39.2	213,514	38.1	274,653	37.2	286,294	37.3	67.7
Medical specialties	25,328	5.8	41,958	7.5	54,877	7.4	57,579	7.5	127.3
Surgical specialties	72,050	16.6	90,052	16.1	101,629	13.8	104,871	13.6	45.6
All other specialties	167,181	38.4	214,464	38.3	306,345	41.5	319,754	41.6	91.3

[a]Includes general practice, family practice, general internal medicine, general pediatrics, and obstetrics/gynecology.

SOURCE: From *Physician Characteristics and Distribution in the U.S., 2004,* 2004, Table 4.1, p. 289, Table 5.2, p. 323, Chicago: Department of Physician Practice and Communications Information, Division of Survey and Data Resources.

not been and do not appear to be closely connected to the graduate medical training system. One result of this has been that students graduating from U.S. medical schools have filled a smaller proportion of available residencies positions, often leaving—as noted earlier—the less desirable positions (Mick & Worobey, 1984; Mick, 1992; Mick, Lee, & Wodchis, 2000). IMGs have had a key role in the provision of medical services in the United States for over a half-century, and there is no evidence that this situation will change.

Trends in Specialty Distribution

Simply increasing physician supply has not guaranteed that necessary medical services would readily be available to the general population. Of particular interest is the availability of primary care—the portal of entry into the health care system where basic medical services are provided. Primary care includes the diagnosis and treatment of common illness and disease, preventive services, home care services, and uncomplicated minor surgery and emergency care.

The increased supply of physicians has also witnessed some change in the proportion of physicians in primary care specialties—general practice, family practice, general internal medicine, and general pediatrics (Table 12.3). There has been substantial growth in primary care specialties both in absolute

numbers and in percent: From 1980 to 2002, the number of primary care physicians has grown to nearly 300,000, an increase of 87 percent. Only growth in the broad category of medical specialties has been greater over this period, reaching to more than 120 percent. On the other hand, the percentage of physicians in any given year who are in primary care has remained fairly constant, with about 38.5 percent of all physicians in these specialties in 1980 and 41.6 percent in 2002. The sources of growth, however measured, in primary care specialties have, interestingly, come disproportionately from IMGs and women. Whereas IMGs constituted 18 percent of all primary care physicians in 1980, they were 29.2 percent of this specialty group by 2003. As for women, they were a mere 13.1 percent of primary care physicians in 1980, but by 2002, they constituted 33.5 percent of the total.

The importance of the concern about whether the nation is producing enough primary care specialists relates to a number of contemporary issues. The rational management of patients with "undifferentiated symptoms," the navigator for the patient through the myriad services available for even the most mundane condition, the least expensive of all specialty services enabling it to be more accessible to the poor and low income portions of the population, and the capacity of primary care to help reduce health disparities, all combine to make the adequate supply of primary care physicians of critical importance (Ferrer, Hambridge, & Maly, 2005). Furthermore, there is some evidence that a higher concentration of primary care providers is correlated with a higher level of health (Starfield & Shi, 2005). If the relationship holds up after more careful scrutiny, there will be a powerful argument for either more growth than there has already been in primary care physicians or a more even distribution between specialists and primary care physicians, or both.

In the 1990s, observers of the managed-care phenomenon noted that high market penetration of such plans was producing change in the specialty composition of physicians in these markets. As managed-care plans used more primary care "gatekeeper" physicians to care for patients and to make referrals to specialists, the demand for the former grew and the latter decreased (Seifer, Troupin, & Rubenfeld, 1996). However, since that time, as managed-care plans have reduced their more stringent controls on physician and enrollee behavior and have opened up direct access to specialty care, the growth in primary care practice appears to have been dampened. Whereas the period 1990–2000 showed a 35.3 percent increase in primary care physicians, the early part of the 2000s experienced a more modest rate of growth of 5.6 percent. It is possible, however, that having two out of five U.S.

physicians in primary care is a sufficient level, and the country may be nearing a balance between primary care physicians and other more specialized medical areas, although there is, and will continue to be, debate about the most desirable mix of these two broad groupings (Whitcomb, 1995).

Geographic Distribution of Physicians

One of the assumptions underlying federal health personnel policy in the 1960s and early 1970s was that a significant increase in the overall supply of physicians would both resolve the problem of a serious shortage and improve the geographic distribution of physicians. It is true that in some rural areas, there has been an increase in the physician-population ratio, but for most rural areas in the United States, there has been only minor improvement: Rural places with no nearby city still have fewer than 100 physicians per 100,000 population whereas large and small cities have over or near three times this ratio, respectively. Figure 12.2 displays the discrepancies in physician to 100,000 population over the period 1940 through 2000: Nonmetro places of 2,500 to 19,000 inhabitants have experienced only a slight increase in the availability of

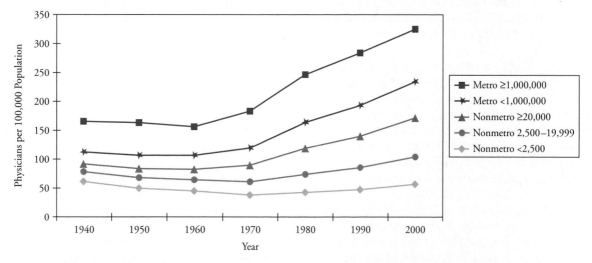

Figure 12.2. Physicians per 100,000 Population for Metro and Nonmetro Places, 1940–2000

SOURCE: Bureau of Health Professions, Health Resources and Services Administration, Area Resource File, 2004 Release.

physicians; nonmetro places of less than 2,500 have actually experienced no improvement in physician availability in 60 years! Furthermore, the disparity between the relative distribution of physicians in urban versus rural localities has increased dramatically from 1970 to 2000: The difference between the ratios of physicians to population in the most urban and rural locations has nearly doubled (Ricketts, 2005). Thus, although there is now debate between adherents of the surplus and shortage hypotheses, there is very little debate about the persistent chronic shortages in rural America, although some argue that actual access by rural dwellers to physician services is not as poor as it may seem because there may be *overuse* of physician services—particularly specialist care—in urban areas by both urban and rural dwellers (Reschovsky & Staiti, 2005). Thus, comparing rural use levels with urban use levels may exaggerate urban-rural differences.

Nevertheless, there has been extensive study of the reasons physicians have been reluctant to locate in rural areas. They include a lack of adequate medical facilities, professional isolation, limited support services, inadequate organizational settings including lack of group practices, excessive workloads and time demands, limits on earnings, lack of social, cultural, and educational opportunities, and spouse's influence (Gordon, Meister, & Hughes, 1992). Efforts to improve the distribution of physicians have tried to address some of these factors.

Federal efforts to improve the distribution of physicians have included loan forgiveness, the National Health Service Corps, Area Health Education Centers (AHECs), and extensive support for the development of family practice training programs, among others (Ricketts, 1994). These programs have experienced a number of difficulties over the past 20 years: Many were severely cut back during the Reagan era and were only partially refunded during the Clinton administration. At the present time, given other budget priorities, there is always danger that these programs will be reduced or eliminated, although a hallmark of the Bush administration has been support for rural health clin-

ics and critical access hospitals, institutions that can attract physicians to rural communities.

At the state level, there have been efforts to improve physician distribution through the authority of Offices of Rural Health in most states. State-level policy has been aimed at increasing the recruitment and retention of health care providers in rural areas as well as cooperative ventures of consortia of states to decentralize medical education programs and coordinate placement of graduates.

Despite the variety of approaches to alter the urban/rural location of physicians, unequal distribution persists. Market forces have altered distribution to some degree, but many rural communities still find it difficult to recruit and retain physicians. The same is true for inner-city locations. Often those locales with the greatest need continue to have the biggest problems attracting physicians. As mentioned earlier, national bodies like the Institute of Medicine (1996) have called for a cutback in IMGs. However, without specific programs aimed at increasing the number of physicians in underserved areas, it is difficult to see how a reduction in the overall number of physicians can do anything but worsen the historic problem of physician maldistribution.

Developing policies to alter physician distribution has therefore turned out to be a difficult undertaking. The limited impact of previous attempts suggests that broader policy options should be considered. The possibilities include changing reimbursement systems to provide a financial reward for physicians practicing in underserved areas. Another remedy might be to modify the admissions policies of medical schools even more than has been done in order to place more emphasis on applicants interested in primary care practice. Or, undergraduate and graduate medical education systems could be changed to ensure that the curriculum, counseling, clinical setting, and role models presented are better related to health needs of the underserved. A revitalized and expanded National Health Service Corps might be one of the best short-term solutions to the distribution problem. Whatever steps are taken, a balance must be found between changing the size and composition of the physician workforce so that goals of improving physician distribution are not forgotten.

Women and Minorities in Medicine

Another important issue in the system of medical education concerns women and minority students. Concerted efforts to increase their enrollment have borne fruit, as noted earlier: Women in medical school are almost half of the total. A more modest, but significant, increase in minority students has been registered: From 1970–1971 to 1999–2000, the percentage of minority students in allopathic medical schools increased from about 9 percent to nearly 35 percent of all first-year students. The greatest increase in minority students has been among Asian Americans, Native Americans, Hispanic Americans, and African Americans, in that order. For example, although African Americans increased their number by 91 percent over the period 1970–2000, Asian Americans increased more than 16-fold. The presence of minority physicians is extremely important because it has been shown that minority patients are four times more likely to receive care from minority physicians than nonminority ones. Low-income patients, Medicaid recipients, and uninsured patients were also more likely to receive care from nonminority physicians (Moy & Bartman, 1995).

Conclusion

In summary, throughout the latter half of the twentieth century and into the early twenty-first century, there has been enormous growth in the number of physicians as well as in the number of physicians per population. The latter ratio has, however, leveled off since the new millennium, raising questions among some observers whether a "new" shortage of physicians may be in the offing. There has also been increasing growth among primary care physicians, and women, and IMGs have contributed disproportionately to this phenomenon. Despite the growth collectively, there continue to be disparities in the availability of physicians

between rural and urban areas. These issues, joined to the debate engendered by the presence of IMGs in U.S. residencies, promise to keep the fundamental problems of the training and deployment of the physician workforce a number-one policy issue in the early twenty-first century.

OSTEOPATHY

Often neglected in discussions of medical personnel is the small but significant number of osteopaths in the United States. Osteopathy differs from allopathic medicine in that osteopaths traditionally emphasize treatments that involve corrections of the position of joints or tissues and they stress diet or environment as factors that might destroy natural resistance. Allopathic medicine views the physician as an active interventionist attempting to neutralize effects of disease by using treatments that produce a counteracting effect. Despite these differences, osteopaths are licensed to practice medicine and perform surgery in all states and are eligible for graduate medical education in either osteopathic or allopathic residencies. In fact, there were 5,675 osteopaths in accredited allopathic residency programs in 2004–2005. Finally, both Medicare and Medicaid, the two major federal financing programs, reimburse osteopaths.

The growth in osteopaths has been great, but this is partially due to the small base number to begin with: In 1970, there were only 12,000 osteopaths; in 2005, there were 50,532, an increase of about 321 percent. The ratio of osteopaths to population was 17 to 100,000. However, this figure is deceptive because osteopaths are unevenly distributed around the country. More than one-half (51.6 percent) of all osteopaths were located in just seven states: Pennsylvania, Michigan, Ohio, New York, Florida, Texas, and New Jersey, in descending order. Hence, in states like these, osteopaths make a contribution to health care disproportionate to their overall number. Finally, historically, osteopaths have been more likely to locate in rural areas than allopathic physicians.

There are now 20 schools of osteopathy, up from 15 schools in the early 1990s. The states with the largest number of osteopaths are also those with schools of osteopathy. From 1975–1976 to 1999–2000, there was an increase in first-year class size of 174 percent. There has been an increasing proportion of first-year female students (14 percent to 47 percent, from 1975–1976 through 2003–2004) as well as an increase in minority first-year students (5 percent to 27 percent over the same period). Since 1987, there have been more osteopaths in allopathic residency programs than in osteopathic programs, underlining the narrow difference between the two groups. Of those osteopaths training in allopathic residencies, about 48 percent select one of the primary care specialties (family medicine, general internal medicine, general pediatrics), whereas only 31 percent of allopathic residents in training were in a primary care area. In 2003, whereas about 40 percent of all allopathic physicians were in primary care specialties, 49 percent of all practicing osteopaths were so engaged. Combining these facts with osteopaths' location in specific states with a tendency to locate in rural areas underscores their importance to health care delivery of primary care medicine.

In short, osteopathic medicine is a small, but important form of medical practice that shares the burden of care with allopathic physicians. It has experienced the same changes, for example, increasing proportion of women and minorities, increasing number of applicants, as its larger cousin has undergone.

DENTISTRY: A PROFESSION IN TRANSITION

In 2000, there were approximately 168,000 active dentists practicing in the United States. The supply of dentists has slowly increased since the 1970s,

as has the ratio of active dentists to population: In 1975 the ratio was 51.6 per 100,000 population and in 1990, 58.7 per 100,000. In 2000, the ratio was 60.6 per 100,000, which indicates a rate just barely exceeding general population growth (Table 12.4). As in medicine, the earlier increases that occurred can be attributed to federal legislation passed in the early 1960s and early 1970s that directly attempted to remedy the perceived shortage. This legislation resulted in increases in the number of dental schools from 47 to 60 in the period 1960 to 1980, and an increase in the number of first-year dental students from 3,600 to more than 6,000 in the same period (Table 12.5). However, since 1980, the total number of dental schools and the first-year class dropped to 55 and 4,327, respectively, by 2000–2001.

Some of the recent trends that are descriptive of medical schools are also descriptive of dental schools. The percentage of female first-year students has soared from a mere 2 percent in 1970–1971 to 39.8 percent in 2000–2001 (Table 12.5). The proportion of underrepresented minority students has also increased dramatically, from 3 percent in 1970–1971 to 10.8 percent in 2000–2001. Dental schools have started to deemphasize their support from federal sources and have increased their state support, dental clinic revenues, and fees from tuition. Also, as with medicine, there was a sizable decrease in the number of applicants to dental school in the 1980s, although the decline started earlier and was steeper for dentistry. Since 1975, when dental school applications peaked at 15,734, there was a steady decline until 1990 when 5,123 persons applied, or one new entrant per 1.3 applicants. Since then applications have increased so that for the 2000–2001 academic year, 7,772 persons applied for dental school, or 1 new entrant per 1.8 applicants.

Unlike their physician counterparts, dentists typically work in solo or small group private practices. However, current economic pressures on the dental profession have initiated changes in the delivery of dental services. Since the 1980s, a variety of nontraditional practice settings have emerged for dentists,

Table 12.4. Total and Active Dentists and Dentist/Population Ratios: Selected Years, 1960 through 2000

Year	Number of Dentists[a] Total	Active	Total Population (Thousands)	Active Dentists per 100,000 Population
1960	105,200	90,120	182,287	49.4
1970	116,250	102,220	206,466	49.5
1975	126,590	112,020	217,095	51.6
1980	147,280	126,240	228,831	55.2
1990	—	147,500	251,340	58.7
2000	—	168,000	276,740	60.7

[a]Includes dentists in federal service.

SOURCES: From *Fourth Report to the President and Congress on the Status of Health Personnel in the United States* (DHHS Pub. No. [HRS]-P-0084.4), 1984, Washington, DC: U.S. Government Printing Office; *Seventh Report to the President and Congress on the Status of Health Personnel in the United States* (DHHS Pub. No. [HRS]-P-OD-90-1), 1990, Washington, DC: U.S. Government Printing Office; *Health Personnel in the United States: Ninth Report to Congress*, 1993, Washington, DC: U.S. Government Printing Office; adapted from "Trends in the Dental Health Work Force," by L. J. Brown, & V. Lazar, 1999, *Journal of the American Dental Association, 130*, pp. 1743–1749; *Health Workforce Factbook*, Bureau of Health Professions, Health Resources and Services Administration, retrieved November 10, 2005, from http://www.hrsa.gov/healthworkforce/reports/factbook02

including HMOs and retail locations in malls, stores, and plazas. Although only a small proportion of dental services is provided in these settings and the number of active private practitioners is expected to grow (Brown & Lazar, 1999), this organizational innovation is an indication of the more competitive environment dentistry is facing in the early 2000s.

The vast majority of dentists are in general practice. Only about one-seventh of all dentists are specialists, and the proportion of specialists has remained stable in recent years. Orthodontists comprise roughly one-third of all dental specialists, with oral surgeons totaling almost another one-fourth of the specialist population.

There is significant variation in the distribution of dentists across the regions of the United States and metropolitan versus nonmetropolitan areas. This variation is caused by the same factors that have led to physician maldistribution, as well as by the lack of reciprocity in the licensing of dentists across states. Those portions of the country that are the most rural have the lowest dentist/population

ratios; for example, in 1999, an urban state like Massachusetts had 81.2 dentists per 100,000 population, whereas a rural state such as Alabama had 43.5 per 100,000. In 2002, there were 2,041 federally designated dental shortage areas in the United States, more than half of which were located in nonmetropolitan areas (Ricketts, 2005).

In addition to the traditional maldistribution of dentists, there is concern that there may be a growing gap between the availability of dentists and the need for their services, especially since the financing of dental services is on a much smaller scale than that for physician services. Currently, less than one-half of the U.S. population has dental insurance, and federal funds pay for less than 2 percent of all dental care (*Health Personnel in the United States*, 1993). Other factors contributing to the gap include the following:

1. Whereas fluoridation of water has reduced the number of dental caries and fillings needing replacement, about 75 percent of dental caries in children are concentrated in about

Table 12.5. Number of Dental Schools, Students, Including Female and Minority Students, and Graduates: Selected Academic Years, 1960–1961 through 2000–2001

Academic Year	Number of Schools	Number of Students[b]		First-Year Female Students	Percent Female of First-Year Students (%)	Total Minority Students[a]	Percent Minority of Total Students (%)	Total Number of Graduates[b]
		Total	First Year					
1960–1961	47	13,580	3,616	—	—	—	—	3,290
1970–1971	53	16,553	4,565	94	2.1	552[c]	3.3	3,775
1980–1981	60	22,842	6,030	1,194	19.8	2,453	10.7	5,550
1990–1991	55	15,951	4,001	1,522	38.0	4,766	29.9	3,995
1997–1998	54	16,926	4,347	1,609	37.0	5,888	34.8	3,930
2000–2001	55	17,349	4,327	1,721	39.8	6,164	35.5	4,171

[a]Includes African American, Hispanic, Native American, Asian American, and, for 1970, "Other Minorities."
[b]Excludes graduates of the University of Puerto Rico for 1960–61 and 1970–71.
[c]Estimated minority enrollment.

SOURCES: From *Minorities and Women in the Health Fields, 1990 Edition* (DHHS Pub. No. [HRSA]-P-DV-90-3), 1990, Washington, DC: U.S. Government Printing Office; *Health Personnel in the United States: Eighth Report to Congress, 1991* (DHHS Pub. No. HRS-P-OD-92.1), 1992, Washington, DC: U.S. Government Printing Office; *Health Personnel in the United States: Ninth Report to Congress, 1993*, Washington, DC: U.S. Government Printing Office; *Minorities and Women in the Health Fields, 1994 Edition* (DHHS Pub. No. HRSA-P-DV-94-2), 1994, Washington, DC: U.S. Government Printing Office; adapted from "Trends in the Dental Health Work Force," by L. J. Brown, & V. Lazar, 1999, *Journal of the American Dental Association, 130,* pp. 1743–1749; *Health Workforce Factbook,* Bureau of Health Professions, Health Resources and Services Administration, retrieved November 10, 2005, from http://www.hrsa.gov/healthworkforce/reports/factbook02

25 percent of the population, with disease levels higher among minority populations.

2. Minority populations where dental problems appear to be concentrated and which have little, if any, dental insurance, are expected to grow between the mid-1990s and 2020, thus potentially widening the gap between ability to pay and receipt of services.

3. The ever-growing adult population—at greater risk for gingivitis and adult-onset periodontis (a major contributor to tooth loss)—will need more dental services.

Auxiliary Personnel

The practice of dentistry has undergone major technological and organizational changes in the past several decades. Of particular importance has been the increased use of dental auxiliary personnel. Two major types of dental auxiliaries are dental hygienists and dental assistants. Dental hygienists provide oral prophylaxis services and dental health education and comprise the only group of auxiliaries that is licensed. Dental assistants have generally supported the dentist at chair side and have had the opportunity in some states to perform expanded functions under the dentist's supervision. In 2000, there were about 112,000 active dental hygienists, and roughly 240,000 dental assistants.

Most dentists employ some dental auxiliary on a full- or part-time basis. The government has supported the training of expanded-function dental auxiliaries (dental hygienists or dental assistants who receive additional education and training that enable them to perform a broader array of clinical functions), as well as the training of dental students to help improve their administrative and organizational skills in managing multiple auxiliary team practices. Support for the auxiliary concept has been due largely to an increase in the productivity of dental practices that employ such persons.

Increasing educational and professional requirements for dental hygienists (they must carry their own malpractice insurance) have made them able to practice without the physical presence of a dentist, something allowed in a majority of the states. There is evidence that these hygienists can provide greater access to dental services in underserved areas, at lower cost and without overall reduction in the quality of care. However, state regulations and the opposition of professional dentists' organizations do not favor the use of dental hygienists, and there is currently a struggle between dentists and dental hygienists over self-regulation and autonomy. This controversy will continue as long as the maldistribution of dentists persists and evidence continues to appear that dental hygienists can perform a variety of functions independently and inexpensively with no loss of quality.

Thus, the dental professions are in transition. The growth of dentists will continue, but probably at a lower rate than other health professions. The financial condition of a number of the remaining 55 dental schools, especially private ones, is poor, and there may be more closures in the next several years, further reducing the growth of dentistry. The role of the expanded function dental auxiliary is still unclear. The demand for dental care is very sensitive to economic conditions (because dental insurance covers only two-fifths of the population and one-third of dental expenditures) and can decrease during periods of recession. Hence, a shortage one year can quickly turn into a surplus the next. Yet, these economic conditions mask the epidemiological and demographic changes that are slowly altering the need for services. How these many factors combine to affect the future of dentistry should be watched closely.

PUBLIC HEALTH: NEW ROLES, NEW POSSIBILITIES

Traditionally, health professionals trained in public health have been sharply demarcated from those involved in the direct delivery of personal health services. Even so, the Institute of Medicine, in its landmark publication *The Future of Public Health* stated that the goal of public health activities was nothing less than assuring the conditions for people to be healthy (Institute of Medicine, 1988). In theory, then, there is a natural affinity between health professionals in public health and those in direct health care delivery.

In practice, public health roles have centered on, among others, administration of local, state, and national public health agencies; on planning, implementing, and evaluating prevention, screening, and health education programs; on surveillance and control of environmental hazards and pollutants; and on the epidemiological description and explanation for the incidence and prevalence of disease and trauma in populations. In certain settings, for example, municipal or county health departments, public health professionals have worked closely with other health professionals such as public health nurses in the delivery of primary care services to special populations such as indigent families, migrant workers, and groups of uninsured persons. But, in general, public health professionals have been a relatively "unseen" group of persons working to maintain a fundamental infrastructure allowing an understanding and an implementation of health-promoting activities at the population level: safe drinking water, adequate sanitary systems, control of infectious diseases, and prevention of disease and injury by reducing behavior such as smoking, high-speed driving, and the like.

The principal training programs for careers in public health are located in the 37 accredited schools of public health (up from about 29 in 2000), as well as a small number of accredited health education programs and community medicine programs.

Nearly 400 other nonaccredited programs exist that offer training in the various subfields of public health such as health administration and environmental health. The primary academic degree is either the master of public health (MPH) or the master of science in public health (MSPH). Other common avenues for careers in public health include the study of medicine with emphasis on and board certification in preventive medicine, the study of public health nursing, dentistry, nutrition, industrial hygiene, and social work among others. Advanced graduate training in some of the fields of public health, for example, epidemiology, environmental health sciences, health services research, health behavior and health education, and biostatistics, is normally obtained through the accredited schools of public health.

Total enrollment in schools of public health has expanded rapidly over the period 1975–1976 to 2004–2005, growing from 6,461 to 19,434, respectively, a 200 percent increase. Of the total students enrolled during the 1981–1982 academic year, 9.9 percent were members of underrepresented minority groups (African American, Hispanic, and Native American); by the 2004–2005 academic year, this proportion had grown to 18.2 percent. The proportion of women in the 1981–1982 total enrollment was 55.4 percent whereas this figure was 69.6 percent by 2001–2002 (Association of Schools of Public Health, 2005). Thus, during a period of major expansion in the number of students studying public health (public health ranked fourth in total enrollment after nursing, allopathic medicine, and pharmacy), there has been significant growth of opportunity for historically underrepresented minorities and women during the past two decades.

New Roles for Public Health Professionals

Two new general roles for public health professionals have arisen in recent years. First, the melding of public health functions with those of professionals in the direct delivery of personal health services is now under way with the expansion of managed-care plans. As explained in other chapters in this text, managed-care plans assume the responsibility for the health care of defined populations of enrollees within a budgetary system constrained by capitation arrangements, that is, a prospectively fixed payment for each enrollee for a defined period of time, usually 1 year. Because the financing system no longer permits an open-ended cost-based billing for services to insurers, the managed-care plan has clear incentives to find ways to deliver health care services efficiently, but more to the point here, to find ways to keep the covered population healthier in the first place.

This function is part of the fundamental mission of public health: Collect information on and monitor disease incidence and prevalence of the plan's enrollees; monitor the outcome of the health care delivery process; and develop, implement, and monitor programs of prevention and other forms of positive intervention into the health habits and behavior of the plan's enrollees (e.g., smoking and diet, receipt of prenatal care, immunization against infectious diseases, and the like). To the extent that managed-care plans emphasize these traditional public health roles, the plans may well be the catalysts for the integration of public health and personal health services that has long been called for in the United States. But, because of traditional insurance schemes based on retrospective cost-based reimbursement, of deep professional fissures between some health professionals and public health professionals, and other reasons, this integration has proceeded very slowly.

The second newer role for public health professionals, one that takes their traditional functions and places them in a new context, resides in bioterrorism surveillance and prevention. Ever since the tragic events of September 11, 2001, the public health community has been called on to develop systems of detection of potential bioterrorism events, including the release of biological and chemical agents into a variety of settings. These efforts have required a reconsideration of the preparedness of local, state, and federal public health organizations and functions to be able to operate in a streamlined, rapid, and effective fashion to identify, isolate, contain, and destroy potentially harmful agents released inadvertently or maliciously. Much more progress must be made in this domain, and public health authorities throughout the nation are working to find appropriate ways to foster this mission.

In short, more than ever, future careers in public health promise to join community-based practice—the historical purview of public health—and the institutional practice of the healing arts. The task of disease prevention and health maintenance promises to bring about integration of these two domains. However, without universal entitlement to health care via a comprehensive health insurance program, there will still continue to be a need for traditional community-based public health specialists involved in meeting needs of disadvantaged groups. At the same time, public health professionals are now called on literally to protect the public's health by prevention of the spread of harmful biological and chemical agents via such things as the food chain, the water supply, and the wider environment.

NURSING

Registered nurses are the largest group of licensed health care professionals in the United States. The supply of registered nurses (RNs) grew from 1,662,382 in 1980 to 2,694,540 in 2000, an increase of 62.2 percent. At the beginning of the twenty-first century, the *active,* that is, employed, supply of RNs increased 72.9 percent (from 1,272,851 in 1980 to 2,201,813 in 2000). An estimated 81.7 percent of RNs were employed in nursing in 2000. This reflects a major feature of the nursing workforce: A substantial number of nurses are not working in nursing or are inactive in the economic workforce.

Profiles show that most nurses are women with 5.4 percent of the RN workforce being men. However, in 2003, nearly 11 percent of enrolled nursing students were men. Twelve percent of the RN population is from minority groups. About 40 percent of RNs are graduates of associate degree programs, with 30 percent holding a nursing diploma,

usually sponsored by hospital programs. The baccalaureate preparation (bachelor of science in nursing) is represented by 30 percent of the RN population. Nursing programs, however, are distributed differently, with baccalaureate 36 percent; associate degree, 59 percent; and hospital diploma programs, 5 percent. The shifting education pattern of RNs, with increasing emphasis on a four-year baccalaureate degree, is discussed in greater detail below.

Despite the overall absolute increase in the number of nurses employed in nursing, a shortage of nurses exists relative to demand. Data from the *National Sample Survey of Registered Nurses* (Health Resources and Services Administration, 2000) indicated that the shortage was estimated at 6 percent in 2000. Based on what is known about trends in the supply of RNs and their anticipated demand, the shortage is expected to grow slowly until 2010, at which time it will have reached 12 percent and by 2015, the shortage is projected to be 20 percent. The cause of the nursing shortage is a confluence of factors. These factors include the declining number of nursing school enrollments, the aging of the RN workforce, nurses not employed in nursing, declines in relative earnings, and the emergence of alternative job opportunities (Health Resources and Services Administration, 2004a).

First, there is the issue of nursing school enrollments. The growth in nursing students during the period 1995 to 2000 experienced an annual decrease in the number of entry-level students in baccalaureate nursing programs. The period 2001 to 2006 saw a reversal of this trend, with increases in entry-level students each of these years, topping at 17 percent (American Association of Colleges of Nursing, 2007). However, the increases have been decreasing steadily since 2003, and this fact combined with the estimate made by the federal government that increases in the number of graduates must be around 90 percent to meet the nursing shortage adequately, means that nursing school production continues to fall short of what will be needed (Health Resources and Services Administration, 2004b).

Second, there is the aging of the RN workforce. The average age for hospital RNs is slightly over 43, the oldest it has ever been (Health Resources and Services Administration, 2004a). Three factors contribute to the aging of the RN workforce: (1) the decline in number of nursing school graduates, (2) the higher average age of recent graduating classes, and (3) the aging of the existing pool of licensed nurses. This slowing of new, young entrants coupled with an accelerating retirement rate for older RNs will produce a national supply of nurses in 2020 that will not only be older, but also no larger than the supply projected for 2005.

Third, there is the phenomenon of nurses not employed in nursing. The number of RNs who gave up their licenses from 1996 to 2000 numbered 175,000, and this is projected to double by 2020. In addition to the number of RNs that gave up their license, there are 500,000 licensed nurses not employed in nursing, with about 69 percent being 50 years or older. Analysis of data from the 2000 *National Sample Survey of Registered Nurses* shows that only 7 percent of the licensed RNs not employed in nursing were actively seeking employment in nursing (Health Resources and Services Administration, 2000).

Fourth, there have been declines in relative earnings. Whereas actual earnings for RNs increased steadily from 1983 through 2000, "real" earnings—the amount available after adjusting for inflation—have been relative flat since 1991 (Health Resources and Services Administration, 2000). In contrast, salaries of elementary school teachers have always been greater than RN salaries, and they are growing at a faster pace. The potential for nurses to increase their salaries decreases over time.

Fifth, there has been an emergence of alternative educational and job opportunities. Women no longer have limited options for education and employment. Medical school and other allied health profession enrollments are seeing increasing numbers of women. In addition, advanced practice nursing opportunities exist that involve independent practice and third-party reimbursement for some services.

As with most other health care professionals, the nursing shortage is not distributed evenly throughout the United States. For example, in 2000, 30 states were estimated to have shortages. By 2020, 44 states and the District of Columbia are projected to have shortages. The maldistribution appears to be due to the geographic immobility of women who are married and are second wage earners in a family. Additionally, rural and inner-city hospitals and other facilities are unable to offer an adequate range of incentives (e.g., flexible working hours, increased salaries, fringe benefits, safe working conditions) to attract nurses.

Rural institutions have found that urban-based education and training programs have not often been relevant to rural needs. Rural hospitals must frequently hire recent nursing graduates with limited skills and often resort to dependence on pool nurses from temporary employment agencies. This problem is of particular concern because of the increased responsibilities and range of skills needed by rural nurses. Rural providers are not likely to improve their chances of attracting well-trained nurses with a broad range of skills.

Nursing Education and Role Changes

The federal government has been largely responsible for increases in nursing school class size during cyclical shortages. Over the period 1960–1980, the federal government spent about $2.0 billion for nursing education, resulting in a more than doubling of admissions to nursing schools. The passage of the Nursing Reinvestment Act (NRA) of 2002 was to infuse money in the education of nurses in response to falling enrollments in nursing schools and to increase the number of admissions. Of particular interest, however, is the switch that has occurred in the control of nursing education from the hospital to nursing educators in colleges and universities.

Three forms of training lead to licensure as an RN: three-year diploma programs that are hospital-based, two-year associate degree programs that are generally in community colleges, and four-year baccalaureate nursing programs in universities or four-year colleges. In 2002–2003 only 6,196 (4.7 percent) of new nursing students were enrolled in diploma programs; in 1960–1961, the percentage had been 78.

In contrast to the other health professions discussed in this chapter, for reasons that are not clear, the supply of RNs had not included as great a proportion of minority group members, although the trend is changing. In 2002–2003, about 24 percent of RN students were members of minority groups. The largest minority group—African Americans—grew from about 7 percent in 1980 to a peak of nearly 13 percent in 2003. Why the field of nursing should lack the appeal to minorities that other health professions appear to have remains an unanswered question, deserving inquiry and remedy.

The major employment patterns now and in the future are shown in Table 12.6. The hospital is and will remain the major locus of employment for RNs, sectioning off about two-thirds of the nursing

workforce. Long-term care and home health nursing employment are expected to increase in importance whereas other areas of employment will show stability over the period 2000–2010. These figures may appear to contradict the notion that non-hospital-based employment is gaining in popularity; however, since many hospitals are themselves involved in owning and operating non-hospital-based services (such as home health and hospice services and ambulatory care sites), these figures may not reveal the true picture. Within these settings, new roles have emerged for the RN. These include clinical nurse specialist, nurse practitioner, nurse anesthetist, and nurse clinician. These positions involve employment in new ambulatory care settings (e.g., insurance companies, ambulatory surgery centers, free-standing urgent care centers, and the like), long-term care facilities, and home health and hospice programs providing care for the elderly and others with chronic and life-limiting illnesses or conditions. Nurses are also finding opportunities in statewide, regional, and hospital-level utilization and quality review roles in which

Table 12.6. Estimated and Projected Requirements for Full-Time Equivalent Registered Nurses by Employment Setting, 1990, 1995, 2000, 2010

Field of Employment	Estimated 1990	Percent (%)	Estimated 1995	Percent (%)	Estimated 2000	Percent (%)	Projected 2010	Percent (%)
Registered Nurse Total	1,466,000	100.0	1,610,200	100.0	2,201,813	100.0	2,344,584	100.0
Hospital	1,009,700	68.9	1,086,600	67.5	1,300,323	59.1	1,451,083	61.9
Nursing Home	105,300	7.2	130,300	8.1	152,894	6.9	223,193	9.5
Home Health	53,000	3.6	57,000	3.5	107,553	4.9	177,583	7.6
Other Community/ Public Health	111,900	7.6	136,700	8.5	175,065	8.0	93,226	4.0
Ambulatory Care	101,200	6.9	107,200	6.7	209,324	9.5	178,272	7.6
Other	84,900	5.8	92,400	5.7	256,654	11.7	221,227	9.4

SOURCES: From *Health Personnel in the United States: Eighth Report to Congress* (DHHS Pub. No. HRS-P-OD-92-1), 1992, Washington, DC: U.S. Government Printing Office; "The Registered Nurse Population," *Findings from the National Sample Survey of Registered Nurses*, U.S. Department of Health and Human Services, Bureau of Health Professions, 2000, Washington, DC: U.S. Government Printing Office; *Projected Supply, Demand, and Shortags of Registered Nurses: 2000–2020*, U.S. Department of Health and Human Services, Bureau of Health Professions, 2002, Washington, DC: U.S. Government Printing Office.

they analyze clinical records describing patient care.

The nursing profession has expanded its boundaries for a broader role in the health care system, including *independent* roles of nurses within institutional settings and the creation of new professional roles outside them. With decreasing numbers of diploma programs sponsored by hospitals and increasing numbers of nurses being educated in academic settings, the result is a decoupling of nursing education from nursing practice. The National League for Nursing (2003) has called for a dramatic reform and innovation in nursing education to create and shape the future of nursing practice. The league recommends new teaching strategies, curriculum changes, and increased collaboration with practitioners to prepare a nursing workforce that practices effectively in new health care environments. Other professional organizations in nursing have also proposed expanded duties through the doctor or nursing practice degree with enhanced duties.

PHARMACISTS

As is the case for all the health professional groups discussed so far, pharmacists are also undergoing extensive change as well as experiencing supply shortages. Until recently, pharmacists performed the traditional role of preparing drug products and filling prescriptions. In the 1980s and 1990s, pharmacists expanded that role to include drug production education and to act as an expert for clients and patients about the effects of specific drugs, drug interaction, and generic drug substitutions for brand-name drugs. In the early twenty-first century, the role has further expanded to include selecting, monitoring, and evaluating appropriate drug regimens, to provide information not only to patients, but also to other health care professionals, and to prevent medication errors. Finally, in their role as businessmen and -women, pharmacists have had to

learn more about the managerial and financial aspects of working in a retail trade.

There has been steady growth in the number of pharmacists during the last quarter century (Table 12.7). From 1973–1974 to 2002–2003, there was a 74 percent increase in the overall number. First-year enrollment in pharmacy schools leveled off during the 1980s, although there was a major increase in the proportion of female first-year students, from about 30 percent in 1973–1974 to about 67 percent of the total pharmacy student enrollment in 2002–2003. The growth of minorities in pharmacy, although not as great, has been steady, increasing from about 12 percent in 1980–1981 to 32 percent in 2002–2003. Another phenomenon of note is the doctorate in pharmacy (PharmD) degree, which was recognized as the entry-level degree in the 1990s, requiring additional clinical training and expanded practice skills, thus preparing pharmacists to take on more complex clinical roles such as counseling patients, advising other health professionals on drug use issues, and participating in disease management programs. Careers for those with the PharmD degree lead not only to research and teaching positions, but also to levels of higher administrative responsibility, often in health care organizations, and insurance and pharmaceutical companies.

Pharmacists are employed in a number of settings, such as pharmacies and drug stores, hospitals and medical centers, retail stores with pharmacies (grocery stores and mass merchandising stores), and other institutional settings such as long-term care facilities. As the 1990s began, about 40 percent of all pharmacists were employed in drug store chains. Estimates are now that at the beginning of the twenty-first century nearly two-thirds of pharmacists practice in retail pharmacies. The remainder of graduates works in hospitals, home health care, insurance companies, consulting groups, and universities.

Forces that may contribute to an increase in the need for pharmacists include the increased use of drugs, especially among the growing aged population, and the pharmacy's expanded role under

Table 12.7. Number of Active Pharmacists and Number of Pharmacy Students, by Gender and Minority Status, Selected Academic Years, 1973–1974, 1980–1981, 1990–1991, and 2002–2003

Academic Year	Total Active Pharmacists	First-Year Students[a]	First-Year Female Students[a]	Percent (%) Female of First-Year Students[a]	Total Graduates	Total Minority Graduates	Percent (%) Minority of Total Graduates
1973–1974	112,600	8,342	2,508	30.1	5,957	—	—
1980–1981	142,400	7,551	3,655	48.4	7,323	891	12.2
1990–1991	161,900	8,356	4,926	59.0	7,122	1,461	20.5
2002–2003	196,011	—	43,047[b]	66.9[b]	7,488	2,391	31.90

[a]Includes students in the first year of the three years of pharmacy education, excluding any students in prepharmacy years.
[b]Includes all students enrolled in pharmacy schools.

SOURCES: From *Minorities and Women in the Health Fields* [DHHS Pub. No. [HRSA]-P-DV-90-3], 1990, Washington, DC: U.S. Government Printing Office; *Health Personnel in the United States: Eighth Report to Congress* [DHHS Pub. No. HRS-P-OD-92-1], 1992, Washington, DC: U.S. Government Printing Office; *Minorities and Women in the Health Fields, 1994, The Pharmacist Workforce: A Study of the Supply and Demand for Pharmacists*, 2000, Department of Health and Human Services, Bureau of Health Professions; American Association of Colleges of Pharmacy 2005, http://www.aacp.org

changes in Medicare and Medicaid programs that require review of patient drug use and patient counseling. Nevertheless, making projections about the future supply of pharmacists in relation to future need or demand is difficult because of the rapidly changing employment circumstances in the field. Further, the aging of the American population would suggest that more medication prescriptions will be written and more work for pharmacists will result. At the same time, because pharmacists are expanding their role to include nontraditional activities, as mentioned, the amount of time an individual pharmacist might spend in traditional "druggist" activities will probably decline. With computerized information procession systems, assistance from pharmacy technicians, and mail-order approaches that pharmacists will be using in increasing numbers, one would expect a positive gain in productivity, and perhaps a diminished need for an increased supply. In short, a number of factors make predicting the future balance of supply and demand difficult, and given the importance of drug therapies for modern medical care, policy makers should watch this important health profession closely.

PHYSICIAN ASSISTANTS AND ADVANCED PRACTICE NURSES

The perceived shortage of physicians in the mid-1960s led to the development of two types of health care providers: physician assistants (PAs) and advanced practice nurses (APNs). PAs are qualified by academic and practical training to provide patient services under the direction and supervision of a licensed physician who is responsible for the performance of the PA. PAs are able to diagnose, manage, and treat common illnesses; provide preventive services; and respond appropriately to common emergency situations. Although PAs are trained as primary care providers, approximately half subsequently serve in specialty roles (Cooper, 2001). All states license or otherwise recognize PAs under a physician's supervision, although as with NPs, that supervision may be intermittent and at a distance, and the actual autonomy of PAs may be substantial.

Forty-two states, as well as the District of Columbia, allow delegation by a physician to the PA the authority to prescribe certain medications (American Academy of Physician Assistants, 2005). The typical PA training program consists of 2 to 3 years of didactic study followed by clinical training. However, programs vary widely in terms of admission requirements, curriculum, and site of educational training. There were 59 accredited PA programs in the early 1990s, and by 2005, the number had more than doubled to 135 (Accreditation Review Commission on Education for the Physician Assistant, 2005), and at the beginning of 2005, there were an estimated 55,061 people in clinical practice as PAs, more than double the number in 1993 (American Academy of Physician Assistants, 2005).

There is a tendency for PAs more often than physicians to serve in rural and medically underserved areas with about 34 percent of PAs working in communities of less than 50,000. Although women represent 60 percent of practicing PAs, this is a trend that has reversed since the mid-1990s. Most PAs are white (88 percent) with the remainder consisting mostly of underrepresented minorities.

In 2004, 57 percent of PAs were employed by solo or multispecialty physician practices, 22 percent were employed by hospitals, 11 percent were not employed in clinical practice, and the remaining 10 percent were employed by other types of organizations. Of practicing PAs, 37 percent report that their "primary" work setting was the hospital (American Academy of Physician Assistants, 2005). In 1990, there were 5,315 PAs practicing in hospitals and by 2004, the number had increased to 7,591. Most PAs work in the private sector (90 percent), and about 10 percent work for government agencies including the Veterans Administration, the Armed Forces, and the U.S. Public Health Service. Finally, the proportion of PAs working in primary care settings has declined over the period 1978 to 2004, from 67 percent to 42 percent. General surgery, surgical subspecialties, intensive care units, orthopedics, and emergency medicine all registered increases.

APNs are nurses with particular skills and credentials, which typically include basic nursing education,

basic licensure, graduate degree in nursing, experience in a specialized area, professional certification from a national certifying body, and—if required in some states—APN licensure (National Council of State Boards of Nursing, 2004). The APN specializes as a nurse practitioner (NP), certified nurse midwife (CNM), certified registered nurse anesthetist (CRNA), or clinical nurse specialist (CNS).

The APN role is defined by seven core competencies or skill performance areas. The first core competency of direct clinical practice is central to and informs all the others, as follows: direct clinical practice; expert guidance and coaching of patients, families, and other care providers; consultation; research skills, including use and implementation of evidence-based practice, evaluation, and conduct; clinical and professional leadership, which includes competence as a change agent; collaboration; ethical decision-making skills (Hamric, 2005).

As with PAs, some states permit certain categories of APNs to write prescriptions for certain classes of drugs. This prescriptive authority varies from one state to another and may be regulated by boards of nursing, pharmacy, or allied health. Of NPs, 97 percent prescribe medications and write an average of 19 prescriptions per day (American Academy of Nurse Practitioners, 2005). Sixty-five percent of NPs are authorized to write prescriptions for controlled substances. Some states require physician supervision of APN practices, although some managed-care plans now include APNs on their lists of primary care providers.

APN Specialization

Certified nurse midwives (CNM) specialize in low-risk obstetrical care, including all aspects of the prenatal, labor and delivery, and postnatal processes. Certified registered nurse anesthetists (CRNAs) complete additional education to specialize in the administration of various types of anesthesia and analgesia to patients and clients. Often, nurse anesthetists work collaboratively with surgeons and anesthesiologists as part of the perioperative care team. Clinical nurse specialists (CNSs) hold masters degrees, have successfully completed a specialty certification examination, and are generally employed by hospitals as nursing "experts" in particular specialties. The scope of the CNS is not as broad as that of the NP; CNSs work with a specialty population under a somewhat circumscribed set of conditions, and the management authority of patients still rests with physicians. In contrast, NPs have developed an autonomous role in which their collaboration is encouraged, and they generally have the legal authority to implement clinical management actions.

As of 2004, there were some 106,000 NPs in the United States, more than double the number in 1992. There is a range of specialties for NPs, including pediatric, family, adult, psychiatric, gerontological, and acute care. Eighty-eight percent of NPs have graduate degrees; 92 percent of NPs maintain national certification; 39 percent of NPs hold hospital privileges; 20 percent of NPs practice in rural or frontier settings; and the average NP is female (95 percent), 48 years old, and has been in practice for nearly 9 years as a family NP (41 percent) (American Academy of Nurse Practitioners, 2005).

There are important differences in the perceptions of the roles of PAs and APNs. The medical profession views PAs as physician "extenders" who can perform many of the usual functions completed by physicians. APNs are nurses in an expanded role. The NP would be the APN specialist with greater supervision of, and responsibility for, primary patient care, with extra emphasis on the traditional nursing competencies of prevention and counseling. Despite these perceptual differences, as well as differences in education, care delivery model, and outlook, many of the performance characteristics of PAs and NPs appear to be similar.

Issues in PA and NP Use

Among the issues that need to be resolved before PAs and NPs can be used to their full capacity and original promise are legal restrictions concerning practice, reimbursement policies, and relationships with physicians. The legal status of PAs and NPs varies considerably across states. As noted in the case of PAs, many states permit considerable delegation of tasks and responsibilities, including prescribing certain drugs. State legislation expanding medical delegation has been unduly restrictive with regard to the scope of practice of qualified nonphysicians, although progress is being made.

Laws and regulations governing the expanded role of the nurse practitioner are also changing rapidly, but inconsistently. Although the majority of states have altered their nurse practice acts to facilitate expanded roles, the constraints on the scope of NP practice continue to vary from state to state. A particular barrier is whether an individual state will authorize prescription practices of NPs. Although most states have explicit regulatory provision for limited prescriptive authority, these authorizations vary in the degree of independence and in the types of drug and devices that may be prescribed. There may also be geographic limitations, for example, more NP discretion in rural than urban settings.

Third-party reimbursement imposes another constraint on the use of PAs and NPs. Current policies generally link their reimbursement directly to the employing physician or institution. Since 1989, federal law requires direct Medicaid reimbursement for pediatric NPs and family NPs whether or not a physician directly supervises the NP. Yet, many states are not yet in compliance with federal legislation. As for the private health insurance sector, some states have laws allowing reimbursement to NPs, but this coverage is usually optional and is not widespread. Some progress has been made in reimbursement of NPs and PAs through the Medicare program. For example, in 1989, the U.S. Congress, in its mandate that a resource-based relative value scale (RBRVS) fee schedule supplant the usual and customary schedule for physician payment under Medicare Part B, called for study of including "nonphysician providers" in the fee schedule. Experimental programs are under review and may lead to a special reimbursement schedule.

A final area of concern is current and future relationships with physicians. In the past, physicians were reasonably accepting of these personnel. Yet, about the time that these midlevel practitioners were becoming popular among those seeking a lower-cost substitute for physician services, the physician surplus was enunciated, and physicians were wary of employing personnel who might take away their work. Further, there was, as noted earlier in this chapter, a tendency for some physicians to move into previously medically underserved areas.

Yet, there has been an increase in NPs and PAs, and much of the current demand has been generated by managed-care plans whose efforts to cut costs, to find flexibility in deployment of caregivers, and to emphasize primary care and prevention coincide with the lower salaries, the broad skill set, and the training that are typical of NPs and PAs. Further, there are many roles that these midlevel professionals have been filling and continue to fill: providing primary care to underserved populations often in underserved areas as well as care to the elderly and the mentally ill, providing preventive care and health education, delivering specialty services in hospitals in lieu of house staff. New practice settings for NPs and PAs include schools, industrial settings, prisons, and nursing homes.

The outcome of the current debate about the physician shortage and the role of IMGs in the physician workforce will be consequential for PAs and NPs. If efforts are successful in increasing the growth of physician supply, the employment of these midlevel health professionals may slow down somewhat throughout the health care system. On the other hand, given the current and projected shortage of nurses, the historic barriers to PAs and NPs may continue to crumble and thus improve the chances for attainment of the full promise of PA and NP service delivery.

THE CHANGING NATURE OF HEALTH PROFESSIONALS

This chapter has summarized trends in the supply of health professionals. From the 1960s into the early 1980s, federal and state support resulted in

large increases in the number of graduates of most health professional occupations. From the mid-1980s to the end of the 1990s, the growth of some occupational groups, for example, PAs, and NPs, was probably affected as much by the workforce requirements of managed-care plans as by any public policy effort. In the early 2000s, the faster than anticipated growth of the U.S. population, the ever-increasing number of elderly persons, the improved effectiveness of and accompanying increase in demand for diagnostic and treatment procedures have led to a searching review of the adequacy of personnel across the spectrum of health occupations, most notably in nursing. Still there has been much growth in the sector, and women and minorities have greatly benefited from this phenomenon. And, in addition to the "standard" health professions discussed in this chapter, there has been steady growth—and popularity with the American public—in numerous less conventional health care occupations like chiropractors, acupuncturists, and naturopaths (Cooper, Laud, & Dietrich, 1998).

The historic federal and state investment in health care personnel has improved access to health care and helped schools training health professionals to remain financially viable. But, current budget deficits have led to reductions in government spending for the health professions, although there have been efforts to increase spending for nursing. Many of the major trends affecting the U.S. health care system, such as restrictive public and private sector reimbursement, growth of alternative delivery systems and managed-care plans, portend continuing pressures against the growth of health professions. Thus, stories are becoming more common of hospitals having potential shortages of not only RNs, but also of pharmacists, in most of the allied health professions, and in certain medical specialists (Steinhauer, 2000).

The increasing number of women in all the health professions also suggests that, on balance, with the rise of single-parent households and the continued disproportionate household and child-rearing responsibilities that married or single working mothers bear, female health professionals, particularly physicians, will probably work fewer hours per week and fewer weeks per year than men. This could add up to a need for more personnel to make up desirable levels of full-time equivalent labor. For example, if the proportion of women entering medicine continues at the current pace, the effective full-time equivalent supply of physician services will decline by about 4 percent between 1986 and 2010, other things being equal (Kletke, Marder, & Silberger, 1990). On the other hand, the effect of managed care plans with their efficient use of health care personnel produces a countervailing force in relation to overall numbers of health care professionals. Such conflicting forces make predicting the balance between need and demand versus supply of health professionals a very difficult enterprise.

THE PUZZLE OF MANAGED CARE

Managed care deserves the final comment in this chapter's conclusion. The rapid growth of managed-care plans and of the number of Americans enrolled in these plans has become a major force reshaping the size and composition of the health care professions' workforce. In the immediate future, there are several important consequences of managed care on the workforce (Council on Graduate Medical Education, 1995b). First, more and more health professionals will have some sort of relationship with managed care. For example, most physicians are now involved in managed care either as full-time employees or as contractors with one or more plans. More than three-fours of all physicians are estimated to have at least one managed-care contract. This trend may have weakened in the early 2000s, but substantial numbers of physicians remain connected to managed care at least through preferred provider organizations and their associated networks.

Second, some observers have felt that continued managed-care growth would only magnify

and exacerbate the problem of a physician surplus. But, the current thinking is that with the weakening of tightly controlled managed-care plans, particularly the classic HMOs, the "managed-care effect" has softened and will not be as powerful an influence on workforce supply as once thought. It remains an open question what impact the organization of health services will have on questions on "shortage" or "surplus" because it is unclear what the future of managed care versus a more fee-for-service-like system of care delivery will be.

SUMMARY

In the longer run, it appears that—one after another—the individual health professions are predicted to be in short supply, and with the potential addition of medicine to the list, there will be great pressure on public and private sources to fund more of the costs of the education health care professionals, including the building of new schools. The phenomenon has already taken place in public health and osteopathy. Official medical associations are calling for increases in allopathic medical education. Nursing educators are striving to increase nursing faculties and class sizes. Some hospital systems, in desperation of finding enough nurses, are actively soliciting nurses from foreign countries and refurbishing long-closed hospital-based, non-university-based, nurse diploma programs. This activity is taking place within the context of an increasingly stringent public and private reimbursement environment, and it is very difficult to see where the funds will come from to support the kind of expansion in health professions for which many are calling. Although what the outcome of these forces will bring is speculative, what is not is the interactive nature of all the health professions and the delivery organizations and the often-surprising outcomes of that interaction. The future presents a vastly different possibility than that predicted at the beginning of the twenty-first century, and the trends that emerge will be of the greatest interest.

REVIEW QUESTIONS

1. Describe the general employment trends in the health care sector.
2. Discuss some of the reasons there may be a physician shortage rather than a surplus.
3. Describe the geographic distribution of physicians across the United States. In addition, list the governmental initiatives taken to improve physician distribution.
4. Discuss the role of osteopathic medicine in the United States.
5. Describe the role of public health professionals.
6. What factors contribute to the nursing shortage?
7. Discuss trends in the pharmacy profession.
8. Discuss the issues associated with the use of physician assistants and nurse practitioners.

REFERENCES & ADDITIONAL READINGS

American Association of Colleges of Nursing. Retrieved April 27, 2007, from http://www.aacn.nche.edu/Media/NewsReleases/065Survey.htm.

Accreditation Review Commission on Education for the Physician Assistant, Inc. (2005). Retrieved February 14, 2005, from http://www.arc-pa.org/General/AccreditedPrograms.html.

Aiken, L. (1982). The impact of federal health policy on nurses. In L. Aiken (Ed.), *Nursing in the 1980s: Crises, opportunities, challenges.* Philadelphia: Lippincott.

American Academy of Family Physicians. (1991). *Report on survey of 1991 graduating family practice residents.* Washington, DC: American Academy of Family Physicians.

American Academy of Nurse Practitioners. (2005). *U.S. nurse practitioner workforce 2004.* Retrieved February 20, 2005, from http://www.aanp.org.

American Academmcy of Physician Assistants. (2005). http://www.aapa.org/.

Association of Schools of Public Health. (2005). *2004 annual data report.* Washington, DC: American Academy of Family Physicians.

Auerbach, D. I., Buerhaus, P. I., & Staiger, D. O. (2000). Associate degree graduates and the rapidly aging RN workforce. *Nursing Economics, 18,* 178–184.

Brown, L. J., & Lazar, V. (1999). Trends in the dental health work force. *Journal of the American Dental Association, 130,* 1743–1749.

Bureau of Health Professions, Health Resources and Services Administration. (1993). *Factbook: Health personnel United States* (DHHS Pub. No. HRSA-P-AM-93-1). Washington, DC: U.S. Government Printing Office.

Carr, P. L., Ash, R. S., Friedman, R. H., Sacramucci, A., Barnett, R. C., Szalacha, L., Paler, A., & Moskowitz, M. A. (1998). Relation of family responsibilities and gender to the productivity and career satisfaction of medical faculty. *Annals of Internal Medicine, 129,* 532–538.

Center for Health Workforce Studies. (2000). *Meeting future nursing needs of New Yorkers: The role of the State University of New York.* Rensselaer, NY: Center for Health Workforce Studies, State University of New York at Albany.

Cooper, R. A. (2001). Health care workforce for the twenty-first century: The impact of nonphysician clinicians. *Annual Review of Medicine, 52,* 51–61.

Cooper, R. A., Getzen, T. E., McKee, H. J., & Laud, P. (2002). Economic and demographic trends signal an impending physician shortage. *Health Affairs, 21,* 140–154.

Cooper, R. A., Laud, P., & Dietrich, C. L. (1998). Current and projected workforce of nonphysician clinicians. *Journal of the American Medical Association, 280,* 788–794.

Council on Graduate Medical Education (1955a). *Seventh report to Congress and the Department of Health & Human Services Secretary: Recommendations for Department of Health and Human Services' programs.* Washington, DC: U.S. Government Printing Office.

Council on Graduate Medical Education. (1995b). *Sixth report to Congress and the Department of Health & Human Services Secretary: Managed health care: Implications for the physician workforce and medical education.* Washington, DC: U.S. Government Printing Office.

Council on Graduate Medical Education. (1999). *COGME physician workforce policies: Recent developments and remaining challenges in meeting national goals.* Washington, DC: U.S. Government Printing Office.

Council on Graduate Medical Education. (2005). *Physician workforce policy guidelines for the United States. 2000–2020* (16th Report). Washington, DC: U.S. Department of Health and Human Services.

Darnay, A. J. (Ed.). (1998). *Statistical record of health & medicine.* Detroit: Gale Research.

Dedobbeleer, N., Contandriopoulous, A. P., & Desjardins, S. (1995). Convergence or divergence of male and female physicians' hours of work and income. *Medical Care, 33,* 796–805.

Dorsey, E. R., Jarjoura, D., & Rutecki, G. W. (2003). Influence of controllable lifestyle on recent trends in specialty choice by U.S. medical students. *Journal of the American Medical Association, 290,* 1173–1178.

Ferrer, R. L., Hambridge, S. J., & Maly, R. C. (2005). The essential role of generalists in health care systems. *Annals of Internal Medicine, 142,* 691–699.

Flexner, A. (1910). *Medical education in the United States and Canada: A report to the Carnegie Foundation for the Advancement of Teaching.* Bulletin no. 4. New York: The Carnegie Foundation.

Gershon, S. K., Cultice, J. M., & Knapp, K. K. (2000). How many pharmacists are in our future? The Bureau of Health Professions Projects Supply to 2020. *Journal of the American Pharmaceutical Association, 40,* 757–764.

Goodman, D. C. (2005). The physician workforce crisis: Where is the evidence? *Health Affairs, 24,* (Suppl.), W5, 108–110.

Gordon, R. J., Meister, J. S., & Hughes, R. G. (1992). Accounting for shortages of rural physicians: Push and pull factors. In W. M. Gesler, & T. C. Ricketts (Eds.), *Health in rural North America: The geography of health care services and delivery.* New Brunswick, NJ: Rutgers University Press, pp. 153–178.

Graduate Medical Education National Advisory Committee. (1980). *Report to the Secretary, DHHS,* Vol. I: *GMENAC summary report* (DHHS Pub. No. [HRA] 81-653). Washington, DC: U.S. Government Printing Office.

Hamric, A. B., Spross, J. A., & Hanson, C. M. (Eds.). (2005). *Advanced Practice Nursing: An Integrative Approach* (3rd ed.). St. Louis: Elsevier Saunders, pp. 95–96.

Health personnel in the United States: Ninth report to Congress, 1993 Edition. (DHHS Pub. No. P-OD-94-1). (1993). Washington, DC: U.S. Government Printing Office.

Health Resources and Services Administration. (2000). *The registered nurse population: Findings from the National Sample Survey of registered nurses.* Washington, DC: U.S. Government Printing Office.

Health Resources and Services Administration. *The registered nurse population: National Sample Survey of registered nurses* (2004a). Washington, DC: U.S. Government Printing Office.

Health Resources and Services Administration. (2004b). *What is behind HRSA's projected supply, demand, and shortage of registered nurses?.* Washington, DC: U.S. Government Printing Office.

Institute of Medicine. (1988). *The future of public health.* Washington, DC: National Academy Press.

Institute of Medicine. (1996). *The nation's physician workforce: Options for balancing supply and requirements.* Washington, DC: National Academy Press.

Kletke, P. R., Marder, W. D., & Silberger, A. B. (1990). The growing proportion of female physicians: Implications for U.S. physician supply. *American Journal of Public Health, 80,* 300–304.

Lesser, C. S., Ginsburg, P. B., Devers, K. J. (2003). The end of an era: What became of the "managed care revolution of 2001"? *Health Services Research, 31,* 337–355.

Levin, E., & Moses, E. (1982). Registered nurses today: A statistical profile. In L. Aiken (Ed.), *Nursing in the 1980s: Crises, opportunities, challenges.* Philadelphia: Lippincott.

Mick, S. S. (1992). *The 1987 career characteristics of foreign and U.S. medical graduates who entered the U.S. medical system between 1969 and 1982.* Report to the Educational Commission for Foreign Medical Graduates, Philadelphia, PA.

Mick, S. S. (2004). The physician "surplus" and the decline of professional dominance. *Journal of Health Politics, Policy and Law, 29,* 907–924.

Mick, S. S., Lee, S.-Y. D., & Wodchis, W. (2000). Variations in geographical distribution of international medical graduates and U.S. medical graduates: "Safety nets" or "surplus exacerbation"? *Social Science & Medicine, 50,* 185–202.

Mick, S. S., & Worobey, J. L. (1984). Foreign and United States medical graduates in practice: A follow-up. *Medical Care, 22,* 1014–1025.

Minnick, A. F. (2000). Retirement, the nursing workforce, and the year 2005. *Nursing Outlook, 48,* 211–217.

Moy, E., & Bartman, B. A. (1995). Physician race and care of minority and medically indigent patients. *Journal of the American Medical Association, 273,* 1515–1520.

National Council of State Boards of Nursing. (2004). Retrieved December 10, 2004, from http://www.ncsbn.org.

National League for Nursing. (2003). Position statement: Innovation in nursing education: A call to reform. New York: National League for Nursing.

Pearse, W. H., Haffner, W. H., & Primack, A. (2001). Effect of gender on the obstetric-gynecologic work force. *Obstetrics and Gynecology, 97,* 794–797.

Pew Health Professions Commission. (2005). *Critical challenges: Revitalizing the health professions for the twenty-first century.*

Philip, M., & Midgley, E. (2006). Immigration: Shaping and reshaping America. *Population Bulletin, 61*(4).

Reschovsky, J. D., Staiti, A. B. (2005). Physician incomes in rural and urban America. *Issue Brief,* No. 92. Washington, DC: Center for Studying Health System Change.

Ricketts, T. C. (1994). Health care professionals in rural America. In J. E. Beaulieu & D. E. Berry (Eds.), *Rural health services: A management perspective.* Ann Arbor, MI: AUPHA Press/Health Administration Press.

Ricketts, T. C. (2005). Workforce issues in rural areas: A focus on policy equity. *American Journal of Public Health, 95,* 42–48.

Seifer, S. D., Troupin, B., & Rubenfeld, G. D. (1996). Changes in marketplace demand for physicians: A study of medical journal recruitment advertisements. *Journal of the American Medical Association, 276,* 695–699.

Society of Hospital Medicine. (2005). Retrieved February 25, 2005, from http://www.hospitalmedicine.Org/Content/NavigationMenu/Media/GrowthofHospitalMedicine/Growth of Hospital Medicine.htm.

Starfield, B., & Shi. L. (2005). Contribution of primary care to health systems and health. *Milbank Memorial Fund Quarterly, 83,* 457–502.

Steinhauer, J. (2000, December 25). Shortage of health care workers keeps growing. *The New York Times,* A1–17.

U.S. Census Bureau. (2007). Retrieved April 25, 2007, from http://www.census.gov.ipc/www/usinterimproj.

Weiner, J. P. (2004). Prepaid group practice staffing and U.S. physician supply: Lessons for workfoce policy. *Health Affairs,* W4-43–59.

Wennberg, J. E. (2004). Practice variations and health care reform: Connecting the dots. *Health Affairs,* (Suppl.), VAR-140–144.

Whitcomb, M. E. (1995). A cross-national comparison of generalist physician workforce data. *Journal of the American Medical Association, 274,* 692–695.

Whitcomb, M. E., & Miller, R. S. (1995). Participation of international medical graduates in graduate medical education and hospital care for the poor. *Journal of the American Medical Association, 274,* 696–699.

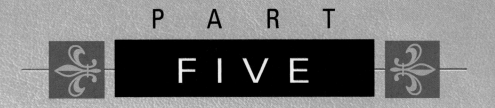

P A R T
FIVE

Assessing and Regulating Health Services

CHAPTER 13

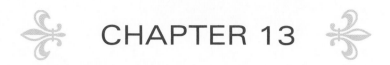

Understanding Health Policy

Paul R. Torrens

CHAPTER TOPICS

❧ The Organizational Form of Health Care in the United States and Its Relation to Health Policy

❧ Types of Health Policy and How They Are Made

❧ How Individual Health Professionals Can Participate in the Development and Implementation of Health Policy

❧ The Major Policy Issues in the Future of Health Care

LEARNING OBJECTIVES

Upon completing this chapter, the reader should be able to

1. Understand the impact of health policies on health care.

2. Gain knowledge of the development of health policy in the United States.

3. Appreciate the roles of government in health policy.

4. Appreciate the competing goals of health policy objectives.

5. Understand the key health policy issues the nation faces.

Throughout this text, references are made to health policy issues that greatly affect health care in the United States at the present time and will continue to affect it in the future (Institute of Medicine of the National Academies, 2003). Unfortunately, for a subject that has such real and potential impacts on health care, many health professionals have little understanding of how policy is made and how it affects the system.

This chapter will discuss several aspects of health policy in the United States: (1) how health care in the United States is organized and how the organizational form influences and, in turn, is influenced by health policy; (2) the different types of health policy and how they are implemented; (3) how individual health professionals can participate in the development and implementation of public policy; (4) the major health policy issues to be addressed in the future.

THE ORGANIZATIONAL FORM OF HEALTH CARE IN THE UNITED STATES AND ITS RELATION TO HEALTH POLICY

The way in which a country chooses to organize its health care and the health policy of that country are closely interrelated, but it is not clear which comes first—which is cause and which is effect. It could be said, for example, that the health care system of a country sets the overall framework in which health policy takes place and in which health policy issues are played out. At the same time, it could just as easily be said that the health policies of a country determine what type of health care system develops and functions; health policy decisions, therefore, are the drivers and shapers of the health care system itself.

In fact, both concepts are true and are actively at play in health care in the United States and in any other country of the world; it is not an "either-or"

situation but rather "both-and." The way a health care system is organized does set the framework for health policy, and at the same time, health policy does influence the way in which a system develops and operates. The famous quote of Winston Churchill holds true: "In the beginning, we shape our institutions and thereafter, they shape us." Therefore, it is important to understand those aspects of our health care system that have important impacts on health policy.

The primary characteristic of health care in the United States has been the general theory of the least government involvement possible. From the beginning, the delivery of health care was not seen as an appropriate government function and was more likely felt to be a personal, private, and local activity. The fact that this country did not have a federal government cabinet-level department for health until 1953 when the Department of Health, Education, and Welfare was created, speaks volumes about this idea. For most of our country's history, government involvement in health was limited to protection of the public's health in more of a policing role against dangers to health, rather than direct involvement in how health services are paid for and delivered.

Directly connected to this idea of least possible government involvement, when health insurance began to be developed, it was primarily a private, employer-based system of financing, not a public system of financing as was the case in many other industrialized countries of the world. Even today, approximately two-thirds of the American population obtains health insurance through their place of employment, not through governmental programs.

At the same time, it must be said that Americans value health care very highly and are quite willing to spend significant amounts of the nation's wealth in support of a system of high excellence and standards. It has always been presumed that health care was a very highly valued social good and that our society would support it fully in economic and political ways.

In line with this idea of health care being seen as high value to the society, there has always been a great degree of trust in science and in physicians. The American people have an almost magical belief in the power of science to eventually solve all health care problems or at least improve the health status of the people. At the same time, people in this country have had extremely strong, positive feeling toward physicians as both the deliverers of that science and as compassionate sources of personal attention.

The increased respect for the benefits of scientific medicine and the already high desire to have close relationships with skilled and compassionate physicians (and hospitals) has led to a great desire for choice in health care options. The American public apparently places significant value on the ability to pick and choose among providers of care, even though they may not actually have appropriate evidence to make well-considered choices. Put another way, the American public does not wish to be locked into limited systems of care and locked out of others.

This respect for science and technology as well as the desire to access the best medical care available have led (at least in part) to a very costly health care system. In 2006, the United States allocated approximately 16 percent of the gross domestic product (GDP) of the United States to health care, with estimates that this percentage will continue to grow in the years ahead. This rapidly rising cost of care has led to greater interest in cost containment and similar efforts to reduce the economic burden of health care.

Unfortunately, the reality is that the American health care system is fragmented, decentralized, and unplanned, making it almost impossible to impose any type of centralized organizational reform that would affect all parts of this increasingly costly enterprise. There is simply no convenient or appropriate authority, let alone organizational structure, from which rational and focused cost-containment measures can be carried forward, and no real policy-making body or group that is acknowledged by everyone in health care as having the responsibility or authority for suggesting organizational reform, let alone to impose it (Mechanic, 2004).

As a result, health care policy in the United States is now driven primarily by financing and health insurance mechanisms, particularly the federal Medicare program and the federal and state Medicaid programs. Because there is no generally accepted central authority over all aspects of the American health care system, those who would try to develop health policy in this country have turned toward the only possible avenue of influence: the source of financing for health care. In particular, because Medicare and Medicaid are now responsible for providing almost half of all the financing of health care in the United States, this is a powerful lever. Also, because these two programs are governmentally organized, legislative bodies on the federal and state levels are able to develop health policy as part of their responsibility to supervise these two governmental programs (Ball, 1995; Moon, 2000). In essence, the major efforts for health care policy in the United States have been carried out through legislative and regulatory oversight of Medicare and Medicaid (Brown & Sparer, 2003).

Finally, since the share of health care financing has increasingly been carried by Medicare and Medicaid, greater and greater responsibility for health care policy development has moved to federal and state governments (and their legislatures). With almost half of all health care financing now being coordinated by one federal government agency, the Centers for Medicare and Medicaid Services (CMS), it is only natural that individuals and organizations throughout the entire country increasingly focus their attention on what happens in Washington, DC.

TYPES OF HEALTH POLICY AND HOW THEY ARE MADE

When discussing "health policy," it is necessary to point out that the term is often used in two different ways, each of which may lead to different conclusions, actions, and impacts. It is important to review the two interpretations, so that health professionals can understand clearly what their objectives and efforts to influence health policy might entail.

On the one hand, "health policy" is a term frequently used to describe an informal and general set of values, ethical standards, legal decisions in court cases, and the like. A statement such as "the policy of this organization will be . . ." lays out general guidelines, directions, and statement of intentions in connection perhaps with a broad statement of mission, vision, and values of a person, an organization, or a society. It has the advantage and strength of being a general summary of a broad set of social, political, and economic truths, but also the disadvantage of perhaps being nonspecific, lacking in detail, and without any means of being carried out by individual actions. It has the strength of being sufficiently broad and general to draw in a broader range of opinions and participants, specifically because it doesn't commit them to a particular set of detailed agreements or details; the weakness is that it does not necessarily force commitment to a particular set of actions. More often than not, health policy of the more formal and detailed variety does not take place until this more informal agreement on general principles and beliefs is solidly developed.

The more frequently used interpretation of "health policy" is the collection of specific laws, programs, entitlements, regulations, administrative directions, and conditions of participation in various aspects of the health care system. In this context, health policy is specific, detailed, and focused and is usually accompanied by descriptions of financing and administration, as well as specific time periods to be covered, assignment of oversight and administrative authority, and other organizational matters.

The formal mechanisms for this interpretation of health policy usually begin with legislative action of some type that creates a broad set of governmental responsibilities, authorities, programs, and financing; this usually follows the more informal and broader consensus building discussed earlier. It may result in the creation of an entirely new area of governmental activities or it may simply mean expansion of an already existing program or orga-

nizational area of activity. The passage of the original Medicare legislation in the 1960s is an example of the first, while the addition of the Part D Medicare drug benefit in 2006 would be an example of the second (Inglehart, 2004).

Often development of a new policy may follow a formal legal or judicial action that either enables or requires development of a new program; often, too, the development of a new policy may be followed by legal or judicial tests of the legislation and programs created by legislative action. An example of the first might be a court ruling stating that the provision of contraceptive materials and information is legal; this might, in turn, require that public insurance programs such as Medicaid include the financing or provision of contraceptive materials to appropriate individuals. An example of the latter might be a program created to provide more information to the public on the quality of care provided to Medicare beneficiaries by specific physicians in specific hospitals that is then challenged by state medical societies claiming the policy impinges on the confidentiality of patient records. No matter whether they precede the passage of specific legislation or follow it, legal and judicial actions play an important role in the development of the specifics of health policy.

Once a law is passed and a particular program or set of organizational activities is put in place, the next phase of health policy development involves the creation of regulations and administrative guidelines and procedures for implementation of that program. These are typically not detailed in the original legislation or in relevant legal actions; they are usually the responsibility of those individuals managing or operating the program or activity. The regulations developed by program staff are designed to tell those involved with the program what specifically is to be done; the administrative guidelines may be less explicit or specific and are designed more to advise how the specific regulations might be carried out in practice. Formal regulations can be the subject of formal investigative actions by the inspector generals of individual government agencies or programs, while administrative guidelines would generally not be the subject of investigative activities.

However, both administrative guidelines and formal regulations play a major role in shaping how health policy is actually carried out.

The conditions of participation, that is, a specific set of health policy activities for a particular program, provide an additional lever or authority in the implementation of health policy. In this set of actions, a governmental program might specify how an organization must be structured and what role it must adopt so as to be allowed to take part in a program. Organizations are not necessarily told they must take part whether they wish to or not, but they are told that if they want to take part, they must meet certain qualifications to participate.

For example, in the case of Medicare, hospitals are never told that they must participate per se, but they are told that if they wish to care for Medicare beneficiaries and subsequently be reimbursed for the care they give, they must be licensed by the appropriate state agency and be accredited by an appropriate accrediting agency. If a hospital decides to apply and meet the conditions of participation, it is then required to follow regulations which provide detailed instructions on specific activities. Together, the conditions of participation, the regulations, and any additional administrative guidelines are significant influences on the majority of what takes place in individual participating organizations.

HOW INDIVIDUAL HEALTH PROFESSIONALS CAN PARTICIPATE IN THE DEVELOPMENT AND IMPLEMENTATION OF HEALTH POLICY

For health care professionals who wish to play a more active part in the development and implementation of health policy, there are a variety of ways in which this can be done and a variety of points at which professional involvement is appropriate. The idea that health policy development is a specialized area of activity and should be left to policy experts, to elected politicians, or to agency administrators is a misleading and potentially dangerous one, since it may remove from the policy development process those people who have most detailed knowledge of the issues at hand. The question then is, How can health care professionals, clinical, administrative, and otherwise, participate more actively in the development of good health care policy for this country?

Going back to the first definition of health policy—the general accumulation and development of values, beliefs, goals, ethics, and social directions—every health care professional can be active in this important early stage by taking part in personal and professional activities to build a consensus. In early value-setting activities, it is continuing strong participation, communication, and education that build the initial groundswell of support for a particular course of action. If a health care professional thinks that smoking is dangerous to the health of the American public, a first level of involvement would on the local level with agencies such as the American Lung Association or the local school district. Opportunities to speak at public gatherings, to influence local and state professional groups, or to contribute written materials to publications of various kinds is not just praiseworthy, but also necessary to build the broad level of support that might eventually lead to formal legislation, court action, or other specific developments. It may be tedious, time consuming, or without immediate results—or all three—but significant formal policy development does not take place unless there is a strong, broad base of public and professional support.

With regard to the development of specific laws and legislative actions, there are two areas in which health care professionals can become directly active: The first involves provision of professional support and energy to the development of ideas that might eventually become legislation, and the second is the personal and professional support of proposed legislation itself.

With regard to the first, there is a great deal of background work that must be done before the possibility of legislation even appears. This background work might be the development of data, research, and experience that can be used in the creation of the idea behind legislative action, since the proposal of a course of action should always be well grounded in facts and genuine experience. Professional organizations and advocacy groups are generally the first place in which to look for opportunities to participate in building a case for particular action. Advocacy groups around specific disease conditions have great potential as motivators for legislative and policy action, and they almost always need professional support for their efforts.

A second way for health care professionals to help generate the demand for health policy in a particular area is by education and communication with political figures and their legislative assistants or adviser. Very few political figures have detailed expertise themselves about specific health matters (unless they have focused on a particular area in the past) and they are dependent on advisers and staff members to bring issues of importance to their attention. Contrary to the idea that political figures may not have great interest in health policy issues, they and their staffs are likely always looking for policy issues of great importance—and health policy matters certainly qualify. Health care professionals can be very helpful in this arena by being available, informative, and supportive to political figures over the long term.

When the health policy development process involves legal or judicial action, health care professionals can play a significant part here as well, even though in a somewhat different manner. Here health professionals can be involved either by assisting in the development of appropriate legal challenges that might eventually require the development of programs or policy, or by supporting challenges to, or expansion of, existing programs or policies. Here the health care professional may act as an individual, but in a more likely scenario, the professional will lend support for appropriate legal actions taken by professional associations or advocacy groups. An important consideration here is that the legal route to influencing health policy is a lengthy process and requires great persistence; it also requires significant resources of personal time and funds.

In the area of regulations and administrative guidelines, the health care professional can help shape the activities of particular organizations or agencies by taking part in the usual public commentary opportunities before regulations are finalized. Although there is often little attention paid to this phase of the development of a health policy, it does provide another opportunity for professional input and can be used to strengthen public opinion and help create a strong case for some particular action or another. The regulatory aspect of health policy is an often neglected area for personal and professional involvement, as is the more informal development of general administrative guidelines. The professional organizations that might be most directly affected by a particular policy are usually very aware of the steps in the development of appropriate regulations and guidelines, and they can usually best decide where individual member or client input is helpful.

If the health care professional wishes to participate in the policy process, there is a wide variety of sites and opportunities for participation, ranging from the development of general consensus building around an issue or a program all the way to active involvement with legislators, the legal process, or the development of regulations. In all these actions, the health care professional who wishes to be involved should understand that the process of health policy development is a long and multifaceted process to which the health care professional must be willing to commit sustained effort over a long period of time. The eventual development of health care policy takes time; the development of good policy takes even longer.

THE MAJOR POLICY ISSUES IN THE FUTURE OF HEALTH CARE

The policy issues facing United States health care in the future are multiple and complex and will require active participation and collaboration from

Table 13.1. Types and Categories of Health Policy Issues

Health System Design and Policy Issues
Financing and Cost Issues
Quality and Access Issues
Specific Disease-Related Issues for Health Policy
Personnel and Workforce Issues
People and Consumer Issues
Global and International Health Issues

all sectors of American society. To achieve maximal success in dealing with these issues, a first step is to understand what they are likely to be. Table 13.1 provides an outline of the types of policy issues that must be dealt with in the years immediately ahead.

Health System Design and Organizational Issues

There are a number of very fundamental system design issues that will eventually be faced by everyone interested in the future of health care in the United States. Certainly the most current design issue is, Should this country move toward universal health insurance coverage? The number of the uninsured is growing in number annually and, as a percentage of the country's population, generating significant concern and effort from many sectors to address this policy challenge.

For the most part, attempts to deal with universal coverage and lack of insurance have not made much progress at the national level, so attempts to address the issue have been taken up at the state government level. A policy question is thus raised: Should the organization of universal health insurance coverage be a state or a national government activity?

Connected with questions about health insurance coverage is the following basic question: Should the health care system in the United States continue to depend so heavily on employer-provided health insurance? In the past, the provision of health insurance to two-thirds of the American

population through their place of work may have been a reasonable approach, but is it still?

Another key design issue to be addressed relates to the model of illness that should shape our future health system's organization. The issue here is, Should the American health system design be shaped around an acute illness or a chronic illness model? The present system design focuses primarily on the acute care model, particularly an acute physical illness model that downplays (to a significant degree) mental illness and its treatment.

Not only is the focus of our present health care system and related public and private insurance structures on the acute physical illness model, but the system also fails to adequately address the issue of chronic illness and care. Given the shifting age demographics of the American population and the unprecedented size of the aging Baby Boomer cohort, a chronic care model may in fact be more appropriate. The present system design focus is for acute curative treatment, rather than a preventive and health protection model. For the future, the role of prevention and health protection, as well as care for the chronic conditions of an aging population destined to live longer and be more active than ever before in history, will need to be closely considered, particularly as the costs of all medical treatment continue to escalate.

One of the most important design changes taking place throughout the country is the rapid adoption of entirely new electronic information systems for health care. This will require standardization of information content and processes, heightened protection of privacy and confidentiality of information, and protection from commercial misuse of data. The new electronic age in health care will also bring new policy concerns that cannot be fully imagined at present; some have emerged already and others are certain to emerge in the future.

Financing and Cost Issues

Numerous financing issues are important to the future of health care in the United States. Principal among them is, How much of its economic resources should the United States invest in health care? At the present, health care's share of the national economy is 16 percent of GDP, or more than one-sixth of the entire economy. Arrival at this figure was not due to any organized intention or economic planning; it has simply happened. The question now becomes, Should this continue and if not, how does a society such as ours intervene?

When this significant megaeconomic issue is discussed, one should not forget that there are a number of specific, localized cost-containment efforts that can be imposed on a short-term basis. The question, of course, is, Which of these cost-containment approaches and efforts make sense, and how can they be imposed effectively?

In specific situations, overall cost-containment efforts may have significant unintended consequences for important segments of the health care system (Ginnsburg, 2004). Hospitals are already operating under relatively tight financial constraints. Thus further cost containment focused on hospitals might raise the question, Where will hospitals obtain the capital needed to meet the increased demands placed on hospitals by the public and their medical and nursing staff? With regard to physicians, the imposition of specific cost-containment methods on their practices will clearly be received badly and may lead to further physician discontent about the future of their profession. The logical policy question here is, How should this society reward and reimburse physicians so as to encourage their positive and constructive involvement in the improvement of the American health system as well as the overall health status of Americans?

One particularly explosive financial issue for the future will be how this country and its health system will handle the unprecedented rises in the cost of new drugs and pharmaceuticals. In the past, the pharmaceutical industry priced its products in a way that seemingly ignored many of the social realities and necessities of drugs and pharmaceuticals in the lives of most Americans. As a result, the public trust in the pharmaceutical industry as a whole has dropped to shockingly low levels, which is probably also unreasonable. In this area, the

question can easily be stated as trying to find an appropriate balance between the economic needs of a very competitive set of business entities and the medical needs of a society whose health may depend in part or entirely on products they cannot purchase (Cogan, Hubbard, & Kessler, 2005).

Quality and Access Policy Issues

In the past, quality and outcome issues were more internal and organizational in form and not matters of public policy, but these issues have increasingly become the subject of health care reform efforts—and they will become even more so in the future.

The key set of health policy issues here is transparency of the health care system, particularly with regard to clinical results and outcomes. Increasingly, health insurance organizations, accreditation and licensing groups, and the general public want to know how well a particular doctor, medical group, hospital, or system of hospitals does with regard to specific procedures and processes of care (Ginnsburg, 2004). Employers want to have more detailed information about outcomes and the quality of care they are paying for and will use that information in health care purchasing decisions. New reimbursement systems that pay on the basis of performance are also appearing with increasing frequency, generating ever-increasing attention as a means for driving quality and process improvement in all manner of health care organizations along a continuum ranging from physician offices to clinics, community hospitals, and on to academic medical centers.

Very specific subsections of these quality concerns are patient safety and accident avoidance in health care, particularly in hospitals (Institute of Medicine, 2001). The exact numbers of injuries and deaths during hospitalization can vigorously be debated, but it is clear that this is a subject about which the general public and leading health care critics express great anxiety and legitimate concerns.

Specific Disease-Related Issues for Health Policy

In a number of specific disease categories, health policy questions will be raised in the future, either because of the seriousness or the high visibility of the particular issues concerned. For example, it is increasingly apparent that there is a significant increase in obesity in the American population (both children and adults), and this will have a serious impact on the long-term health status of Americans. Partially connected with this, but also partially separate, there is great concern about the increasing incidence of diabetes, particularly among some minority group populations (Steinbrook, 2004). Also on the future health policy agenda will be the need to expand mental health services, both as part of the overall health care system and as an item requiring increased insurance coverage.

Additionally, while the already recognized women's health issues of breast, ovarian, and uterine cancer are still important, there has recently been much greater appreciation that heart disease is the leading cause of mortality in women. Nearly twice as many women die from heart disease and stroke as from all forms of cancer, including breast cancer. Previously, heart disease was considered a man's disease and certainly it is, but attention to the fact that it is the number-one killer of women needs much greater consideration from policy makers.

Personnel and Workforce Issues

The key personnel and workforce issue for the future is the short supply of well-trained and well-respected nurses in the American health care system. There is no other single workforce issue comes close in importance, and the shortage crisis requires innovative and immediate solutions.

At the same time other professional groups have workforce concerns, such as the availability of reasonably priced malpractice insurance for physicians (Kessler, Sage, & Becker, 2005). Although it is unclear exactly what impact the fear of malpractice legal actions has on physician behavior and rising health care costs, it is absolutely clear that the cost of malpractice insurance and the fear of legal actions have a significant impact on morale and the professional's sense of value to our society.

Another potentially important set of health policy issues for the future center around the role of labor unions in the organization and management of health care, not so much as a good or bad influence, but rather as a new organizational player. Health care has not had extensive experience with labor organization among its professional workers, nor have labor unions had much experience with the unique circumstances of health care itself; this means that both parties may have a great deal to learn and that the entire interaction may become the focus of specific policy actions.

Public and Consumer Issues

The role of the public and consumers in health care has already changed and will continue to do so in major ways in the future. These role changes will bring significant health policy questions. How should direct-to-consumer advertising for drugs and medical procedures be handled in the future? With regard to the costs of care, how can consumers obtain comparative costs for medical procedures, drugs and pharmaceuticals, and other items about which the consumer must make decisions (Herzlinger & Parsa-Parsi, 2004)? In the arena of quality, what sort of information should the public have available on a regular basis about the outcomes of care provided by specific physicians and hospitals? With regard to online sources of information about diseases and treatment, how should the accuracy and completeness of information be monitored and regulated so that the public can be assured it is getting correct and reliable information in an unbiased presentation?

The overwhelming issue for the public in the future will likely be related to the uncertainty of health insurance coverage and concerns about whether insurance carriers will serve the best interests of the beneficiaries and not the more limited interests of the insurance carrier itself (Rosenthal & Milstein, 2004). Consumers increasingly see themselves in an adversarial relationship with insurance carriers—even those they have dealt with for years. Consumer protection in this area will certainly be a health policy concern in the future (Enthovan & Fuchs, 2006; Robinson, 2004).

Global and International Health Issues

The most obvious and pressing international health issue is the threat of terrorist activities carried out via health-related actions. Fortunately, at present, terrorist activities have not involved viable health threats, but the potential is real and will require continuous attention.

A more probable global health concern is the rapid transmission of infectious disease from one corner of the world to another in very short time spans (Tilson & Berkowitz, 2006). In a world in which the time and mileage difference between various parts of the world are shrinking rapidly, the ability of illness in one part of the world to affect people in a distant part of the world is very real and will require surveillance and protection processes that are not well formalized now.

SUMMARY

Health policy development is an important aspect of all health care professions and institutions. The policy decisions have the potential to shape what everyone in health care does and how they do it. To participate, health care professionals need to understand the health system we have and how health policy affects that system. Professionals have to understand how health policy is made at different levels of public and private action and must develop a desire to take part (Fuchs & Emanuel, 2005). Finally, they should understand that there is a wide variety of potentially important policy challenges ahead in the future and should actively

decide which are important to them and to their organizations. Involvement in health policy development should not be a spectator sport, engaged in at a distance, but should instead involve the best talents and energies of all professionals, so that the best possible policies finally emerge.

REVIEW QUESTIONS

1. What is health policy?
2. Briefly describe the health policy development process.
3. How can health care professionals, clinical, administrative, and otherwise, participate more actively in the development of good health care policy?
4. List some of the key policy issues that will affect the organization and design of the U.S. health care system.
5. List some of the key health policy issues that will directly affect consumers.

REFERENCES & ADDITIONAL READINGS

Ball, R. M. (1995). What medicare's architects had in mind. *Health Affairs, 14*(4), 62–72.
Brown, L. D., & Sparer, M. S. (2003). Poor program's progress: The unanticipated politics of medicaid policy. *Health Affairs, 22*(1), 31–44.
Cogan, J. F., Hubbard, G., & Kessler, D. P. (2005). Making markets work: Five steps to a better health care system. *Health Affairs, 293*(21), 1447–1457.
Enthovan, A., & Fuchs, V. (2006). Employment-based health insurance: Past, present and future. *Health Affairs, 25*(6), 1538–1547.
Fuchs, V., & Emanuel, E. (2005). Health care reform: Why? What? When? *Health Affairs, 24*(6), 1399–1414.
Ginnsburg, P. B. (2004). Controlling health care costs. *New England Journal of Medicine, 351*(16), 1591–1593.
Herzlinger, R. E., & Parsa-Parsi, R. (2004). Consumer-driven health care: Lessons from Switzerland. *Journal of the American Medical Association, 292*(10), 1213–1220.

Inglehart, J. K. (2004). The new medicare prescription-drug benefit—a pure power play. *New England Journal of Medicine, 350*(8), 826.

Institute of Medicine. (2001). Crossing the quality chasm: A new health system for the 21st century. Washington DC: National Academies Press.

Institute of Medicine of the National Academies. (2003). *Informing the future: Critical issues in health,* 2nd ed., Washington, DC: National Academies Press.

Kessler, D., Sage, W., & Becker, D. (2005). Impact of malpractice reforms on the supply of physician services. *Journal of the American Medical Association, 293*(21), 2618–2625.

Mechanic, D. (2004). The rise and fall of managed care. *Journal of Health and Social Behavior, 45,* 76–86.

Moon, M. (2000). Medicare matters: Building on a record of accomplishments. *Health Care Financing Review, 22*(1), 9–22.

Robinson, J. C. (2004). Reinvention of health insurance in the consumer era. *Journal of the American Medical Association, 291*(15), 1880–1886.

Rosenthal, M., & Milstein, A. (2004). Awakening consumer stewardship of health benefits: Prevalence and differentiation of new health plan models. *Health Services Research, 39*(4), 1055–1070.

Steinbrook, R. (2004). Disparities in health care—from politics to policy. *New England Journal of Medicine, 350*(15), 1486–1488.

Tilson, H., & Berkowitz, B. (2006). The public health enterprise: Examining our twenty-first-century policy challenges. *Health Affairs, 25*(4), 900–910.

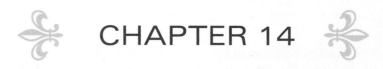

CHAPTER 14

The Quality of Health Care*

Stephen J. Williams and Paul R. Torrens

CHAPTER TOPICS

🙢 Origins of the Quality Movement

🙢 The Theoretic Underpinnings of Quality Improvement Efforts

🙢 Types of Quality Improvement Strategies

🙢 Traditional Measures of Quality

🙢 Quality and Health Care Disparities

LEARNING OBJECTIVES

Upon completing this chapter, the reader should be able to

1. Appreciate the complexity of defining and measuring the quality of care.

2. Understand how measuring and monitoring quality can result in improved outcomes.

3. Define how quality is assessed and ensured.

4. Appreciate strategies that now exist for influencing physician behavior.

*Adapted in part from *Closing The Quality Gap: A Critical Analysis of Quality Improvement Strategies*, Volume 1: *Series Overview and Methodology* [Technical Review 9 (Contract No. 290-02-0017 to the Stanford University—UCSF Evidence-based Practices Center), AHRQ Publication No. 04-0051-1], by K. G. Shojania, K. M. McDonald, R. M. Wachter, and D. K. Owens, August 2004, Rockville, MD: Agency for Healthcare Research and Quality.

Assuring the quality of health care services in the United States represents one of the greatest challenges for the nation's health services system over the coming decades. Quality enhancement has undergone a revolution over the past 10 years with an increasing recognition that quality enhancing saves lives and dollars. Payers, particularly employers and insurance companies, are also increasingly demanding higher quality and more efficient services. Consumers, of course, have the greatest expectation for enhancement of quality and have traditionally held their providers to perhaps unrealistically high standards.

The continuing evolution of computerized information systems is the principal vehicle through which quality improvement standards will be met. Both hardware and software have advanced to the point where it is now realistic to expect that institutional providers will implement programs with quality measurements, assessment, improvement, and recording. The increasing use of computerized medical records, clinical algorithms, and increasingly sophisticated data analysis techniques greatly facilitates these trends. Adverse consequences of poor medical practice have many costs and the human toll alone justifies full remediation where possible.

Expectations for quality enhancement range from protecting against inappropriate procedures to medication errors. Monitoring and improving systems, personnel behaviors, patient reactions, and provider judgments have all been incorporated within these systems. Practical aspects of data entry, physician and other professional personnel use, and acceptance of new technologies and appropriate feedback mechanisms for continued improvement in quality are also essential. Only through a comprehensive approach to the application of technology for quality improvement, including the human side of the implementation of these systems, can our goals be achieved. Improving the quality of care has the potential to substantially improve the nation's health care system and to more rationally utilize our scarce resources. These issues have long been a major challenge for the system. But the emergence

of new technologies, cost incentives, and demands for quality improvement from all participating parties suggests that now is the time to move to full implementation and acceptance.

ORIGINS OF THE QUALITY MOVEMENT

Although humans have long been intrigued and moved by the complex science of healing others, the science of measuring and improving the quality of delivered care is a relatively recent undertaking. Boston surgeon Ernest A. Codman (1869–1940) began his "end results system" a century ago to track surgical outcomes and to improve surgical practice. Codman's work in this area ultimately led to the creation of the Joint Commission.

Despite Codman's pioneering work and several other individuals and organizations whose efforts extended through the middle of the twentieth century, the science of health care quality improvement truly took root only a generation ago. Several forces catalyzed this transformation. First, medicine transcended its status as an anecdotal, non-evidence-based enterprise to one in which good data led to the discovery of improved treatment practices. For example, in the mid-1960s, 100 clinical trials were published each year. Thirty years later, that number had grown to more than 10,000.

Second, as the public's interest and investment in the "miracles" of modern medicine grew—particularly in high-technology specialties such as cardiac surgery and transplantation—so, too, did the public's demand for greater provider accountability and positive patient outcomes. Although public awareness of patient safety and quality increased with the Institute of Medicine's (IOM's) seminal publication in 2000 of *To Err Is Human: Building a Safer Health Care System*, and the broader indictment of health care quality in *Crossing the Quality Chasm* (Kohn et al., 2001), the trend had already been established. In an increasingly consumerist society, people had become less inclined to simply trust that their caregivers would deliver the highest quality care. And the public's skepticism only grew with the cost-driven growth of managed care.

Third, the expense of medical technology and the highly trained personnel needed to deliver that technology required the expansion of third-party payment systems, many of which were employer based. These costs became a disproportionately large part of annual operating budgets and so employers, accustomed to making purchasing decisions based on *value* (quality and cost), found themselves without any information from the quality dimension of this equation. Their unwillingness to take it on faith that medicine's "product" was of the highest quality only grew with the published evidence of huge regional variations in the numbers of common procedures (coronary bypass grafting, hysterectomies, transurethral prostate resections) that could not be explained by differences in patient populations or justified by differences in outcomes. Other studies showed unacceptably high rates of "inappropriate" surgical procedures such as carotid endarterectomy, further fueling the skepticism regarding the quality of health care in America and increasing demands for accountability.

These pressures were mounting during the same time that tools for measuring the quality of evidence supporting clinical practice, such as clinical epidemiology, decision- and cost-effectiveness-analysis, meta-analysis, and the like, were becoming more robust. Driven in part by sizable congressional allocations to the National Institutes of Health and by private investments on the part of pharmaceutical companies and others, the clinical research knowledge base grew as well. The use of computer-assisted health care management systems led to the creation of large databases that could be mined to provide information on the quality of care, as large and complex clinical trials became commonplace. Before long, specialties such as cardiology, for example, were transformed. Cardiologists witnessed a shift in the cultural context, their focus drawn away from the art of medicine and redirected toward the dozens of regularly published clinical trials and emerging evidence on best practice treatments and heart disease prevention.

Today's Challenge

By the mid-1990s, the powerful influences of clinical treatment information, skepticism of the medical community's ability to ensure high-quality health care, increased consumer and purchaser knowledge, and the science of quality measurement had come together. More and more studies revealed large gaps between the findings of scientific studies and their practical implementation, even in areas of medicine where the optimal clinical approach was ensured. Several large and recent studies have confirmed sizable quality of care gaps in areas spanning preventive medicine, acute and chronic care, and care of elders. These and other studies emphasized the notion that research into quality health care does not, in itself, ensure the clinical patient will receive the highest quality care. A new area of inquiry—how best to translate research into practice—was born.

There are many reasons for the gaps that exist between the best evidence-based understanding of high-quality treatment practices, and the actual practices themselves. First, there may be a gap in the dissemination of knowledge. The large and growing number of clinical trials underway at any given time makes it impossible for any individual physician or system of care to stay fully abreast. There is an inevitable time lag between the publication of studies that demonstrate an effective practice and its implementation. There is sometimes a need for a consensus to emerge among specialists, or a diffusion from specialists to generalists.

Second, providers may be aware of a best practice but fail to implement it because of skepticism surrounding the cost-effectiveness of the practice (in terms of dollars or time needed to educate patients or adapt work processes). Or, they may have reservations regarding their treatment environment and the systems support (people or equipment) or changes in organizational culture needed to implement the practice.

Finally, while the treatment practice may have been proven effective in a special research setting, it may not be applicable to an individual provider's setting. Clinical trials differ in many ways from real-life practice: Staff members are attentive to the research protocols, personnel with specialized training may have been hired to provide additional support or patient education, patient selection may be related to the research protocol, and additional safety measures may be built into the trial. In addition, research studies are often carried out in specialized settings that may bear little resemblance to the smaller treatment setting of a physician considering the practice. This gap between efficacy (how well the practice works in the research environment) and effectiveness (how well it works in clinical practice—generalized to include a wide range of treatment settings, with providers who may not be committed to or expert in its application, and a broader array of patients) has been well appreciated in recent years.

As the quality gap has become more widely acknowledged, investigators have focused on its genesis and possible strategies for closing it. Six possible interventions to improve adoption of improved treatment practices are education, feedback, participation by physicians in efforts to bring about change, administrative rules, financial incentives, and financial penalties. In addition to those interventions that focus largely on the clinical behavior of individual providers (mostly physicians), more attention is being given to systematic changes in the practice environment, some of which (e.g., computerized rules and checklists, automatic stop orders) may bypass physicians entirely. A parallel movement is focusing on patients as the guardians of their own health care quality.

Whatever the method used to achieve the desired change, there is little doubt that the movement to base accountability and competition on metrics of quality has just begun. Business coalitions including the Pacific Business Group on Health and the Leapfrog Group are partnering with accreditation groups such as the Joint Commission to develop new quality-of-care standards. These standards will be made available to the public and can be used as the foundation for purchasing or payment decisions. The National Committee for Quality Assurance (NCQA) publishes its own "Report Card" for use by government agencies, employers, and consumers. As the case for improved quality in health care grows, so too does the realization that the best way to improve patient outcomes is a strict adherence to well-researched and respected quality improvement practices.

THE THEORETIC UNDERPINNINGS OF QUALITY IMPROVEMENT EFFORTS

Medicine has a long history of investigating what works in the clinical realm and why. At the same time, we have a fairly limited understanding of the causal mechanisms of interventions to improve health care quality. Theories abound with regard to changing the behavior of patients, clinicians, and organizations for the better. These theories are often drawn from studies that try to isolate the effect of a single varied element or combinations of setting, interventions, and targets for change. The challenge for researchers rests in the accurate interpretation of this diverse literature regarding implementation.

Various theories, including those from disciplines outside of health care, may be marshaled to design interventions for health care protocols in need of modification. Such theories have been applied in many ways—often borrowing techniques from industry such as those promoted by Joseph Juran and W. Edwards Deming—with varying degrees of success. The methods generally emphasize the importance of identifying a process with less-than-ideal outcomes, measuring the key performance attributes, using careful analysis to devise a new approach, integrating the redesigned approach with the process, and reassessing performance to determine if the change in process is successful.

The mixed results produced by industry-oriented quality improvement programs [such as total quality management (TQM) and continuous quality improvement (CQI) have taught managers and others the need to exercise caution before assuming that strategies drawn from other industries automatically will work in health care settings. These forces are an outgrowth of human needs and desires: the altruism of most health care professionals, their desire for success and peer respect, their preference for avoiding embarrassment, and the goal of financial independence, to name but a few. These inspirations have prompted a more recent movement, in which the traditional quality improvement sensibilities of programs such as TQM or CQI are coupled with more modern approaches to behavior modification, such as performance auditing and feedback. An audit will often measure provider adherence to a specific process or treatment practice, and the providers being studied will receive comparative data after the fact about their performance and how they stack up against their peers. In other types of audits, providers might receive financial rewards for their strict adherence to desired behaviors, or information regarding their performance and standing might be forwarded on to their patients (who can influence nonconforming providers to make the appropriate behavioral change, or choose to seek care elsewhere).

Even for common disorders like diabetes, hypertension, and cancer care—areas in which research has successfully demonstrated that some best practices can save tens of thousands of lives—there has been only modest systematic study of the techniques and strategies shown to close the quality gap. Moreover, in those few areas that have benefited from such studies, little consideration has been given to crosscutting practices (i.e., how a practice that closes the quality gap in asthma, might be applicable to congestive heart failure).

Definitions

Quality of health care is defined as the degree to which health services for individuals and patient populations increase the likelihood of desirable health outcomes and are consistent with current professional knowledge. The quality gap is the difference between health care processes or outcomes observed in practice and those thought to be achievable with the most current and effective professional knowledge. The difference must be attributable in whole or in part to a deficiency that could be addressed by the health care system. An example of a process-level quality gap for hypertension involves the 62 percent of clinical visits during which physicians failed to introduce evidence-based, guideline-concordant drug therapy to patients with a systolic blood pressure of 140 mm/HG or higher. An example of an outcome-level quality gap for myocardial infarctions involves a disparity in survival rates. Despite numerous new therapies that have substantially decreased mortality over the past 25 years, survival gains have occurred mainly in males and in younger patients, with less gain in women and the elderly.

TYPES OF QUALITY IMPROVEMENT STRATEGIES

Nine examples of quality improvement (QI) strategies are outlined in Table 14.1. These categories are broad, and in some cases, combine multiple interventions.

Provider reminder systems are any patient or clinical encounter-specific information, provided verbally, in writing, or by computer, to prompt a clinician to recall information or intended to prompt consideration of a specific process of care (i.e., "This patient last underwent screening mammography 3 years ago"). The reminder may also include information prompting the clinician to follow evidence-based care recommendations (e.g., to make medication adjustments, or to order appropriate screening tests). The phrase "clinical encounter-specific" in the definition serves to distinguish reminder systems from audit and feedback,

Table 14.1. Taxonomy of Quality Improvement Strategies with Examples

Strategy	Examples
Provider reminder systems	■ Reminders in charts for providers ■ Computer-based reminders for providers ■ Computer-based decision support
Facilitated relay of clinical data to providers	■ Transmission of clinical data from outpatient specialty clinic to primary care provider by means other than medical record (e.g., phone call or fax)
Audit and feedback	■ Feedback of performance to individual providers ■ Quality indicators and reports ■ National/state quality report cards ■ Publicly released performance data ■ Benchmarking—provision of outcomes data from top performers for comparison with provider's own data
Provider education	■ Workshops and conferences ■ Educational outreach visits (e.g., academic detailing) ■ Distributed educational materials
Patient education	■ Classes ■ Parent and family education ■ Patient pamphlets ■ Intensive education strategies promoting self-management of chronic conditions
Promotion of self-management	■ Materials and devices promoting self-management
Patient reminder systems	■ Postcards or calls to patients
Organizational change	■ Case management, disease management ■ TQM, CQI techniques ■ Multidisciplinary teams ■ Change from paper to computer-based records ■ Increased staffing ■ Skill mix changes
Financial incentives, regulation, and policy	*Provider directed* ■ Financial incentives based on achievement of performance goals ■ Alternative reimbursement systems (e.g., fee-for-service, capitated payments) ■ Licensure requirements *Patient directed* ■ Co-payments for certain visit types ■ Health insurance premiums, user fees *Health system directed* ■ Initiatives by accreditation bodies (e.g., residency work hour limits) ■ Changes in reimbursement schemes (e.g., capitation, prospective payment, salaried providers)

where clinicians typically receive performance summaries relative to a process or outcome of care spanning multiple encounters (e.g., all Type 2 diabetic patients seen by the clinician during the past 6 months).

Facilitated relay of clinical data to providers is used to describe the transfer of clinical information collected directly from patients and relayed to the provider, in instances where the data are not generally collected during a patient visit, or using some format other than the existing local medical record system (i.e., the telephone transmission of a patient's blood pressure measurements, from a specialist's office).

Audit and feedback is any summary of clinical performance for health care providers or institutions performed for a specific period of time and reported either publicly or confidentially to the clinician or institution (e.g., the percentage of a provider's patients who achieved or did not achieve some clinical target, such as blood pressure control, over a certain period). Benchmarking is a term referring to the provision of performance data from institutions or providers regarded as leaders in the field. These data serve as performance targets for other providers and institutions.

Provider education includes a variety of interventions such as educational workshops, meetings [e.g., traditional continuing medical education (CME)], lectures (in person or computer based), educational outreach visits (by a trained representative who meets with providers in their practice settings to disseminate information with the intent of changing the providers' practice). The same term is also used to describe the distribution of educational materials (electronically published or printed clinical practice guidelines and audiovisual materials).

Patient education is centered on in-person patient education, either individually or as part of a group or community, and through the introduction of print or audio-visual educational materials. Patient education may be the sole component of a particular quality improvement strategy, or it can be one part of a multifaceted strategy.

Promotion of self-management includes the distribution of materials (i.e., devices for blood pressure or glucose self-monitoring) or access to a resource that enhances the patient's ability to manage his or her condition, the communication of useful clinical data to the patient (e.g., most recent lipid panel levels), or follow-up phone calls from the provider to the patient, with recommended adjustments to care.

Patient reminders are any effort directed by providers toward patients that encourages them to keep appointments or adhere to other aspects of the self-management of their condition.

Organizational change is any intervention having features consistent with at least one of the following: disease management or case management (the coordination of assessment, treatment, and referrals by a person or multidisciplinary team in collaboration with, or supplementary to, the primary care provider; team or personnel changes); adding new members to a treatment team (e.g., the addition of a diabetes nurse, a clinical pharmacist, or a nutritionist to a clinical practice); creating multidisciplinary teams within a practice, or revising the roles of existing team members (e.g., a clinic nurse is given a more active role in patient management), or the simple addition of more nurses, pharmacists, or physicians to a clinical setting; communications, case discussions and the exchange of treatment information between distant health professionals (i.e., telemedicine); total quality management (TQM) or continuous quality improvement (CQI) techniques for measuring quality problems, designing interventions and their implementation, along with process remeasurements; changes in medical records systems—adopting improved office technology (e.g., computer-based records, patient tracking systems).

Financial, regulatory or legislative incentives include positive or negative financial incentives directed at providers (e.g., regarding adherence to some process of care or achievement of target patient outcome); positive or negative financial incentives directed at patients; systemwide changes in reimbursement (e.g., capitation, prospective payment, shift from fee-for-service to salary); changes to provider licensure requirements; and changes to institutional accreditation requirements.

Report Cards

Among the quality-related feedback mechanisms that have gained some traction recently are provider report cards. Report cards have been utilized for health plans, provider organizations, and individual professionals. Health plan report cards have been issued for example, by the National Committee for Quality Assurance (http://www.ncqa.org). Data for health plan analysis is obtained from HEDIS® (Health Plan Employer Data and Information Sets). HEDIS data are collected from health plans using a formal protocol and established data collection instruments. NCQA report card evaluations are based on such factors as access to needed services, qualification providers, planned promotions of appropriate preventive services, tests, screenings, health plan evaluation of new medical procedures and drugs for currency, and patient assistance living with chronic conditions including provision of appropriate services and educational information.

Report cards, especially on individual providers, are complicated to devise and evaluate. Differentiating between the role of the provider, the organization, and the patient in achieving compliance with medical regimens and outcomes of care is a particularly difficult and complicated issue. However, the general concept of enhanced accountability, if formed in a consistent and reliable manner, holds some attributes.

Any evaluation information on professional service providers must be consistent and reliable, accurate and appropriate, and easily interpreted by consumers to be broadly useful. Even mass media has gotten into the act with many magazines reporting on the best hospitals and doctors in the nation. Among those publications doing so, *US News and World Report* has published hospital listings for more than a decade. The Medicare program has also chimed in in recent years to provide consumers

with information about hospital quality. Again, this program is not without some degree of controversy.

Ultimately, report cards and other mechanisms for informing consumers and purchasers about the quality of health care provided involve complex issues ranging from accuracy of measures to attribution of outcomes. The movement toward increased consumer enlightenment through the provision of more complex information related to quality boils down to providing relatively succinct indicators that consumers can use to make discretionary health care decisions.

Small Area Variations

For many, the modern quality of care movement had its origins with the innovative work of John Wennberg and Allan Gittelsohn in the 1960s and 1970s. These two scientists were among the first to epidemiologically examine differences in patterns of care provided in different geographic regions and originally focused on the states of Vermont and New Hampshire.

Their work created a ground swell of concern since they revealed tremendous differences in how medical care was provided between relatively similar populations. In some instances, such as for certain elective surgical procedures, the differences were quite pronounced and alarming. Their work represented a defining moment in the quality improvement arena. Many other researchers over the years have elaborated in various ways on their groundbreaking efforts. Significant research has uncovered vast examples of inappropriate care provided to patients, duplication of services, lack of patient compliance, drug interactions resulting in adverse consequences, and many other quality and utilization-related deficiencies in the health care system.

What has followed as a result of these investigations has been an increasing emphasis on standardization of care and compliance with professionally accepted practice patterns. These efforts have taken many forms and have continued to evolve over the years, particularly with the availability of more sophisticated computerized information systems and through the initiatives of professional medical organizations and quality-oriented voluntary groups. The federal Agency for Health care Research and Quality (AHRQ) has also promoted these efforts through funding and other forms of sponsorship. Medicare, Medicaid, private insurers, and employers have lent their support to these efforts as well.

Many approaches to standardization of quality have been developed. These include, for example, benchmarking, which compares performance criteria in hospitals and other settings against established, better performing, institutions. The use of clinical assessments such as those included in the HEDIS measures of quality, the use of clinical protocols for assessing physician practice behaviors, the increased emphasis on outcome measures, including patient satisfaction, and improvement in health status as reflected in functional ability and morbidity are all examples of these efforts.

Quality of care mechanisms are gravitating toward evidence-based methodologies that are formulated as a result of scientific studies that provide empirical support for various practice approaches and guidelines. Clinical protocols, quality assessments, practice guidelines, and clinical pathways rely on measurable improvements in morbidity, mortality, functional status, quality of life, and other documented parameters of improvement resulting from the medical care that is provided. The overall objective is to base clinical practice on scientifically supported approaches and then to evaluate for quality assessment and compliance with such scientifically based criteria. Medical education is also enhanced with the use of scientifically documented guidelines. Continued refinement of the guidelines through further scientific investigation strengthens this approach. Medical student, and postgraduate and continuing medical education instruction can also be facilitated through this route.

The implementation of quality assurance mechanisms is dependent on provider education. In particular, providing practitioners with clinical information and comparing their practices and procedures to establish scientifically valid guidelines is a powerful form of education and feedback for enhancement of quality in clinical practice. Feedback, provided after the fact, and concurrent feedback, provided while care is rendered, both have valid educational and evaluative importance. The increasing availability of real-time computer information systems facilitates more rapid and critical feedback to practitioners, especially when combined with larger databases of appropriate care patterns and other relevant information such as drug interactions.

From a broader perspective, care management, evaluation of preventive services, and other approaches and mechanisms that provide a more comprehensive and prospective approach can be particularly beneficial for patient outcomes and quality of care. Ultimately, scientifically based real-time active surveillance combined with comprehensive databases and patient clinical information should provide guidance to practitioners as well as nearly instant evaluation of the care process. These longer-term goals will provide the ultimate in quality assurance for our nation's population.

TRADITIONAL MEASURES OF QUALITY

Much of the groundbreaking progress in measuring quality can be traced to the pioneering work of Avedis Donabedian who defined the dimensions of quality. Quality of care must be viewed in the context of clinical knowledge and professional and consumer expectations.

Quality can be measured with the unit of analysis being an institutional setting such as a hospital or nursing home, or an individual provider such as a physician. Quality can be measured in a variety of organizations such as institutional providers (hospitals and physician groups) or in insurance plans such as a commercial insurance HMO or PPO, or in a government managed health care system such as the British National Health Service. Quality can be measured prospectively or retrospectively. Quality can measure the direct provision of clinical services, what is termed technical quality of care focusing on the actual care provided, or more broadly on patient assessment of the ambience and interactive experiences within the system, reflected in various measures of patient satisfaction. Quality can be measured explicitly against specific established standards or implicitly, a more descriptive representation of the care provided. Quality assessments can relate many multirelational variables or can be focused on a limited number of specific attributes of care.

In assessing quality of care, measurement and data availability are key concerns. Reliability of data as well as their consistency and replicability are all key elements in accuracy and provider acceptance. In quality assessment, nondirect observational data collection, particularly from medical records and insurance claims data, always raises the issue of the extent to which the assessment is measuring the accuracy of data collection versus the actual care provided. Without accurate data, valid quality conclusions cannot be drawn.

Assuming the availability of accurate and appropriate data, Donabedian devised three dimensions of measurement for quality assessment. The first is the structure of care. Structure reflects the environment within which care is provided, such as the appropriateness of the facilities or certification of the providers. Donabedian's second dimension is process of care. Process relates to what is done to the patient, such as specific tests or procedures performed. While measuring structure represents a more static dimension, process becomes more dynamic by assessing the appropriateness of the care that is provided particularly, when available, compared to accepted clinical guidelines. Professionally developed clinical protocols from national professional organizations provide a powerful tool against which process measures can be assessed.

The final dimension of quality as defined by Donabedian is outcome of care. Outcome reflects what happened to the patient. Outcome can include morbidity, mortality, functional status, and other measures reflecting clinical outcomes, quality of life, patient satisfaction, and related issues. Outcome measures may philosophically be the most valid indicator of quality. However, outcomes can be difficult to measure. Patient follow-up may preclude the collection of accurate outcome data, and outcomes result from not only the care provided, but also such factors as patient compliance and environment issues. The determination of causal relationships between medical care and patient outcomes is a challenge. Outcome measures are highly dynamic, continually changing as the patient's condition evolves, and are vastly more complex to assess than structure and process measures.

Among the most important outcome measures is mortality. Physiological evidence to attribute mortality to the medical care provided may not be easy to collect, especially in the absence of a definitive postpartum evaluation. One of the most significant concerns in assessing mortality rates is that some organizations and some providers attract more ill patients, such as in the case of academic medical centers and teaching hospitals. Thus, mortality rates have to be adjusted for case severity, multiple illnesses, and the nature of highly complex tertiary care provided to very ill patients.

Quality assessment and assurance have also increasingly focused on the relationship of health services to life and the quality of life. Again, many of these variables have highly complex measurement issues. Ideally, pursuing assessments through these channels could yield valuable measures of system and clinical successes. Measuring health status and quality of life has tremendous appeal since medical care functions not only to cure disease but also to improve patients' survival and functioning, an excellent example being certain types of arthritis.

Quality assessment based in part on patient satisfaction is desirable, but complicated. Patient perceptions typically focus on ambience and interaction with providers and organizations rather than technical aspects of care. While these indicators are important, and they enhance patient compliance with medical regimens, they are still less significant than the technical quality of care provided.

Pressure from payers, including employers, health plans, and voluntary accreditation agencies, has promoted assessment of patient satisfaction with care. Provider financial incentives are increasingly tied to patient satisfaction, quality achievement goals, and other measurable indicators such as pay-for-performance schemes.

QUALITY AND HEALTH CARE DISPARITIES

Disparity reflects being unequal, as regards such factors as age, rank, or degree. There are several potential reasons for the differences observed at the individual level. For example, a patient may receive fewer medications because of differences in underlying disease processes, individual choice, systemic barriers to obtaining needed medications, or some combination of these reasons.

Disparities are most easily identified when there is a clear reference point for what is appropriate and reasonable to expect. While there may be uncertainty regarding many aspects of clinical care, quality measures have been developed around health care interventions for which there is sound scientific evidence of effectiveness and for which there is a professional consensus and expectation that these services will be provided to all patients. Even after consideration of variation in patients' medical conditions and severity of illness, there should be little deviation from specific quality measures associated with population.

Access to health care is a prerequisite to obtaining quality care. However, dimensions of access vary in predicting an individual's likelihood of receiving care that has been shown to improve health outcomes. For use of services, patient-reported experience of care, and structural issues such as transportation, there is limited scientific consensus regarding which measures are most responsive to system improvements. In addition, the most important factors may not be consistent across communities and populations.

Many factors may lead to differences in health care, especially with respect to aggregate measures of use. These include different underlying rates of illness due to genetic predisposition, local environmental conditions, or lifestyle choices. There are differences in the care-seeking behavior of patients, which vary due to differing cultural beliefs, linguistic barriers, degree of trust of health care providers, or variations in the predisposition to seek timely care. In addition, the availability of care is dependent upon such factors as the ability to pay for care (directly or through insurance coverage), the location, management and delivery of health care services, clinical uncertainty, and health care practitioner beliefs, among others.

A vital step in the effort to eliminate health care disparities is the systematic collection and analysis of health care data. This will help policy makers and researchers discern the areas of greatest need, monitor trends over time, and identify successful programs for addressing those needs.

Racial, ethnic, and socioeconomic disparities are national problems that affect health care at all points in the process, at all sites of care, and for all medical conditions—in fact, disparities are pervasive in our health care system.

While disparities in health care potentially affect all Americans and individuals from of any group, they are not uniformly distributed across populations. Geography can play an important mitigating role in health care disparities. Remote rural populations, for example, are clearly at risk for having worse access and receiving poorer quality care. Some examples of disparities related to patient's quality of care follow.

- Minorities are more likely to be diagnosed with late-stage breast cancer and colorectal cancer compared with whites.

- Patients of lower socioeconomic position are less likely to receive recommended diabetic services and more likely to be hospitalized for diabetes and its complications.

- When hospitalized for acute myocardial infarction, Hispanics are less likely to receive optimal care.

- Many racial and ethnic minorities and persons of lower socioeconomic position are more likely to die from HIV.

- The use of physical restraints in nursing homes is higher among Hispanics and Asian/Pacific Islanders compared with non-Hispanic whites.

- Blacks and poorer patients have higher rates of avoidable hospital admissions (i.e., hospitalizations for health conditions that, in the presence of comprehensive primary care, rarely require hospitalization).

Health care disparities are costly. Poorly managed care or missed diagnoses result in expensive and avoidable complications. The personal cost of disparities can lead to significant morbidity, disability, and lost productivity at the individual level. For example, end-stage renal disease may result from longstanding poorly controlled diabetes.

Without screening, cancers may not be detected until they grow large or metastasize to distant sites and cause symptoms. Such late-stage cancers are usually associated with more limited treatment options and poorer survival. Minorities and persons of lower socioeconomic status are less likely to receive cancer screening services and more likely to have late-stage cancer when the disease is diagnosed.

Many racial and ethnic minorities and persons of lower socioeconomic position are less likely to receive recommended immunizations for influenza and pneumococcal pneumonia, the most common type of pneumonia. Once hospitalized, some ethnic and racial minorities, as well as lower income patients, suffer worse quality of care for pneumonia. These differential rates of vaccination and hospitalization present opportunities for provider-based and community-based interventions to reduce disparities.

Access to health care is an important prerequisite to obtaining quality care. Some access barriers, whether perceived or actual, can result in adverse health outcomes. Patients may perceive barriers to delay seeking needed care, resulting in presentation of illness at a later, less treatable stage of illness. For example, a usual source of care can serve as a navigator to the health care system and an advocate to obtain needed evidence-based preventive and health care services. Of the major measures of access, the lack of health insurance has significant consequences. Avoidable hospitalizations are a good example of the link between access and disparities in quality of care. When health care needs are not met by the primary health care system, rates of avoidable admissions may rise. Hispanics and people of lower socioeconomic status are more likely to report unmet health care needs. While most of the population has health insurance, racial and ethnic minorities are less likely to report health insurance compared with whites. Lower income persons are also less likely to report insurance compared with higher income persons.

Blacks and persons of lower socioeconomic status tend to have higher rates of death from cancer. While rates of cancer death may reflect a variety of factors not associated with health care such as genetic disposition, diet, and lifestyle, screening and early treatment of cancers can lead to reductions in mortality. Many racial and ethnic minorities and persons of lower socioeconomic position are less likely to receive screening and treatment for cardiac risk factors. The combination of lower screening and effective treatment of risk factors, such as smoking among the uninsured, lend themselves to quality improvement initiatives that can potentially reduce heart disease disparities among populations at risk.

SUMMARY

Quality of care has markedly improved; the vast majority of patients are getting the care they need in many areas. For people with diabetes, most have their blood sugar and cholesterol levels checked. Most people have their blood pressure and cholesterol levels checked to help prevent or control heart disease, and 85 percent of people experiencing a heart attack receive aspirin on arrival at the hospital. Women are being screened for breast cancer with mammography. For child health, more than 73 percent of children aged 19 to 35 months have all recommended vaccinations. Seniors receive influenza immunization at very high rates.

Health care is improving in many areas. For cancer patients, more cancers are being detected at earlier stages. As a result of investments in biomedical research, new treatment options now exist to extend the lives of individuals with cancer. For diabetic patients, there are fewer unnecessary admissions to the hospital. For maternal and child health care, the percent of women using prenatal care in their first trimester has increased over the past 30 years. For adult asthma patients, fewer are admitted to hospitals. In nursing homes, progress has been made in reducing use of physical restraints. In patient safety, there has been significant progress in reducing infection rates in certain types of hospital intensive care units.

In other areas, improvement can be made. Despite the sophisticated diagnostic and therapeutic options now available, rates remain low for provision of some basic and cost-effective preventive care (e.g., colorectal cancer screening and checking for high cholesterol levels). Only 23 percent of persons with hypertension have it under control. Control of hypertension is essential to continued successes in reducing mortality from heart disease, stroke, and complications of diabetes. Half of the people with depression stop using their medicines within the first month, a far shorter time period than recommended by experts and scientific evidence. In terms of patient safety, about one in five elderly Americans is prescribed medications that may be inappropriate for him or her and thus are potentially harmful.

More focus on prevention can save more lives and resources. For example, while smoking remains the single most preventable cause of mortality, rates of smoking cessation counseling of patients, both in the hospital and during office visits, are only 40 percent and 60 percent, respectively. Likewise, data on screening for high cholesterol show that 67 percent of adults have had their cholesterol checked within the past 2 years and can state whether it is normal or high. Screening for high cholesterol—which is

also a risk factor for diabetes—can prevent the development of heart disease.

Limitations in the availability of data constrain the ability to track certain conditions. Data can come from several different sources: medical charts, patient surveys, facility surveys, vital statistics, surveillance systems, and administrative and claims records. The degree to which data are collected from any of these sources varies widely. Expected gains in information technology, including the adoption of electronic medical records, will address this dearth of data by providing one data source without imposing any additional burden on providers. The quality future is bright.

REVIEW QUESTIONS

1. What is quality?
2. How do we measure quality?
3. Define structure, process, and outcome in the context of quality assurance.
4. What are the six possible interventions to improve adoption of improved treatment practices?
5. Describe the taxonomy of quality-improvement strategies.
6. What types of disparities exist within the U.S. health care system, and how can we eliminate them?
7. What are report cards?
8. Describe the improvements that can be made to increase the quality of health care services.

REFERENCES & ADDITIONAL READINGS

Agency for Healthcare Research and Quality (AHRQ). http://www.ahrq.gov/qual/qualix.htm.

Berwick, D. M., & Leape, L. I. (1999). Reducing errors in medicine. *British Medical Journal, 319,* 136–137.

Clancy, C., & Eisenberg, J. W. (1998). Outcomes research: Measuring the end results of health care. *Science, 282,* 245–246.

Donabedian, A. (1966, July). Evaluating the quality of medical care. *Milbank Memorial Fund Quarterly, 44*(Suppl., Part 2), 166–206.

Institute of Medicine, Committee on the Quality of Health Care in America. (2001). *Crossing the quality chasm: A new health care system for the 21st century.* Washington, DC: National Academy Press.

Kohn, L. T., Corrigan, J., Richardson, W. C., & Donaldson, M. S. (2000). *To err is human: Building a safer health system.* Washington, DC: National Academy Press.

Leapfrog Group. http://www.leapfroggroup.org/.

Leatherman, S., Berwick, D. M., Lies, D., et al. (2003). The business case for quality: Case studies and an analysis. *Health Affairs, 22,* 17–30.

Lohr, K. N. (2004). Rating the strength of scientific evidence: Relevance for quality improvement programs. *International Journal of Quality in Health Care, 16,* 9–18.

Lohr, K. N., & Steinwachs, D. M. (2002). Health services research: An evolving definition of the field. *Health Services Research, 37,* 7–10.

McLaughlin, C. P., & Kaluzny, A. D. (1999). *Continuous quality improvement in health care: Theory, implementation, and applications.* Gaithersburg, MD: Aspen Publishers.

McNeil, B. J. (2001). Shattuck Lecture: Hidden barriers to improvement in the quality of care. *New England Journal of Medicine, 345,* 1612–1620.

National Quality Measures Clearinghouse (NQMC). http://www.qualitymeasures.ahrq.gov.

Rosenthal, M. B., Fernandopulle, R., Song HyunSook, R., & Landon, B. (2004). Paying for quality: Provider's incentives for quality improvement. *Health Affairs, 23,* 127–141.

Wennberg, J., & Gittelsohn, A. (1973). Small area variations in health care delivery. *Science, 182,* 1102–1108.

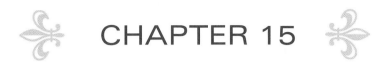

CHAPTER 15

Ethical Issues in Public Health and Health Services*

Pauline Vaillancourt Rosenau and Ruth Roemer

CHAPTER TOPICS

❧ Overarching Public Health Principles: Our Assumptions

❧ Ethical Issues in Developing Resources

❧ Ethical Issues in Economic Support

❧ Ethical Issues in Organization of Services

❧ Ethical Issues in Management of Health Services

❧ Ethical Issues in Delivery of Care

❧ Ethical Issues in Assuring Quality of Care

❧ Mechanisms for Resolving Ethical Issues in Health Care

LEARNING OBJECTIVES

Upon completing this chapter, the reader should be able to

1. Appreciate the central role of public health ethical concerns in health policy and management.

2. Understand ethics issues with regard to the development and distribution of, and payment for, services, and with regard to the organization, management, assessment, and delivery of services.

3. Acquire a framework for ethical analysis of issues within health services systems.

4. Be a humanistic as well as technically adept participant in the health services field.

*From *Changing the U.S. Health Care System*, 3rd Ed. (pp. 643–673), by R. M. Andersen, T. H. Rice, and G. F. Kominski, 2007, San Francisco: Jossey-Bass. Copyright 2007 by John Wiley & Sons, Inc. Reprinted with permission of John Wiley & Sons, Inc.

The cardinal principles of medical ethics[1]—autonomy, beneficence, and justice—apply in public health ethics but in somewhat altered form. Personal autonomy and respect for autonomy are guiding principles of public health practice as well as of medical practice. In medical ethics, the concern is with the privacy, individual liberty, freedom of choice, and self-control of the individual. From this principle flows the doctrine of informed consent. In public health ethics, autonomy, the right of privacy, and freedom of action are recognized insofar as they do not result in harm to others. Thus, from a public health perspective, autonomy may be subordinated to the welfare of others or of society as a whole.[2]

Beneficence, which includes doing no harm, promoting the welfare of others, and doing good, is a principle of medical ethics. In the public health context, beneficence is the overall goal of public health policy and practice. It must be interpreted broadly, in light of societal needs, rather than narrowly, in terms of individual rights.

Justice—whether defined as equality of opportunity, equity of access, or equity in benefits—is the core of public health. Serving the total population, public health is concerned with equity among various social groups, with protecting vulnerable populations, with compensating persons for suffering disadvantage in health and health care, and with surveillance of the total health care system. As expressed in the now-classic phrase of Dr. William H. Foege, "Public health is social justice."[3]

This chapter concerns public health ethics as distinguished from medical ethics. Of course, some overlap exists between public health ethics and medical ethics, but public health ethics, like public health itself, applies generally to issues affecting populations, whereas medical ethics, like medicine itself, applies to individuals. Public health involves a perspective that is population-based, a view of conditions and problems that gives preeminence to the needs of the whole society rather than exclusively to the interests of single individuals.[4]

Public health ethics evokes a number of dilemmas, many of which may be resolved in several ways, depending on one's standards and values. The authors' normative choices are indicated. Data and evidence are relevant to the normative choices involved in public health ethics. We refer the reader to health services research wherever appropriate.

To illustrate the concept of public health ethics, we raise several general questions to be considered in different contexts in this chapter[5]:

- What tensions exist between protection of the public health and protection of individual rights?
- How should scarce resources be allocated and used?
- What should the balance be between expenditures and quality of life in the case of chronic and terminal illness?
- What are appropriate limits on using expensive medical technology?
- What obligations do health care insurers and health care providers have in meeting the right-to-know of patients as consumers?
- What responsibility exists for the young to finance health care for older persons?
- What obligation exists for government to protect the most vulnerable sectors of society?

We cannot give a clear, definitive answer that is universally applicable to any of these questions. Context and circumstance sometimes require qualifying even the most straightforward response. In some cases, differences among groups and individuals may be so great and conditions in society so diverse and complex that no single answer to a question is possible. In other instances, a balance grounded in a public health point of view is viable. Sometimes there is no ethical conflict at all because one solution is optimal for all concerned: for the individual, the practitioner, the payer, and society: For example, few practitioners would want to perform an expensive, painful medical act that was without benefit and might do damage. Few patients would demand it, and even fewer payers would reimburse for it. But in other circumstances, competition for resources poses a dilemma. How does one choose, for example, between a new, effective, but expensive drug of help to only a few, or use of a less-expensive but less-effective drug for a larger number of persons? The necessity for a democratic, open, public debate about rationing in the future seems inevitable.

Even in the absence of agreement on ethical assumptions, and facing diversity and complexity that prohibit easy compromises, we suggest mechanisms for resolving the ethical dilemmas in health care do exist. We explore these in the concluding section of this chapter.

A word of caution: space is short and our topic complex. We cannot explore every dimension of every relevant topic to the satisfaction of all readers. We offer here, instead, an introduction whose goal is to awaken readers—be they practitioners, researchers, students, patients, or consumers—to the ethical dimension of public health. We hope to remind them of the ethical assumptions that underlie their own public health care choices. This chapter, then, is limited to considering selected ethical issues in public health and the provision of personal health services. We shall examine our topic by way of components of the health system: (1) development of health resources, (2) economic support, (3) organization of services, (4) management of services, (5) delivery of care, and (6) assurance of the quality of care.[6]

OVERARCHING PUBLIC HEALTH PRINCIPLES: OUR ASSUMPTIONS

We argue for these general assumptions of a public health ethic:

- Provision of care on the basis of health need, without regard to race, religion, gender, sexual orientation, or ability to pay

- Equity in distribution of resources, giving due regard to vulnerable groups in the population (ethnic minorities, migrants, children, pregnant women, the poor, the handicapped, and others)

- Respect for human rights—including autonomy, privacy, liberty, health, and well-being—keeping in mind social justice considerations

Central to the solution of ethical problems in health services is the role of law, which sets forth the legislative, regulatory, and judicial controls of society. The development of law in a particular field narrows the discretion of providers in making ethical judgments. At the same time, law sets guidelines for determining policy on specific issues or in individual cases.[7]

ETHICAL ISSUES IN DEVELOPING RESOURCES

When we talk about developing resources, we mean health personnel, facilities, drugs and equipment, and knowledge. Choices among the kinds of personnel trained, the facilities made available, and the commodities produced are not neutral. Producing and acquiring each of these involve ethical assumptions, and they in turn have public health consequences.

The numbers and kinds of personnel required and their distribution are critical to public health.[8] We need to have an adequate supply of personnel and facilities for a given population in order to meet the ethical requirements of providing health care without discrimination or bias. The proper balance of primary care physicians and specialists is essential to the ethical value of beneficence so as to maximize health status. The ethical imperative of justice requires special measures to protect the economically disadvantaged, such as primary care physicians working in health centers. The imperfect free market mechanisms employed in the United States to date have resulted in far too many specialists relative to generalists. Other modern western countries have achieved some balance, but this has involved closely controlling medical school enrollments and residency programs.

At the same time, the ethical principle of autonomy urges that resource development also be diverse enough to permit consumers some choice of providers and facilities. Absence of choice is a form of coercion. It also reflects an inadequate supply. But it results, as well, from the absence of a range of personnel. Patients should have some—though not unlimited—freedom to choose the type of care they prefer. Midwives, chiropractors, and other effective and proven practitioners should be available if health resources permit it without sacrificing other ethical considerations. The ethical principle of autonomy here might conflict with that of equity, which would limit general access to specialists in the interest of better distribution of health care access to the whole population. The need for ample public health personnel is another ethical priority, necessary for the freedom of all individuals to enjoy a healthful, disease-free environment.

Physician assistants and nurses are needed, and they may serve an expanded role, substituting for primary care providers in some instances to alleviate the shortage of primary care physicians, especially in underserved areas. But too great a reliance on these providers might diminish quality of care if they are required to substitute entirely for physicians, particularly with respect to differential diagnosis.[9] The point of service is also a significant consideration. For example, effective and expanded health care and dental care for children could be achieved by employing the school as a geographic point for monitoring and providing selected services.

Health personnel are not passive commodities, and freedom of individual career choice may conflict with public health needs. Here autonomy of the individual must be balanced with social justice and beneficence. In the past, the individual's decision to become a medical specialist took precedence over society's need for more generalists. A public health ethic appeals to the social justice involved and considers the impact on the population. A balance between individual choice and society's needs is being achieved today by restructuring financial compensation for primary care providers.

Similarly, in the United States an individual medical provider's free choice as to where to practice medicine has resulted in underserved areas, and ways to develop and train health personnel for rural and central city areas are a public health priority. About 20 percent of the U.S. population lives in rural communities, and four in ten do not have adequate access to health care. Progress has been made in the complex problem of assuring rural health clinics, but providing for the health care of rural America remains a problem. It challenges efforts at health care reform as well.[10] Foreign medical graduates are commonly employed in underserved urban centers and rural areas in the US today but this raises other ethics questions. Is it just to deprive the citizens of the country of origin of these practitioners of their services?[11]

An important issue in educating health professionals is the need to assure racial and ethnic diversity in both the training and practice of health professionals. A series of court decisions and state initiatives have, with one exception, seriously limited admissions of minority students to professional schools.

In 1978, the US Supreme Court in the Bakke case invalidated a quota system in admissions to medical schools, but provided that race could be considered as one factor among various criteria for admission.[12] In 1996, the Court of Appeals for the Fifth Circuit in the Hopwood case, in considering admission policies for the University of Texas Law School, held unconstitutional an preference based on race.[13] In 2003, the US Supreme Court made a sharp turn and in two cases involving affirmative action policies at the University of Michigan upheld an individualized policy of admission to the Law School but struck down an undergraduate admission policy based on a point system. It held that the Law School had a compelling interest in attaining a diverse student body and that its affirmative action policies were legally sound as evaluating each candidate as an individual.[14] At the same time, the court invalidated the undergraduate admission policy as not providing for individualized consideration of each candidate.[15]

The ethical issues of beneficence and justice involved in these decisions also plague initiatives at the state level. In California, Proposition 209, passed in 1996, banned consideration of race, gender, or national origin in hiring and school admissions. In the state of Washington, Initiative 200 adopted by the voters in 1998 eliminated all preferential treatment based on race or gender in government hiring and school admissions. In Florida, the Governor's Cabinet enacted in 2000 the "One Florida" program that ended consideration of race in university admissions and state contracts.[16] These state actions have significant ethical effects on the health system and underserved communities. They contribute to a shortage of physicians in minority communities, and they deny many minority candidates admission to medical school.[17]

Similar ethical public health dilemmas are confronted with respect to health facilities. From a public health point of view, the need for equitable access to quality institutions and for fair distribution of health care facilities takes priority over an individual real estate developer's ends or the preferences of for-profit hospital owners. Offering a range of facilities to maximize choice suggests the need for both public and private hospitals, community clinics and health centers, and inpatient and outpatient mental health facilities, as well as long-term care facilities and hospices. At the same time, not-for-profit providers, on several performance variables, do a better job than the for-profit institutions. Overall, studies since 1980 suggest that non profit providers out perform for profit providers on cost, quality, access, and charity care.[18] For example, the *medical loss ratio* is much higher in nonprofit health care providers compared to for-profit health care providers. The higher the medical loss ratio, the greater the proportion of revenue received that goes for health care rather than administration and management. In 1995, for example, Kaiser Foundation Health Plan in California "devoted 96.8 percent of its revenue to health care and retained only 3.2 percent

for administration and income."[19] They have lower disenrollment rates,[20] offer more community benefits,[21] feature more preventive services,[22] too. How long this can continue to be the case in the highly competitive health care market is unknown because not-for-profits may have to adopt for-profit business practices to survive.[23]

The financial crisis facing public hospitals throughout the nation poses an ethical problem of major proportions. At stake is the survival of facilities that handle an enormous volume of care for the poor, that train large numbers of physicians and other health personnel, and that make available specialized services—trauma care, burn units, and others—for the total urban and rural populations they serve.

Research serves a public health purpose too. It has advanced medical technology, and its benefits in new and improved products should be accessible to all members of society. Public health ethics also focuses on the importance of research in assessing health system performance, including equity of access and medical outcomes. Only if what works and is medically effective can be distinguished from what does not work and what is medically ineffective, are public health interests best served. Health care resources need to be used wisely and not wasted. Health services research can help assure this goal. This is especially important in an era in which market competition appears, directly or indirectly, to be having a negative influence on research capacity.[24]

Research is central to developing public health resources. Equity mandates a fair distribution of research resources among the various diseases that affect the public's health because research is costly, resources are limited, and choices have to be made. Research needs both basic and applied orientation to assure quality. There is a need for research on matters that have been neglected in the past,[25] as has been recognized in the field of women's health. Correction of other gross inequities in allocating research funds is urgent. Recent reports indicate that younger scientists are not sufficiently consulted in the peer review process, and they do not receive their share of research funds. Ethical implications involving privacy, informed consent, and equity affect targeted research grants for AIDS, breast cancer, and other special diseases. The legal and ethical issues in the human genome project, and now stem cell research, involve matters of broad scope—wide use of genetic screening, information control, privacy, and possible manipulation of human characteristics—it is no surprise that Annas has called for "taking ethics seriously."[26]

Federal law in the United States governs conduct of biomedical research involving human subjects. Ethical issues are handled by ethics advisory boards, convened to advise the Department of Health and Human Services on the ethics of biomedical or behavioral research projects, and by institutional review boards of research institutions seeking funding of research proposals. Both kinds of board are charged with responsibility for reviewing clinical research proposals and for ensuring that the legal and ethical rights of human subjects are protected.[27] Finding researchers to serve on IRBs is a growing problem because about half of all researchers have serious conflicts of interest due to the fact that they serve as industry consultants.[28]

An overarching problem is the conflict of interest of scientists who are judging the effectiveness of treatments and drugs and, at the same time, may be employed by or serving as consultants to a pharmaceutical or biotechnology firm. In 2005, several scientists at the National Institutes of Health resigned in the wake of a new regulation banning NIH scientists from accepting funding from pharmaceutical firms.[29]

Among the principal concerns of these boards is assurance of fully informed and unencumbered consent, by patients competent to give it, in order to assure the autonomy of subjects. They are also concerned with protecting the privacy of human subjects and the confidentiality of their relation to the project. An important legal and ethical duty of researchers, in the event that a randomized clinical trial proves beneficial to health, is to terminate the trial immediately and make the benefits available to the control group and to the treated group alike.

The ethical principles that should govern biomedical research involving human subjects are a high priority, but criticism has been leveled at the operation of some institutional review boards. Some say they lack objectivity and are overly identified with the interests of the researcher and the institution. Recommendations to correct this type of problem include appointing patient and consumer advocates to review boards, in addition to physicians and others affiliated with the institution and along with the sole lawyer who is generally a member of the review board; having consumer advocates involved early in drawing up protocols for the research; having third parties interview patients after they have given their consent to make sure that they understood the research and their choices; requiring the institution to include research in its quality assurance monitoring; and establishing a national human experimentation board to oversee the four thousand institutional review boards in the country.[30] Others say the pendulum has moved in the other direction and that IRBs excessively limit researchers ability to do their studies and that they increase the cost of research, perhaps making it impossible to carry it out at all in some cases.

Correction of fraud in science and the rights of subjects are important ethical considerations in developing knowledge. Ethical conflict between the role of the physician as caregiver and as researcher is not uncommon inasmuch as what is good for the research project is not always what is good for the patient. Certainly, in some instances society stands to benefit at the expense of the research subject, but respect for the basic worth of the individual means that he or she has a right to be informed before agreeing to participate in an experiment. Only when consent is informed, clear, and freely given can altruism, for the sake of advancing science and humanity, be authentic.

Policy makers concerned with developing resources for health care thus confront tensions between protecting public health and protecting the rights of individual patients and providers. They face issues concerning allocation of scarce resources and use of expensive medical technology.

We trust that in resolving these issues their decisions are guided by principles of autonomy, beneficence, and justice as applied to the health of populations.

ETHICAL ISSUES IN ECONOMIC SUPPORT

Nowhere is the public health ethical perspective clearer than on issues of economic support. Personal autonomy and respect for privacy remain essential, as does beneficence. But a public health orientation suggests that the welfare of society merits close regard for justice. It is imperative that everyone in the population have equitable access to health care services with dignity, so as not to discourage necessary utilization; in most cases, this means universal health insurance coverage. Forty-five million Americans lack health insurance, which makes for poorer medical outcomes even though individuals without health insurance do receive care in hospital emergency rooms and community clinics. Most of the uninsured are workers in small enterprises whose employers do not offer health insurance for their workers or dependents.[31] The uninsured are predicted to rise to 56 million or 27.8% by 2013.[32] The Institute of Medicine has provided an up-to-date and thorough analysis of the scope of uninsurance and underinsurance in America.[33] The underinsured, those with coverage that is not sufficient and leaves bills that the individual cannot pay, are also on the rise. This happens when employers shift health insurance costs to employees with greater deductibles and co-pays for example.[34]

From a public health perspective, financial barriers to essential health care are inappropriate. Yet they exist to a surprising degree. Witness the fact that the cost reached $5,670 per person in the US in 2003.[35] If each and every human being is to develop to his or her full potential, to participate fully as a productive citizen in our democratic society, then preventive health services and alleviation of pain and suffering due to health conditions that can be effectively treated must be available without financial barriers. Removing economic barriers to health services does not mean that the difference in health status between rich and poor will disappear. But it is a necessary, if not sufficient, condition for this goal.

Economic disparity in society is a public health ethical issue related to justice. Increasing evidence suggests that inequality in terms of income differences between the rich and the poor has a large impact on a population's health.[36] This may be due to psychosocial factors,[37] or a weakened societal social fabric,[38] or loss of social capital,[39] or a range of other factors.[40] Whatever the cause, "income inequality, together with limited access to health care, has serious consequences for the working poor."[41]

From a public health point of view, the economic resources to support health services should be fair and equitable. Any individual's contribution should be progressive, based on ability to pay. This is especially important because the rise of managed care has made it increasingly difficult to provide charity care.[42] This may be because of funding restrictions for a defined population. Although some individual contribution is appropriate—no matter how small—as a gesture of commitment to the larger community, it is also ethically befitting for the nation to take responsibility for a portion of the cost. The exact proportion may vary across nation and time, depending on the country's wealth and the public priority attributed to health services.[43]

Similarly, justice and equity suggest the importance of the ethical principle of social solidarity in any number of forms.[44] By definition, social insurance means that there is wisdom in assigning responsibility for payment by those who are young and working to support the health care of children and older people no longer completely independent. A public health orientation suggests that social solidarity forward and backward in time, across generations, is ethically persuasive. Those in the most productive stages of the life cycle today were once dependent children, and they are likely one day to be dependent older persons.

Institutions such as Social Security and Medicare play a moral role in a democracy. They were established to attain common aims and are fair in that they follow agreed-upon rules.[45] Proposals to privatize them undermine these goals. Financing of the Social Security system in part by individual investment accounts, favored by the Bush Administration, carries serious risks in case of market failure and certainly does not assure the subsidy for low-income workers contained in the current government system. With respect to Medicare, the Bush Administration's support of a voucher system enabling the beneficiary to buy private insurance will induce healthy and affluent elderly to opt out of Medicare, leaving Medicare as a welfare program for the sick and the poor. With less income, Medicare will be forced to cut services.

Social solidarity between the young and the elderly are critical. As members of a society made up of overlapping communities, our lives are intricately linked together. No man or woman is an island; not even the wealthiest or most "independent" can exist alone. The social pact that binds us to live in peace together requires cooperation of such a fundamental nature that we could not travel by car (assuming respect for traffic signals) to the grocery store to purchase food (or assume it is safe for consumption) without appealing to social solidarity. These lessons apply to health care as well.

In 1983, the President's Commission for the Study of Ethical Problems in Medicine and Biomedical and Behavioral Research made as its first and principal recommendation on ethics in medicine that society has an obligation to assure equitable access to health care for all its citizens.[46] Equitable access, the commission said, requires that all citizens be able to secure an adequate level of care without excessive burden. Implementation of this principle as an ethical imperative is even more urgent all these years later, as an increasing number of people become uninsured and as the prices of pharmaceuticals dramatically increase.[47]

ETHICAL ISSUES IN ORGANIZATION OF SERVICES

The principal ethical imperative in organization of health services is that services be organized and distributed in accordance with health needs and the ability to benefit. The problem with rationing on the basis of ability to pay is that it encourages the opposite.[48] The issues of geographic and cultural access also illustrate this ethical principle.

To be fair and just, a health system must minimize geographic inequity in distributing care. Rural areas are underserved, as are inner cities. Any number of solutions have been proposed and tried to bring better access in health services to underserved areas. They include mandating a period of service for medical graduates as a condition of licensure, loan forgiveness and expansion of the National Health Service Corps, rural preceptorships, creating economic incentives for establishing a practice in a rural area, and employing physician assistants and nurse practitioners.[49] Telemedicine may make the best medical consultants available to rural areas in the near future,[50] but the technology involves initial start-up costs that are not trivial. Higher Medicare payments to rural hospitals also ensure that they will remain open.[51]

Similarly, the principles of autonomy and beneficence require health services to be culturally relevant to the populations they are designed to serve.[52] This means that medical care professionals need to be able to communicate in the language of those they serve and to understand the cultural preferences of those for whom they seek to provide care.[53] The probability of success is enhanced if needed health professionals are from the same cultural background as those they serve. This suggests that schools of medicine, nursing, dentistry, and public health should intensify their efforts to reach out and extend educational and training opportunities to qualified and interested members of such populations. To carry out such programs, however, these schools must have the economic resources required to offer fellowships and teaching assistant positions.

The development of various forms of managed care—health maintenance organizations, prepaid group practices, preferred provider organizations, and independent practice associations—raise another set of ethical questions. As experienced in the United States in recent years, managed care is designed more to minimize costs than to ensure that health care is efficient and effective. If managed care ends up constraining costs by depriving individuals of needed medical attention (reducing medically appropriate access to specialists, for instance), then it violates the ethical principle of beneficence because such management interferes with doing good for the patient.[54] If managed care is employed as a cost-containment scheme for Medicaid and Medicare without regard to quality of care, it risks increasing inequity. It could even contribute to a two-tiered health care system in which those who can avoid various forms of managed care by paying privately for their personal health services will obtain higher-quality care.

Historically, the advantages of staff-model managed care are clear: team practice, emphasis on primary care, generous use of diagnostic and therapeutic outpatient services, and prudent use of hospitalization. All contribute to cost containment. At the same time, managed care systems have the disadvantage of restricted choice of provider. Today's for-profit managed care companies run the risk of under-serving; they may achieve cost containment through cost shifting and risk selection.[55]

The ethical issues in the relationships among physicians, patients, and managed care organizations include denial of care, restricted referral to specialists, and gag rules that bar physicians from telling patients about alternative treatments (which may not be covered by the plan) or from

discussing financial arrangements between the physician and the plan (which may include incentives for cost containment).[56] Requiring public disclosure of information about these matters has been proposed as a solution, but there is little evidence that disclosure helps the poor and illiterate choose a better health plan or a less-conflicted health care provider.

The ethical issues in managed care are illustrated most sharply by the question of who decides what is medically necessary: the physician or others, the disease management program, the insurer, the employer, or the state legislature.[57] This question is not unique to managed care; it has also arisen with respect to insurance companies and Medicaid.[58] On the one hand, the physician has a legal and ethical duty to provide the standard of care that a reasonable physician in the same or similar circumstances would. On the other hand, insurers have traditionally specified what is covered or not covered as medically necessary in insurance contracts. The courts have sometimes reached different results, depending on the facts of the case, the character of the treatment sought (whether generally accepted or experimental), and the interpretation of medical necessity. With the rise of managed care, the problem becomes even more of an ethical dilemma because, as even those highly favorable to managed care agree, there is a risk of too little health care.[59]

Malpractice suits against managed care organizations in self-insured plans are barred by the provision in the Employee Retirement Income Security Act that preempts or supersedes "state laws that contain provisions involving any type of employee benefit plan." As a result of the preemption, employees covered by such plans are limited to the relief provided by ERISA—only the cost of medical care denied—with no compensation for lost wages and pain and suffering. Self-insured health insurance plans that cause injury by denying care or providing substandard care have immunity from suit in state courts because of legal interpretation of ERISA by the US Supreme Court. In view of the fact that 140 million people receive their health care through plans sponsored by employers and covered by ERISA, it is a serious matter of equity to bar them from access to the state courts for medical malpractice.[60]

In June of 2004, the Supreme Court "immunized employer-sponsored health plans against damage suits for wrongful denial of coverage." It thus voided laws that allowed such suits in 10 states. This will mean that the legal risk to health plans for denying coverage will be reduced. The poor will be the greatest losers as they cannot afford to fight such denials through the now available reviews mandated in 40 of the states. This law is also likely to make for high malpractice claims as physicians and hospital do not have legal shelter from responsibility.[61]

As more and more integrated health care delivery systems are formed, as more mergers of managed care organizations occur, as pressure for cost containment increases, ethical issues concerning conflict of interest, quality of care choices, and patients' rights attain increasing importance. The principles of autonomy, beneficence, and justice are severely tested in resolving the ethical problems facing a complex, corporate health care system.

If medicine is "for-profit," as seems to be the case today and for the near future in the United States, then the ethical dilemma between patients' interests and profits will be a continuing problem.[62] Sometimes the two can both be served, but it is unlikely to be the case in all instances. Surveys of business "executives admit and point out the presence of numerous generally accepted practices in their industry which they consider unethical."[63] As Fisher and Welch conclude, "Stakeholders in the increasingly market-driven U.S. health care system have few incentives to explore the harms of the technologies from which they stand to profit."[64] That both consumers and employers are concerned about quality of care is clear from Paul Ellwood's statement expressing disappointment in the evolution of HMOs because "they tend to place too much emphasis on saving money and not enough on improving quality—and we now have the technical skill to do that."[65]

ETHICAL ISSUES IN MANAGEMENT OF HEALTH SERVICES

Management involves planning, administration, regulation, and legislation. The style of management depends on the values and norms of the population. Planning involves determining the population's health needs (with surveys and research, for example) and then ensuring that programs are in place to provide these services. A public health perspective suggests that planning is appropriate to the extent that it provides efficient, appropriate health care (beneficence) to all who seek it (equity and justice). Planning may avoid waste and contribute to rational use of health services. But it is also important that planning not be so invasive as to be coercive and deny the individual any say in his or her health care unless such intervention is necessary to protect public health interests. The ethical principle of autonomy preserves the right of the individual to refuse care, to determine his or her own destiny, especially when the welfare of others is not involved. A balance between individual autonomy and public health intervention that affords benefit to the society is not easy to achieve. But in some cases the resolution of such a dilemma is clear, as in the case for mandatory immunization programs. Equity and beneficence demand that the social burdens and benefits of living in a disease-free environment be shared. Therefore, for example, immunization requirements should cover all those potentially affected.

Health administration has ethical consequences that may be overlooked because they appear ethically neutral: organization, staffing, budgeting, supervision, consultation, procurement, logistics, records and reporting, coordination, and evaluation.[66] But all these activities involve ethical choices. Faced with a profit squeeze, the managed care industry is pressuring providers to reduce costs and services.[67] The result has been downsizing, which means more unlicensed personnel are hired to substitute for nurses.[68] California is the first state to mandate nurse-to-patient staffing ratios.[69] Surveys of doctors suggest patients do not always get needed care from HMOs.[70] Denial of appropriate needed health care is an ethical problem related to beneficence. In addition, the importance of privacy in record keeping (to take an example) raises once again the necessity to balance the ethical principles of autonomy and individual rights with social justice and the protection of society.[71]

Distribution of scarce health resources is another subject of debate. The principle of first come, first served may initially seem equitable. But it also incorporates the "rule of rescue," whereby a few lives are saved at great cost, and this policy results in the "invisible" loss of many more lives. The cost-benefit or cost-effectiveness analysis of health economics attempts to apply hard data to administrative decisions. This approach, however, does not escape ethical dilemmas because the act of assigning numbers to years of life, for example, is itself value-laden. If administrative allocation is determined on the basis of the number of years of life saved, then the younger are favored over the older, which may or may not be equitable. If one factors into such an analysis the idea of "quality" years of life, other normative assumptions must be made as to how important quality is and what constitutes quality. Some efforts have been made to assign a dollar value to a year of life as a tool for administering health resources. But here, too, we encounter worrisome normative problems. Does ability to pay deform such calculations?[72]

Crucial to management of health services are legal tools—legislation, regulations, and sometimes litigation—necessary for fair administration of programs. Legislation and regulations are essential for authorizing health programs; they also serve to remedy inequities and to introduce innovations in a health service system. Effective legislation depends on a sound scientific base, and ethical questions are especially troubling when the scientific evidence is uncertain.

For example, in a landmark decision in 1976, the Court of Appeals for the District of Columbia upheld a regulation of the Environmental Protection Agency restricting the amount of lead additives in gasoline based largely on epidemiological evidence.[73] Analysis of this case and of the scope of judicial review of the regulatory action of an agency charged by Congress with regulating substances harmful to health underlines the dilemma the court faced: the need of judges trained in the law, not in science, to evaluate the scientific and epidemiological evidence on which the regulatory agency based its ruling.[74] The majority of the court based its upholding of the agency's decision on its own review of the evidence. By contrast, Judge David Bazelon urged an alternative approach: "In cases of great technological complexity, the best way for courts to guard against unreasonable or erroneous administrative decisions is not for the judges themselves to scrutinize the technical merits of each decision. Rather, it is to establish a decision making process that assures a reasoned decision that can be held up to the scrutiny of the scientific community and the public."[75]

The dilemma of conflicting scientific evidence is a persistent ethical minefield, as reflected by a 1993 decision of the U.S. Supreme Court involving the question of how widely accepted a scientific process or theory must be before it qualifies as admissible evidence in a lawsuit. The case involved the issue of whether a drug prescribed for nausea during pregnancy, Bendectin, causes birth defects. Rejecting the test of "general acceptance" of scientific evidence as the absolute prerequisite for admissibility, as applied in the past, the Court ruled that trial judges serve as gatekeepers to ensure that pertinent scientific evidence is not only relevant but reliable. The Court also suggested various factors that might bear on such determinations.[76]

It is significant for the determination of ethical issues in cases where the scientific evidence is uncertain that epidemiological evidence, which is the core of public health, is increasingly recognized as helpful in legal suits.[77] Of course, it should be noted that a court's refusal (or an agency's) to act because of uncertain scientific evidence is in itself a decision with ethical implications.

Enactment of legislation and issuance of regulations are important for management of a just health care system, but these strategies are useless if they are not enforced. For example, state legislation has long banned the sale of cigarettes to minors, but only recently have efforts been made to enforce these statutes rigorously through publicity, "stings" (arranged purchases by minors), and penalties on sellers, threats of license revocation, denial of federal funds under the Synar Amendment, and banning cigarette sales from vending machines.[78] A novel case of enforcement involves a Baltimore ordinance prohibiting billboards promoting cigarettes in areas where children live, recreate, and go to school, enacted in order to enforce the minors' access law banning tobacco sales to minors. The Baltimore ordinance has not been overturned despite the fact that a Massachusetts regulation restricting advertising of tobacco and alcohol near schools was struck down as unconstitutional by the US Supreme Court on the ground of preemption.[79]

Thus, management of health services involves issues of allocating scarce resources, evaluating scientific evidence, measuring quality of life, and imposing mandates by legislation and regulations. Although a seemingly neutral function, management of health services must rely on principles of autonomy, beneficence, and justice in its decision-making process.

ETHICAL ISSUES IN DELIVERY OF CARE

Delivery of health services—actual provision of health care services—is the end point of all the other dimensions just discussed. The ethical considerations of only a few of the many issues pertinent to delivery of care are explored here.

Resource allocation in a time of cost containment inevitably involves rationing. At first blush, rationing by ability to pay may appear natural, neutral, and inevitable, but the ethical dimensions for delivery of care may be overlooked. If ability to pay is recognized as a form of rationing, the question of its justice is immediately apparent. The Oregon Medicaid program (Oregon Health Plan) is another example. It is equitable by design and grounded in good part in the efficacy of the medical procedure in question, thus respecting the principle of ethical beneficence. It is structured to extend benefits to a wider population of poor people than those entitled to care under Medicaid. It has been tested for more than 10 years in its effort to provide a basic level of care deemed effective and appropriate without over-treatment. The Prioritized List of Health Services continues to be re-evaluated and updated in light of new evidence by the Health Services Commission of the Department of Administrative Services' Office for Oregon Health Policy and Research. The Legislature continues to set the funding level to cover the services on the prioritized list without having re-arranged them.[80]

The plan does not qualify as equitable and fair, however, because it does not apply to the whole population of Oregon, but only to those on Medicaid. It denies some services to some persons on Medicaid in order to widen the pool of beneficiaries. It has, therefore, not resolved all the ethical problems in this respect.[81]

Rationing medical care is not always ethically dubious; rather, it may conform to a public health ethic. In some cases, too much medical care is counterproductive and may produce more harm than good. Canada, Sweden, the United Kingdom, and the state of Oregon, among others, have rationing of one sort or another.[82] For example, Canada rations health care, pays one-third less per person than the United States, and offers universal coverage; yet health status indicators do not suggest that Canadians suffer. In fact, on several performance indicators Canada surpasses the United States.[83] If there were better information about medical outcomes and the efficacy of many medical procedures, rationing would actually benefit patients if it discouraged the unneeded and inappropriate treatment that plagues the U.S. health system.[84]

Rationing organ transplants, similarly, is a matter of significant ethical debate because fewer organs are available for transplant than needed for the 85,000 people on waiting lists. Rationing, therefore, must be used to determine who is given a transplant. Employing tissue match makes medical sense and also seems ethically acceptable. But to the extent that ability to pay is a criterion, ethical conflict is inevitable. It may, in fact, go against scientific opinion and public health ethics if someone who can pay receives a transplant even though the tissue match is not so good as it would be for a patient who is also in need of a transplant but unable to pay the cost. Rationing on this basis seems ethically unfair and medically ill advised. It is no surprise, then, that the National Organ Transplant Act, adopted in 1984, made it illegal to offer or receive payment for organ transplantation. Yet the sale of organs for transplantation still exists. It has even been advocated as a market-friendly, for-profit solution to the current supply problems.[85]

One solution would be to make more organs available through mandatory donation from fatal automobile accidents, without explicit consent of individuals and families. A number of societies have adopted this policy of presumed consent because the public health interest of society and the seriousness of the consequences are so great for those in need of a transplant that it is possible to justify ignoring the individual autonomy (preferences) of the accident victim's friends and relatives. Spain leads other nations regarding organ donation with 33.8 donors pmp in 2003 by interpreting an absence of prohibition to constitute a near-death patient's implicit authorization for organ transplantation.[86] This has not been the case in the United States to date.[87]

Delivery of services raises conflict-of-interest questions for providers that are of substantial public health importance. Criminal prosecution of fraud in the health care sector increased threefold between 1993 and 1997.[88] In today's market-driven health system, about half of all doctors report that they have "exaggerated the severity of a patient's condition to get them care they think is medically necessary."[89] Hospitals pressed by competitive forces strain to survive and in some cases do so only by less-than-honest cost shifting—and even direct fraud. A recent survey of hospital bills found that more than 99 percent included "mistakes" that favored the hospital.[90]

Class action suits claim that HMOs are guilty of deceiving patients because they refuse to reveal financial incentives in physician payment structures.[91] Physicians have been found to refer patients to laboratories and medical testing facilities that they co-own to a far greater extent than can be medically justified.[92] As the trend to make medicine a business develops, the AMA's Council on Ethical and Judicial Affairs has adopted guidelines for the sale of nonprescription, health-related products in physicians' offices, but problems remain.[93] The purpose is to "help protect patients and maintain physicians' professionalism."[94] The public health ethic of beneficence is called into question by unnecessary products and inappropriate medical tests.

The practice of medicine and public health screening presents serious ethical dilemmas. Screening for diseases for which there is no treatment, except where such information can be used to postpone onset or prevent widespread population infection, is difficult to justify unless the information is explicitly desired by the patient for personal reasons (life planning and reproduction). In a similar case, screening without provision to treat those discovered to be in need of treatment is unethical. Public health providers need to be sure in advance that they can offer the health services required to provide care for those found to be affected. These are the ethical principles of beneficence and social justice.

The tragic epidemic of HIV/AIDS has raised serious ethical questions concerning testing, reporting, and partner notification. The great weight of authority favors voluntary and confidential testing, so as to encourage people to come forward for testing, counseling, and behavior change. A study by the U.S. Centers for Disease Control and Prevention (CDC) concludes that confidential names-based reporting of HIV has not deterred testing and treatment.[95] Nevertheless, concern about violation of privacy and possible deterrence of testing and treatment with confidential names-based reporting of HIV persists.

This issue raises sharply the ethical conflict between the individual's right to confidentiality and the needs of public health. Some guidance for resolving ethical questions in this difficult sphere is presented by Stephen Joseph, former commissioner of health for New York City, who states that the AIDS epidemic is a public health emergency involving extraordinary civil liberties issues—not a civil liberties emergency involving extraordinary public health issues.[96]

Partner notification was at first generally disapproved on grounds of nonfeasibility and protection of privacy, but in accordance with CDC guidelines, some states have enacted legislation permitting a physician or public health department to notify a partner that a patient is HIV-positive if the physician believes that the patient will not inform the partner.[97]

With the finding that administration of AZT during pregnancy to an HIV-positive woman reduces the risk of transmission of the virus to the infant dramatically, CDC recommends that all pregnant women be offered HIV testing as early in pregnancy as possible because of the available treatments for reducing the likelihood of perinatal transmission and maintaining the health of the woman. CDC also recommends that women should be counseled about their options regarding pregnancy by a method similar to genetic counseling.[98]

The field of reproductive health is a major public health concern, affecting women in their reproductive years. Here the principles of autonomy, beneficence, and justice apply to providing contraceptive services, including long-acting means of contraception, surgical abortion, medical abortion made possible by development of Mifepristone, sterilization, and use of noncoital technologies for reproduction. The debate on these issues has been wide, abrasive, and divisive. Thirty-two years after abortion was legalized by the U.S. Supreme Court's decision in Roe v. Wade,[99] protests against abortion clinics have escalated. Violence against clinics and murders of abortion providers threaten access to abortion services and put the legal right to choose to terminate an unwanted pregnancy in jeopardy. The shortage of abortion providers in some states and in many rural areas restricts reproductive health services. The mergers of Catholic hospitals with secular institutions and the insistence that the merged hospital be governed by the Ethical and Religious Directives for Catholic Health Care Services means that not only abortion services are eliminated but also other contraceptive and counseling services (except for "natural family planning"), sterilization procedures, infertility treatments, and emergency postcoital contraception (even for rape victims).[100] The Food and Drug Administration's refusal to approve over-the-counter sales of emergency contraception, despite the approval of two scientific committees, is a particularly troubling ethical decision.

We state our position as strongly favoring the pro-choice point of view in order to ensure autonomy of women, beneficence for women and their families faced with unwanted pregnancy, and justice in society. In the highly charged debate on teenage pregnancy, we believe that social realities, the well-being of young women and their children, and the welfare of society mandate access to contraception and abortion and respect for the autonomy of young people. The ethics of parental consent and notification laws, which often stand as a barrier to abortions needed and wanted by adolescents, is highly questionable. Economists estimate the cost of such laws to be around $150 million in Texas alone.[101]

Many other important ethical issues in delivering health care have not been discussed extensively in this chapter because of space limitations. There are three such issues that we want to mention briefly.

First, the end-of-life debate is generally considered a matter of medical ethics involving the patient, his or her family, and the physician. But this issue is also a matter of public health ethics because services at the end of life entail administrative and financial dimensions that are part of public health and management of health services. The Terri Shiavo

Case is an example where the potential alternative use of societal resources brings to mind the contradictions involved in end-of-life issues.[102]

Second, in the field of mental health, the conflict between the health needs and legal rights of patients on the one hand and the need for protection of society on the other illustrates sharply the ethical problems facing providers of mental health services. This conflict has been addressed most prominently by reform of state mental hospital admission laws to make involuntary admission to a mental hospital initially a medical matter, with immediate and periodic judicial review as to the propriety of hospitalization-review in which a patient advocate participates.[103] The Tarasoff case presents another problem in providing mental health services: the duty of a psychiatrist or psychologist to warn an identified person of a patient's intent to kill the person, despite the rule of confidentiality governing medical and psychiatric practice.[104] In both instances, a public health perspective favors protection of society as against the legal rights of individuals.

Third, basic to public health strategies and effective delivery of preventive and curative services are records and statistics. The moral and legal imperative of privacy to protect an individual's medical record gives way to public health statutes requiring reporting of gunshot wounds, communicable diseases, child abuse, and AIDS.[105] More generally, the right of persons to keep their medical records confidential conflicts with society's need for epidemiological information to monitor the incidence and prevalence of diseases in the community and to determine responses to this information. At the same time, it is essential, for example, that an individual's medical records be protected from abuse by employers, marketers, etc.[106] A common resolution of this problem is to make statistics available without identifying information.

Congress has adopted HIPAA (Health Insurance Portability and Accountability Act) in 1996 to protect the privacy of medical records. Only in 2003 did these aspects of the law take effect, HIPAA limits who may see medical records, how the records

are stored, and even how they are disposed of when no longer needed. Compliance costs have been enormous.[107]

ETHICAL ISSUES IN ASSURING QUALITY OF CARE

If a public health ethic requires fair and equitable distribution of medical care, then it is essential that waste and inefficiency be eliminated. Spending scarce resources on useless medical acts is a violation of a public health ethic.[108] To reach this public health goal, knowledge about what is useful and medically efficacious is essential.

As strategies for evaluating the quality of health care have become increasingly important, the ethical dimensions of peer review, practice guidelines, report cards, and malpractice suits—all methods of quality assurance—have come to the fore. Established in 1972 to monitor hospital services under Medicare to ensure that they were "medically necessary" and delivered in the most efficient manner, professional standards review organizations came under attack as over-regulatory and too restrictive.[109] Congress ignored the criticism and in 1982 passed the Peer Review Improvement Act, which did not abolish outside review but consolidated the local peer review agencies, replaced them with statewide bodies, and increased their responsibility.[110] In 1986, Congress passed the Health Care Quality Improvement Act, which established national standards for peer review at the state and hospital levels for all practitioners regardless of source of payment.[111] The act also established a national data bank on the qualifications of physicians and provided immunity from suit for reviewing physicians acting in good faith.

The functions of peer review organizations (PROs) in reviewing the adequacy and quality of care necessarily involve some invasion of the patient's privacy and the physician's confidential relationship with his or her patient. Yet beneficence and justice in an ethical system of medical care mandate a process that controls the cost and quality of care. Finding an accommodation between protection of privacy and confidentiality on the one hand and necessary but limited disclosure on the other has furthered the work of PROs. Physicians whose work is being reviewed are afforded the right to a hearing at which the patient is not present, and patients are afforded the protection of outside review in accordance with national standards.

Practice guidelines developed by professional associations, health maintenance organizations and other organized providers, third-party payers, and governmental agencies are designed to evaluate the appropriateness of procedures. Three states— Maine, Minnesota, and Vermont—have passed legislation permitting practice guidelines to be used as a defense in malpractice actions under certain circumstances.[112] Defense lawyers are reluctant to use this legislation, however, because they fear their case will be caught up in a lengthy constitutional appeal. Such a simplistic solution, however, avoids the question of fairness: whose guidelines should prevail in the face of multiple sets of guidelines issued by different bodies, and how should accommodation be made to evolving and changing standards of practice?[113]

Beneficence and justice are involved in full disclosure of information about quality to patients. Health plan report cards aim to fulfill this role.[114] Employers, too, could use report cards to choose health plans for their employees, though some studies suggest that many employers are interested far more in cost than quality.[115] How well reports actually measure quality is itself subject to debate.[116] These are discussed in Part 3 of this book.

Malpractice suits constitute one method of regulating the quality of care, although an erratic and expensive system. The subject is fully discussed elsewhere in this volume. Here we raise only the ethical issue of the right of the injured patient to compensation for the injury and the need of society for a system of compensation that is more equitable and more efficient than the current system.

The various mechanisms for ensuring quality of care all pose ethical issues. Peer review requires some invasion of privacy and confidentiality to conduct surveillance of quality, although safeguards have been devised. Practice guidelines involve some interference with physician autonomy but in return afford protection for both the patient and the provider. Malpractice suits raise questions of equity, since many injured patients are not compensated. In the process of developing and improving strategies for quality control, the public health perspective justifies social intervention to protect the population.

MECHANISMS FOR RESOLVING ETHICAL ISSUES IN HEALTH CARE

Even in the absence of agreement on ethical assumptions, and in the face of diversity and complexity that prohibit easy compromise, mechanisms for resolving ethical dilemmas in public health do exist. Among these are ombudsmen, institutional review boards, ethics committees, standards set by professional associations, practice guidelines, financing mechanisms, and courts of law. Some of these mechanisms are voluntary. Others are legal. None is perfect. Some, such as financing mechanisms, are particularly worrisome.

Although ethics deals with values and morals, the law has been very much intertwined with ethical issues. In fact, the more that statutes, regulations, and court cases decide ethical issues, the narrower is the scope of ethical decision making by providers of health care.[117] For example, the conditions for terminating life support for persons in a persistent vegetative state are clearer, when the patient has an up-to-date living will. The scope of decision making by physicians and families is constrained. A court of law, therefore, is an important mechanism for resolving ethical issues in such cases.

The law deals with many substantive issues in numerous fields, including that of health care. It also has made important procedural contributions to resolving disputes by authorizing, establishing, and monitoring mechanisms or processes for handling claims and disputes. Such mechanisms are particularly useful for resolving ethical issues in health care because they are generally informal and flexible and often involve the participation of all the parties. Administrative mechanisms are much less expensive than litigation and in this respect potentially more equitable.

Ombudsmen in health care institutions are a means of providing patient representation and advocacy. They may serve as channels for expression of ethical concerns of patients and their families.

Ethics committees in hospitals and managed care organizations operate to resolve ethical issues involving specific cases in the institution. They may be composed solely of the institution's staff, or they may include an ethicist specialized in handling such problems.

Institutional review boards, discussed earlier, are required to evaluate research proposals for their scientific and ethical integrity.

Practice guidelines, also discussed earlier, offer standards for ethical conduct and encourage professional behavior that conforms to procedural norms generally recognized by experts in the field.

Finally, financing mechanisms that create incentives for certain procedures and practices have the economic power to encourage ethical conduct. Perhaps the highest ethical priority in health care in the United States is the achievement of universal coverage of the population by health insurance. At the same time, financing mechanisms may function to encourage the opposite behavior.[118]

As the health care system continues to deal with budget cuts, greater numbers of uninsured persons, and restructuring into managed care and integrated delivery systems, ethical questions loom large, Perhaps their impact can be softened by imaginative and rational strategies to finance, organize, and deliver health care in accordance with the ethical principles of autonomy, beneficence, and justice.

Ethical issues in public health and health services management are likely to become increasingly complex in the future. New technology and advances in medical knowledge challenge us and raise ethical dilemmas. In the future they will need to be evaluated and applied in a public health context and submitted to a public health ethical analysis. Few of these developments are likely to be entirely new and without precedent, however. Already, current discussions, such as that presented here, may inform these new developments.

ENDNOTES

1 Beauchamp, T. L., & Childress, J. F. (1989). *Principles of Biomedical Ethics*. New York: Oxford University Press, especially chapters 3, 4, and 5; Beauchamp, T. L., & Walters, L. (1999). *Contemporary Issues in Bioethics*. Belmont, Calif.: Wadsworth, (chapter 1).

2 Burris, S. (1997). The Invisibility of Public Health: Population-Level Measures in a Politics of Market Individualism. *American Journal of Public Health*, 87(10), 1607–1610.

3 Foege, W. H. (1987). Public Health: Moving from Debt to Legacy. 1986 Presidential Address. *American Journal of Public Health*, 77(10), 1276–1278.

4 Annas, G. J. (2004). *American Bioethics: Crossing Human Rights and Health Law*. Oxford University Press, p. 244.

5 Another public health question is how threats to the environment should be reconciled with the need for employment. We acknowledge that issues in environmental control have an enormous impact on public health. Here; however, our focus is on the ethical issues in policy and management of personal health services. For a discussion of equity and environmental matters, see Paehlke, R., & Vaillancourt, R. P. (1993). Environment/Equality: Tensions in North American Politics. *Policy Studies Journal*, 21(4), 672–686.

6 This outline is taken from Roemer, M. I. *National Health Systems of the World*, Vol. 1: *The Countries*. (New York: Oxford University Press, 1991). Financial resources are treated later in the section on economic support.

[7] For an example of the symbiotic relationship between ethics and law, see Annas, G. J. (1998). *Some Choice: Law, Medicine, and the Market.* New York: Oxford University Press; and Annas, G. I. (2004). *American Bioethics: Crossing Human Rights and Health Law Boundaries.* New York: Oxford University Press.

[8] Gebbie, Kristine, Merrill, Jacqueline, & Tilson, Hugh, H. (2002). The Public Health Workforce. *Health Affairs, 21*(6), 57–68.

[9] Roemer, M. I. (1977). Primary Care and Physician Extenders in Affluent Countries. *International Journal of Health Services, 7*(4), 545–555.

[10] Moscovice, I., & Rosenblatt, R. (1999). *Quality of Care Challenges for Rural Health.* Published by Rural Health Research Centers at University of Minnesota and University of Washington. Retrieved October 17, 1999, from http://www.hsr.umn.edu/centers/rhrc/rhrc.html.

[11] McMahon, G. T. (2004). Coming to America—International Medical Graduates in the United States. *New England Journal of Medicine, 10;* McMahon, G. T. (2002). Outward Bound: Do Developing Countries Gain or Lose When Their Brightest Talents Go Abroad? *Economist, 28.*

[12] *Regents of University of California* v. *Bakke,* 438 U.S. 265, 1978.

[13] *University of Texas* v. *Hopwood,* 78 F.3d 932 (5th Cir. 1996), cert, denied, 116 S.Ct. 2581, 1996.

[14] *Gruntter* v. *Bellinger et al.* no 02-241, 2003, The U.S. Court of Appeals for the 6th circuit.

[15] *Gratz* v. *Bollinger.*

[16] The New York Times. June 24, 2003, National, p. A25.

[17] Komaromy, M. Affirmative Action and the Health of Californians, UCLA Center for Health Policy Research, Policy Brief, October 1996.

[18] Rosenau, P. V., & Linder, S. (2003). Two Decades of Research Comparing For-Profit and Nonprofit Health Provider Performance. *Social Science Quarterly, 84*(2), 219–241; Rosenau, P. V., & Linder, S. A Comparison of the Performance of For-Profit and Nonprofit U.S. Psychiatric Care Providers since 1980. *Psychiatric Services, 54*(2), 183–187; Rosenau, P. V. Performance Evaluations of For-Profit and Nonprofit Hospitals in the U.S. since 1980. *Nonprofit Management & Leadership, 13*(4), 401–423.

[19] Bell, J. E. (1996). Saving Their Assets: How to Stop Plunder at Blue Cross and Other Nonprofits. *The American Prospect, 26,* 60–66.

[20] Dallek, G., & Swirsky, L. (1997). *Comparing Medicare HMOs: Do They Keep Their Members?* Washington, DC: Families USA Foundation.

[21] Claxton, G., Feder, J., Shactman, D., & Altman, S. (1997). Public Policy Issues in Nonprofit Conversions: An Overview. *Health Affairs, 16*(2), 9–27.

[22] Himmelstein, D. U., Woolhandler, S., Hellander, I., & Wolfe, S. M. (1999). Quality of Care in Investor-Owned vs. Not-for-Profit HMOs. *Journal of the American Medical Association, 282*(2), 159–163.

[23] Melnick, G., Keeler, E., & Zwanziger, J. (1999). Market Power and Hospital Pricing: Are Nonprofits Different? *Health Affairs, 18*(3), 167–173.

[24] Moy, E., et al. (1997). Relationship Between National Institutes of Health Research Awards to US Medical Schools and Managed Care Market Penetration. *Journal of the American Medical Association, 278*(3), 217–221.

[25] Gross, C. P., Anderson, G. F., & Powe, N. R. (1999). The Relation Between Funding by the National Institutes of Health and the Burden of Disease. *New England Journal of Medicine, 340,* 1881–1887; Varmus, H. (1999). Evaluating the Burden of Disease and Spending the Research Dollars of the National Institutes of Health. *New England Journal of Medicine, 340,* 1914–1915.

[26] Annas, G. J. (1989). Who's Afraid of the Human Genome? *Hastings Center Report, 19*(4), 19–21.

[27] 422 USCS Secs. 289, 289a-1-6, 1994, 21 CFR Secs. 56-58, 1994. See Ladimer, I., & Newman, R. W. (Eds.). *Clinical Investigation in Medicine: Legal, Ethical and Moral Aspects, An Anthology and Bibliography.* Boston: Law-Medicine Research Institute, Boston University, 1963.

[28] Campbell, E. G., Weissman, J. S., Clarridge, B. et al. (2003). Characteristics of Medical School Faculty Members Serving on Institutional Review Boards: Results of a National Survey. *Academic Medicine, 78,* 831–836.

[29] Rosenwald, M. S., & Rick, W. (2005). New Ethics Rules Cost NIH Another Top Researcher. *Washington Post,* 2 April, p. A01.

[30] Hilts, P. J. (1995). Conference Is Unable to Agree on Ethical Limits of Research: Psychiatric Experiment Helped Fuel Debate. *New York Times,* 15 January, p. 12.

31 Schauffler, H. H., Brown, E. R., & Rice, T. (1997). *The State of Health Insurance in California, 1996.* Los Angeles: Health Insurance Policy Program, University of California Berkeley School of Public Health, and UCLA Center for Health Policy Research.

32 Gilmer, T., & Kronick, R. (2005). It's the Premiums, Stupid: Projections of the Uninsured through 2013. *Health Affairs Web Special,* pp. 143–151.

33 Institute of Medicine (U.S.). (2004). *Committee on the Consequences of Uninsurance.* Insuring America's health: principles and recommendations/Committee on the Consequences of Uninsurance, Board on Health Care Services, Institute of Medicine of the National Academies. Washington, DC: National Academies Press.

Institute of Medicine (U.S.). (2003). *Committee on the Consequences of Uninsurance.* Hidden costs, value lost: uninsurance in America/Committee on the Consequences of Uninsurance, Board on Health Care Services, Institute of Medicine of the National Academies. Washington, DC: National Academies Press.

Institute of Medicine (U.S.). (2003). *Committee on the Consequences of Uninsurance.* Institute of Medicine (U.S.). Committee on the Consequences of Uninsurance. A Shared destiny: community effects of uninsurance/Committee on the Consequences of Uninsurance, Board on Health Care Services, Institute of Medicine. Washington, DC: National Academy Press.

Institute of Medicine (U.S.). (2002). *Committee on the Consequences of Uninsurance.* Care without coverage: too little, too late/Committee on the Consequences of Uninsurance, Board on Health Care Services, Institute of Medicine. Washington, DC: National Academy Press.

Institute of Medicine (U.S.). (2002). *Committee on the Consequences of Uninsurance.* Institute of Medicine (U.S.). Committee on the Consequences of Uninsurance. Health insurance is a family matter/Committee on the Consequences of Uninsurance, Board of Health Care Services, Institute of Medicine. Washington, DC: National Academy Press.

Institute of Medicine (U.S.). (2001). *Committee on the Consequences of Uninsurance.* Institute of Medicine (U.S.). Committee on the Consequences of Uninsurance. Coverage matters: insurance and health care/Committee on the Consequences of Uninsurance, Board on Health Care Services, Institute of Medicine. Washington, DC: National Academy Press.

34 Finkelstein, J. B. (2005). Underinsured and overlooked: The Growing Problem of Inadequate Insurance. A Med News.com: The Newspaper for America's Physicians. Retrieved April 18, 2005, from www.ama-assn.org/amednews/2005/04/04/gusa0404.htm.

35 Smith, Cynthia, et al. (2003). Health Spending Growth Slows in 2003. *Health Affairs, 24*(1), 155–194.

36 Wilkinson, R. G. (1996). *Unhealthy Societies: The Afflictions of Inequality.* London: Routledge.

37 Kawachi, I., Kennedy, B. P., Lochner, K., & Prothrow-Stith, D. (1997). Social Capital, Income Inequality, and Mortality. *American Journal of Public Health, 87,* 1491–1498; Kawachi, I., & Kennedy, B. P. (1999). Income Inequality and Health: Pathways and Mechanisms, *Health Services Research, 34*(1), 215–228.

38 Wilkinson (1996).

39 Putnam, R. D. (1995). Bowling Alone: America's Declining Social Capital. *Journal of Democracy, 6*(1), 65–78.

40 Evans, R. G., Barer, M. L., & Marmor, T. R. (1994). *Why Are Some People Healthy and Others Not? The Determinants of Health of Populations.* Hawthorne, NY: Aldine de Gruyter.

41 Lynch, J. W., Kaplan, G. A., & Shema, S. J. (1997). Cumulative Impact of Sustained Economic Hardship on Physical, Cognitive, Psychological, and Social Functioning. *New England Journal of Medicine, 337*(26), 1889–1895.

42 Winslow, R. (1999). Rise in Health-Care Competition Saps Medical-Research Funds, Charity Care. *Wall Street Journal,* 24 March, p. B6; Cunningham, P. J., Grossman, J. M., St. Peter, R. F., & Lesser, C. S. (1999). Managed Care and Physicians' Provision of Charity Care. *Journal of the American Medical Association, 281*(12), 1087–1092; Preston, J. (1996). Hospitals Look on Charity Care as Unaffordable Option of Past. *New York Times,* 14 April, pp. A1 and A15.

43 Roemer (1991).

44 For an explanation of the communitarian form of social solidarity, see The Responsive Communitarian

Platform: Rights and Responsibilities: A Platform. *Responsive—Community,* (Winter 1991/1992): 4–20. Robert Bellah, Richard Madsen, William Sullivan, Ann Swindler, & Steven Tipton take a similar view in *Habits of the Heart* (New York: Harper-Collins, 1985). See also Minkler, M. Intergenerational Equity: Divergent Perspectives, paper presented at the annual meeting of the American Public Health Association, Washington, DC:, Nov. 1994; also Minkler, M., & Robertson, A. (1991). Generational Equity and Public Health Policy: A Critique of 'Age/Race War' Thinking. *Journal of Public Health Policy, 12*(3), 324–344.

45 Bellah, R., et al. (1991). *The Good Society.* New York: Knopf.

46 President's Commission for the Study of Ethical Problems in Medicine and Biomedical and Behavioral Research (A. M. Capron, exec. dir.). *Securing Access to Health Care: The Ethical Implications of Differences in the Availability of Health Services,* Vol. 1. Washington, DC: U.S. Government Printing Office, 1983.

47 Soumerai, S. B., & Ross-Degnan, D. (1999). Inadequate Prescription-Drug Coverage for Medicare Enrollees—A Call to Action. *New England Journal of Medicine, 340,* 722–728.

48 Maynard, A., & Bloor, K. (1998). Our Certain Fate: Rationing in Health Care. (ISBN 1 899040 70U6) London: Office of New Health Economics.

49 Lewis, C. E., Fein, R., & Mechanic, D. (1976). *The Right to Health: The Problem of Access to Primary Medical Care.* New York: Wiley.

50 Wheeler, S. V. TeleMedicine, *BioPhotonics* (Fall 1994): 34–40; and Smothers, R. 150 Miles Away, the Doctor Is Examining Your Tonsils, *New York Times,* 16 September, 1992 (late edition final), p. C14.

51 Moscovice, I., Wellever, A., & Stensland, J. (1999). *Rural Hospitals: Accomplishments and Present Challenges, July 1999.* Rural Health Research Center, School of Public Health, University of Minnesota. Retrieved on October 18, 1999, from [www.hsr.umn.edu/centers/rhrc/rhrc.html].

52 Marin, G., & VanOss, M. B. (1992). *Research with Hispanic Populations* (Thousand Oaks, CA: Sage, 1991), Chapter 3. See, for example, Orlandi, M. (Ed.), *Cultural Competence for Evaluators.* Rockville, MD: U.S. Department of Health and Human Services.

53 Rafuse, J. (1993). Multicultural Medicine. *Canadian Medical Association Journal, 148,* 282–284; Maher, J. (1993). Medical Education in a Multilingual and Multicultural World. *Medical Education, 27,* 3–5.

54 There is no evidence that HMOs, prior to 1992, offered reduced quality of care. Miller, R. H., & Luft, H. S. (1997). Does Managed Care Lead to Better or Worse Quality of Care? *Health Affairs, 16*(5), 7–25. The evidence on HMOs and quality of care in the context of today's market competition is still out. The not-for-profit HMOs seem to provide better quality than do the for-profit HMOs. How Good Is Your Health Plan? *Consumer Reports,* August 1996, pp. 40–44; Kuttner, R. (1998). Must Good HMOs Go Bad? The Commercialization of Prepaid Group Health Care. *New England Journal of Medicine, 338*(21), 1558–1563; Kuttner, R. (1998). Must Good HMOs Go Bad? The Search for Checks and Balances. *New England Journal of Medicine, 338*(22), 1635–1639; Himmelstein, Woolhandler, Hellander, & Wolfe (1999).

55 Rice, T. (1998). *The Economics of Health Reconsidered.* Chicago: Health Administration Press.

56 Miller, T. E., & Sage, W. M. (1999). Disclosing Physician Financial Incentives. *Journal of the American Medical Association, 281*(15), 1424–1430.

57 Rosenbaum, S., Frankford, D. M., Moore, B., & Borzi, P. (1999). Who Should Determine When Health Care Is Medically Necessary? *New England Journal of Medicine, 340,* 229–232. *Fox v. Health Net of California,* California Superior Court, no. 219692, Dec. 23 and 28, 1993.

58 *Pinneke v. Preisser,* 623 F.2d 546 (8th Cir. 1980); *Bush v. Barham,* 625 F.2d 1150 (5th Cir. 1980).

59 Danzon, P. M. (1997). Tort Liability: A Minefield for Managed Care? (Part 2). *Journal of Legal Studies, 26*(2), 491–519.

60 Rosenbaum, Frankford, Moore, & Borzi. (1999).

61 *Aetna Health Inc.* v. *Davila,* 124 S. Ct 2488 (2004), Bloche, H. G. (2004). Back to the 90s—The Supreme Court Immunizes managed Care. *The New England Journal of Medicine,* 23 September, pp. 1277–1279.

62 Emanuel, E. J. (1999). Choice and Representation in Health Care. *Medical Care Research and Review, 56*(1), 113–140.

63 Baumhart, R. C. (1961). How Ethical Are Businessmen? *Harvard Business Review* (July/August), pp. 6–19, 156–176.

64 Fisher, E. S., & Welch, H. G. (1999). Avoiding the Unintended Consequences of Growth in Medical Care: How Might More Be Worse? *Journal of the American Medical Association, 281*(5), 452; Deyo, R. A., et al. (1997). The Messenger Under Attack: Intimidation of Researchers by Special-Interest Groups. *New England Journal of Medicine, 336*(16), 1176–1180.

65 Ellwood quoted in Noble, H. B. (1995). Quality Is Focus for Health Plans. *New York Times,* 3 July, pp. 1, 7. For discussion of problems in business ethics, see Cederblom, J., & Dougherty, C. J. *Ethics at Work* (Belmont, CA: Wadsworth, 1990); Iannone, A. P. (Ed.), *Contemporary Moral Controversies in Business.* (New York: Oxford University Press, 1989); Bayles, M. D. *Professional Ethics,* 2nd ed. (Belmont, CA: Wadsworth, 1989); Callahan, J. C. *Ethical Issues in Professional Life* (New York: Oxford University Press, 1988).

66 Roemer. (1991).

67 Kuttner, R. (1999). The American Health Care System: Wall Street and Health Care. *New England Journal of Medicine, 340,* 664–668.

68 Shindul-Rothschild, J., Berry, D., & Long-Middleton, E. (1996). Where Have All the Nurses Gone? Final Results of Our Patient Care Survey. *American Journal of Nursing, 96,* 25–39.

69 Rundle, R. L. (1999). California Is the First State to Require Hospital-Wide Nurse-to-Patient Ratios. *Wall Street Journal,* p. B6.

70 Kaiser Family Foundation and Harvard University School of Public Health, *Survey of Physicians and Nurses: Randomly Selected Verbatim Descriptions from Physicians and Nurses of Health Plan Decisions Resulting in Declines in Patients' Health Status* (Menlo Park, CA: Kaiser Family Foundation, July 1999).

71 See, for example, *Whalen* v. *Roe,* 429 U.S. 589, 1977, upholding the constitutionality of a state law requiring that patients receiving legitimate prescriptions for drugs with potential for abuse have name, address, age, and other information reported to the state department of health.

72 Hillman, A. L., et al. (1991). Avoiding Bias in the Conduct and Reporting of Cost-Effectiveness Research Sponsored by Pharmaceutical Companies. *New England Journal of Medicine, 324,* 1362–1365.

73 *Ethyl Corporation* v. *Environmental Protection Agency,* 541 F.2d 1, 1976.

74 Silver, L. (1980). An Agency Dilemma: Regulating to Protect the Public Health in Light of Scientific Uncertainty. In R. Roemer & G. McKray (Eds.), *Legal Aspects of Health Policy: Issues and Trends.* Westport, CT: Greenwood Press.

75 Silver. (1980), p. 81, quoting this passage from Judge Bazelon's concurring opinion in *International Harvester Company* v. *Ruckelshaus,* 478 F.2d 615, 652, 1973.

76 *Daubert* v. *Merrell Dow Pharmaceuticals, Inc.,* 509 U.S. 579, 113 S. Ct. 2786, 125 L.Ed. 2d 469, 1993.

77 Ginzburg, H. M. (1986). Use and Misuse of Epidemiologic Data in the Courtroom: Defining the Limits of Inferential and Particularistic Evidence in Mass Tort Litigation. *American Journal of Law and Medicine, 12*(3&4), 423–439.

78 Roemer, R. (1993). *Legislative Action to Combat the World Tobacco Epidemic* (2nd ed.). Geneva, Switzerland: World Health Organization; U.S. Department of Health and Human Services (1989). *Reducing the Health Consequences of Smoking: 25 Years of Progress. A Report of the Surgeon General.* (DHHS publication no. CDC 89-8411.) Washington, DC: Office on Smoking and Health, Center for Chronic Disease Prevention and Health Promotion, Centers for Disease Control, Public Health Service, U.S. Department of Health and Human Services.

79 Penn Advertising of Baltimore, Inc. v. Mayor of Baltimore, 63 F.3d 1318 (4th Cir. 1995) aff'g 862 F. Supp. 1402 (D. Md. 1994), discussed by Garner, D. W. Banning Tobacco Billboards: The Case for Municipal Action. Journal of the American Medical Association, 1996, 275(16), 1263–1269. But Lorillard Tobacco Company v. Thomas Riley, Attorney General of Massachusetts, 533 US 525 (2001).

80 http://egov.oregon.gov/DAS/OHPPR/HSC/docs/ InterMod4-05.pdf and http://www.oregon.gof/ DHS/healthplan/priorlist/main.shtml.

81 Annas, G. J. (1993). *The Standard of Care: The Law of American Bioethics.* New York: Oxford University Press; Rosenbaum, S. (1992). Mothers and Children Last: The Oregon Medicaid Experiment. *American Journal of Law and Medicine, 18*(1&2), 97–126; see also Lamb, E. J. (2004). Rationing of Medical Care: Rules of Rescue, Cost-Effectiveness, and the Oregon Plan. *American Journal of Obstetrics and Gynecology, 190,* 1636–1641.

82 Maynard and Bloor (1998).

83 Anderson, G. F., & Poullier, J. P. (1999). Health
    Spending, Access, and Outcomes: Trends in Indus-
    trialized Countries. *Health Affairs, 18*(3), 178–182.
84 Schuster, M. A., McGlynn, E. A., & Brook, R. H.
    (1999). How Good Is the Quality of Health Care
    in the United States? *Milbank Quarterly, 76*(4),
    517ff.
85 Kaserman, David L., & Barnett, A. H. (2002). The
    US Organ Procurement System: A Prescription For
    Reform, American Enterprise Institute. *The New
    England Journal of Medicine* published a "sounding
    board" article strongly opposed to the sale of
    organs. Delmonico, F. et al. financial Incentives-Not
    Payment-For Organ Donation *New England Journal
    of Medicine, 346*(25):2002–2005.
86 Bosch, X. (1999). Spain Leads World in Organ Do-
    nation and Transplantation. *Journal of the American
    Medical Association, 282*, 17–18.
87 "Legislation, Practice, and Donor Rates," Council
    of Europe: National Transplant Organization in
    Parliamentary office of Technology Postnote.
    October, 2004, no. 231 p. 2.
88 Define, T. (1999). Mediscare. *Healthcare Business,
    2*(3), 60–70.
89 Kaiser Family Foundation, pp. 7, 16.
90 The GAO estimate is quoted in Rosenthal, E.
    (1993). Confusion and Error Are Rife in Hospital
    Billing Practices. *New York Times;* see also Kerr, P.
    (1992). Glossing over Health Care Fraud. *New York
    Times*, p. F17; U.S. General Accounting Office.
    *Health Insurance: Remedies Needed to Reduce
    Losses from Fraud and Abuse Testimony* (GAO/
    T-HRD-9308) (Washington, DC: General Account-
    ing Office, 1993). Alan Hillman, director of the
    Center for Health Policy at the University of Penn-
    sylvania, suggests that hospital records are so de-
    formed and manipulated for billing and reimburse-
    ment purposes that they are no longer of any use
    for outcomes research (quoted in *New York Times*,
    9 August, 1994, p. A11.)
91 Pear, R. (1999). Stung by Defeat in House, HMO's
    Seek Compromise. *New York Times*, 9 October,
    p. A9.
92 Hillman, B., et al. (1992). Physicians' Utilization
    and Charges for Outpatient Diagnostic Imaging in
    a Medicare Population. *Journal of the American
    Medical Association, 268*, 2050–2054; Mitchell, J.,
    & Scott, E. (1992). Physician Ownership of Physi-
    cal Therapy Services: Effects on Charges, Utiliza-

tion, Profits, and Service Characteristics. *Journal
of the American Medical Association, 268*,
2055–2059; Kolata, G. (1994). Pharmacists Help
Drug Promotions; Pharmacists Paid by Companies
to Recommend Their Drugs. *New York Times*, pp. A1,
D2; Hilts, P. J. (1994). FDA Seeks Disclosures by
Scientists: Financial Interests in Drugs Are at Issue.
New York Times, p. 7; Winslow, R. (1994). Drug
Company's PR Firm Made Offer to Pay for Edito-
rial, Professor Says. *Wall Street Journal*, p. B12; U.S.
General Accounting Office. (1994). Medicare:
Referrals to Physician-Owned Imaging Facilities
Warrant HCFA's Scrutiny. (GAO/HEHS-95-2.)
Washington, DC: General Accounting Office.
93 Krimsky, S. (2003). *Science in the Private Interest:
    Has the Lure of Profits Corrupted Biomedical
    Research?* Lanham, MD: Rowman & Littlefield,
    pp. 247.
94 Prager, L. O. (1999). Selling Products OK—But Not
    for Profit. *American Medical News*, July 12, p. 1.
95 WHO Consultation on Testing and Counseling for
    HIV Infection. (WHO/GPA/NF/93.2.) Geneva,
    Switzerland: Global Programme on AIDS, World
    Health Organization, 1993; Field, M. A. Testing for
    AIDS: Uses and Abuses. *American Journal of Law
    and Medicine, 16*(1 & 2), 33–106; Fluss, S. S., &
    Zeegers, D. (1989). AIDS, HIV, and Health Care
    Workers: Some International Perspectives. *Mary-
    land Law Review, 48*(1), 77–92.
96 Joseph, S. C. (1992). *Dragon Within the Gates: The
    Once and Future AIDS Epidemic.* New York: Carroll
    and Graf.
97 1998 Guidelines for Treatment of Sexually Transmit-
    ted Diseases. *Morbidity and Mortality Weekly Report*,
    23 January, 1998, 47, RR-1, 16. See California
    Health and Safety Code, sec. 199.25 (1990) and the
    insightful analysis of Bayer, R. (1992). HIV Preven-
    tion and the Two Faces of Partner Notification.
    American Journal of Public Health, 82, 1156–1164.
98 1998 Guidelines . . . (1998). Public Health Service
    Task Force Recommendations for the Use of
    Antiretroviral Drugs in Pregnant Women Infected
    with HIV-1 for Maternal Health and for Reducing
    Perinatal HIV-1 Transmission in the United States.
    Morbidity and Mortality Weekly Report, 30 January,
    1998, 47, RR-2.
99 410 U.S. 113, 1973.
100 United States Conference of Catholic Bishops. *Ethi-
    cal and Religious Directives for Caltholic Health*

Care Services, 4th Ed., 2001 at http://www.usccb
.org/bishops/directives.htm. See especially directives 36, 45, 48, 53, and 54.

101 Franzini, Luisa, Marks, Elena, Cromwell, Polly F.,
et al. (2004). Projected Economic Costs Due to
Health Consequences of Teenagers' Loss of Confi-
dentiality in Obtaining Reproductive Health Care
Services in Texas. *Archives of Pediatric Adolescent
Medicine, 158,* 1140–1146.

102 Kitzhaber, J. (2005). Congress' Implicit Healthcare
Rationing. *The Christian Science Monitor,* 4 April.
For an insightful analysis of how a society's cultural
beliefs, concept of autonomy, and informed consent
laws influence resource allocation at the end of life,
see Annas, G. J., & Miller, F. H. (1994). The Em-
pire of Death: How Culture and Economics Affect
Informed Consent in the U.S., the U.K., and Japan.
American Journal of Law and Medicine, 20(4),
359–394.

103 See, for example, N.Y. Mental Hygiene Law, Article
9, Secs 9.01-9.59, 1988 and Supp. 1995; Special
Committee to Study Commitment Procedures of
the Association of the Bar of the City of New York,
in cooperation with the Cornell Law School. *Mental Illness and Due Process: Report and Recommendations on Admission to Mental Hospitals Under
New York Law.* Ithaca, NY: Cornell University
Press, 1962.

104 *Tarasoff* v. *Regents of the University of California,*
17 Cal. 3d 425, 551 P. 2d 334, 131 Cal. Rptr. 14,
1976.

105 Grad, F. P. (1990). *The Public Health Law Manual.*
(2nd ed.). Washington, DC: American Public
Health Association.

106 Starr, P. (1999). Health and the Right to Privacy.
American Journal of Law and Medicine, 25(2 & 3),
193–201.

107 Conkey, C. (2003). Doctors, Hospitals Act to Safeguard Medical Data. *The Wall Street Journal,* 21
April, p. D2.

108 McGlynn, E. A., & Brook, R. H. (1996). Ensuring
Quality of Care. In R. M. Andersen, T. H. Rice, &
G. F. Kominski (Eds.), *Changing the U.S. Health
Care System.* San Francisco: Jossey-Bass; Chassin,
M. R., & Galvin, R. W. (1998). The Urgent Need to
Improve Health Care Quality: Institute of Medicine
National Roundtable on Health Care Quality. *Jour-
nal of the American Medical Association, 280*(11),
1000–1005; Detsky, A. S. (1995). Regional

Variation in Medical Care. *New England Journal of
Medicine, 333*(9), 589–590; Leape, L. L. (1994).
Error in Medicine. *Journal of the American Medical
Association, 272,* 1851–1857.

109 For a thoughtful discussion of peer review organizations under the law as it existed in November
1979, see Price, S. J. (1980). Health Systems Agencies and Peer Review Organizations: Experiments
in Regulating the Delivery of Health Care. In
Roemer & McKray. For a more recent analysis, see
Luce, G. M. (1986). The Use of Peer Review Organizations to Control Medicare Costs. *ALI-ABA
Course Materials-Journal, 10,* 111–120; Pear, R.
(1999). Clinton to Unveil Rules to Protect Medical
Privacy. *New York Times,* 27 October, p. A1.

110 42 U.S.C. Sec. 1320c et seq.

111 42 U.S.C. Sec. 11101 et seq.

112 U.S. Congress, Office of Technology Assessment.
(1993). *Impact of Legal Reform on Medical
Malpractice Costs* (OTA-BP-H-19). Washington,
DC: U.S. Government Printing Office.

113 For analysis of various aspects of practice guide-
lines, see Capron, A. M. (1995). Practice Guide-
lines: How Good Are Medicine's New Recipes?
Journal of Law, Medicine and Ethics, 23(1), 47–56;
Parker, C. W. (1995). Practice Guidelines and Pri-
vate Insurers. *Journal of Law, Medicine and Ethics,
23*(1), 57–61; Kane, R. L. (1995). Creating Prac-
tice Guidelines: The Dangers of Over-Reliance on
Expert Judgment. *Journal of Law, Medicine and
Ethics, 23*(1), 62–64; Pauly, M. V. (1995). Practice
Guidelines: Can They Save Money? Should They?
Journal of Law, Medicine and Ethics, 23(1), 65–74;
Halpern, J. (1995). Can the Development of Prac-
tice Guidelines Safeguard Patient Values? *Journal of
Law, Medicine and Ethics, 23*(1), 75–81.

114 The Joint Commission on Accreditation of Healthcare Organizations is going to make available to
consumers information about provider performance
or outcomes. The National Committee on Quality
Assurance, a national agency located in Washington, DC, will undertake similar activities. See
http://www.ncqa.org/Pages/Main/index.htm.
Consumer Reports, Newsweek, and *U.S. News &
World Report* publish HMO assessments from time
to time.

115 McLaughlin, C. G., & Ginsburg, P. B. (1998).
Competition, Quality of Care, and the Role of the
Consumer. *Milbank Quarterly, 76*(4), 737–743;

Weinstein, M. M. (1999). Economic Scene: The Grading May Be Too Easy on Health Plans' Report Cards. *New York Times,* 19 August, p. C2.

116   Hofer, T. P. et al. (1999). The Unreliability of Individual Physician 'Report Cards' for Assessing the Costs and Quality of Care of a Chronic Disease. *Journal of the American Medical Association, 281*(22), 2098–2105.

117   Grad, F. P. (1978). Medical Ethics and the Law. *Annals of the American Academy of Political and Social Science, 437,* 19–36.

118   See the references in note 90 on conflict of interest and referral.

REVIEW QUESTIONS

1. What are the cardinal principles of medical ethics?
2. What is the difference between medical ethics and public health ethics?
3. What overarching public health principles and assumptions are basic in approaching a discussion of public health ethics?
4. What are the ethical issues in developing resources?
5. What are the ethical issues in economic support?
6. What are the ethical issues in the organization of services?
7. What are the ethical issues in management of health services?
8. What are the ethical issues in the delivery of care?
9. What are the ethical issues in ensuring quality of care?
10. What are some mechanisms for resolving ethical issues in health care?

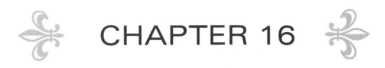

CHAPTER 16

The Future of Health Services

Stephen J. Williams and Paul R. Torrens

CHAPTER TOPICS

- The Diseases That Challenge Us
- Health Disparities Continued
- Paying for Health Care
- The Uninsured and Disenfranchised
- Public Health Services
- Ambulatory Care Services
- Hospital and Health Systems
- The Future of Long-Term Care
- Mental Health Services
- Future of the Pharmaceutical Industry
- Health Care Personnel
- Health Care Policy and Politics
- Quality of Care
- International Health
- The Future of Health Care

LEARNING OBJECTIVES

Upon completing this chapter, the reader should be able to

1. Understand the challenges facing the nation in each major area of health care.
2. Establish criteria for a future health care system.
3. Want to address the nation's health care challenges.

The nation's health care system is tremendously complex in its component parts and operations. The chapters of this book have highlighted not only the structure and function of those component parts, but also many of the key issues faced by the system's constituencies: payers, providers, and consumers.

This chapter seeks to identify and further elucidate many of the key issues that appear as unifying themes and challenging issues throughout the book. This chapter builds on the discussions of the individual chapters and also provides an opportunity to raise additional concerns, challenges, and policy issues facing the nation's health care system. The sections of this chapter are designed to parallel the individual chapters of the book, while at the same time addressing key core unifying themes.

The challenges involved in the health care system are so complex and, to an extent, overwhelming, that the discussion in this chapter should be viewed as a starting point for the reader to pursue his or her own strategic and analytical assessments and investigations of health care in the United States. That, indeed, is the principal mission of this book.

THE DISEASES THAT CHALLENGE US

Overall, United States mortality continues to decline as our successes in disease prevention and intervention mount. At the same time, there are many serious concerns involved in assessing long-term disease, illness, and injury patterns in the United States. Although the total mortality rate continues to drop and life expectancy continues to increase, these macrotrends mask concerns involving specific illnesses, diseases, injuries, and population groups. Differential morbidity and mortality between men and women, among different ethnic groups, in different age groups within the population, by geographic region, and in other important population comparisons raise red flags about our limited successes for certain populations, and the challenges that we face.

Even among the middle and upper socioeconomic classes, serious health concerns abound. These include hypertension, obesity, inactivity, chronic diseases, accidents, and injuries. International comparisons further support the notion that even with access to health care, knowledge about health and health services, and adequate health insurance, most populations have much to improve in terms of health behaviors and status.

Among our top concerns in differential morbidity and mortality are significant race differences. These data, when combined with data related to differential measurements of access to, and quality of, care suggest that limits exist in the availability and use of health services to many individuals and groups within our population, especially those who are most vulnerable.

Low-income population groups, particularly those in inner-city and rural areas, certain minority groups, and individuals with less are among those of greatest concern. Access considerations for these population groups are broad based and include financial access, such as the availability of individual financial resources, insurance plans, and entitlement programs; serious access limits, including physical access to care, transportation, availability of specialty and often even primary care services; and effective patient flow and referral systems.

Patient education, clinical preventive services, and targeted interventions to alleviate the long-term adverse consequences associated with preventable health conditions such as hypertension and obesity are also in short supply for these populations. Many successful intervention programs have demonstrated positive outcomes, including lower morbidity and mortality, when targeted to higher-risk population groups. Often such programs are not widely available, are underfunded, or are poorly coordinated in areas of local need. The lack of a broad-based and consistent financing and distribution system for patient education and preventive services is a particular national concern.

Within disease categories, demonstrated differentials in clinical services provided to at-risk and disadvantaged populations are also a concern. Physicians may provide clinical care differently and less aggressively to these populations, members of these population groups may be less receptive to clinical interventions, and patient compliance may suffer from less patient understanding and awareness as compared to better educated and higher income populations. The lack of adequate health insurance or other financial support for accessing services, combined with structural defects in the health care system to facilitate a comprehensive approach to the delivery of care for many of these population groups, further complicates the challenge faced by our nation, particularly when considering these issues in a cumulative context over an individual's entire lifetime.

Certain disease categories present us with a sobering reality and contrast sharply with the successes that we have achieved in such areas as cardiovascular and cerebrovascular disease. Formidable challenges remain, including most types of cancers, certain infectious diseases, particularly HIV/AIDS, and influenza, accidents, injuries and violence, mental illness, and emerging diseases. The threats accruing from potential terrorist's actions, new forms of virulent disease or the outbreak of previously dormant diseases, and even potential unknown and undetermined threats lurk in the future. Recent epidemics and threats including SARS, avian bird flu, hemorrhagic fevers, and a host of endemic infectious diseases, which have long vanished from our shores, such as diphtheria, malaria, and polio, challenge us on the international scene.

Then there are the truly global issues in all senses of the term. These will affect the health and well-being of our population and of all people worldwide. Included in these concerns are such issues as global warming, natural disasters, food and agriculture yields and diseases, global population trends in migration and fertility, and broad economic trends, such as changing standards of living, real economic growth, and other indicators of prosperity, or lack thereof. Major political and security threats also pose health and welfare chal-

lenges, ranging from the impact of potential terrorism to political instability in raw materials rich countries. All of these and many other concerns have the potential to severely affect our health, directly and indirectly, in many ways.

HEALTH DISPARITIES CONTINUED

Differential access to health care services and concerns about the implications for health status have significantly heightened awareness of, and attempts to address, health disparities in our nation's population since the 1960s. Examples of the implications of health disparities have been presented in this book. Differences in access to health care and how individuals are treated within the system are measurable through physical, financial, and attitudinal indicators. Reducing disparities, particularly those that could potentially be associated with poorer outcomes of care, should be a high priority for our nation's health care system.

In recent years, recognition that differences in treatment modalities and even specific pharmacological agents may be warranted to reflect differences in genetic and ethnic composition has further heightened the need to address the full range of disparities involved in health care delivery. Potential reductions in adverse consequences, enhancement of continuity of care, and better outcomes of the care process can all result from reducing these disparities.

Disparities in the health care system are so widespread, and the potential benefits from reducing them so well accepted, that most participants in the system concur about the need to make progress in this area. The more complex issues are how to proceed and who will pay for implementation of these improvements.

Disparities in health status, disease patterns, and access to care have received heightened media attention in recent years. Poignant episodes such as patient dumping, literally, from emergency rooms, and other instances of really poor treatment of people in need of help have been picked up by the national media, frequently leading to calls for action. Various states have passed legislation, or as in California, have proposed legislation to address issues of access and equity. The presidential election campaign of 2008, perhaps more than most other prior national elections, has thrust the issues surrounding health care into the spotlight.

Disparities truly affect all segments of our nation's population. There are few, if any, segments in our population that could not benefit from a more efficient system that removes or minimalizes disparities of all types. Race, language, genetics, age, sex, income, and many other social demographic variables are correlated with one type of disparity or another. A more equitable, integrated, and comprehensive health care system can benefit everyone.

PAYING FOR HEALTH CARE

For many individuals, the health care system that they utilize is defined in large measure by their insurance plan or entitlement program. Understanding how the design and function of health insurance plans and programs work and the impact of various mechanisms are critical to improving the operation of the system. Even revolutionary change would require an understanding of past lessons and the knowledge of the impact of various insurance and health plan mechanisms. The issues involved in the payment mechanisms for health care are tremendously complex and involve critical data and information as well as policy, ethical, psychological, and economic factors.

Reforming Health Insurance

Short of a national health care system in one form or another, the evolution of health care in the United States typically follows an incremental approach with modest short-term changes and occasional dramatic realignments. Every year witnesses a wide range of changes associated with the former. The shift from indemnity to service insurance and the introduction and widespread adoption of various forms of managed care are examples of the latter. Looking toward the future, opportunities for at least incremental change and improvement in health insurance plans and operations are likely. Further changes in national entitlement programs, particularly Medicare and Medicaid, are also probable, following on the heels of the implementation of Medicare, Part D, the prescription drug benefit.

Voluntary health insurance in the United States has permanently adopted the utilization of managed-care mechanisms to structure, monitor, and control most individuals' health care systems. Control mechanisms under managed care such as gatekeepers and prior authorization have had their ups and downs since they were introduced. Other parameters of health plans ranging from premium increases to coinsurance and provider reimbursement methods to quality assessment have also experienced primarily incremental changes.

Recently, the development of mechanisms designed to entice consumers to be more cost aware and discriminating when purchasing health care services has grown dramatically. Consumer-driven health plans, which essentially involve large deductibles in one form or another, often combined with health savings accounts or other financial mechanisms, attempt to encourage consumers to be more discriminating. However, consumers often do not have direct control over much of their health care utilization. These mechanisms may have longer term effects, such as lower health status as a result of not seeking needed care earlier.

It has proven extremely difficult to design mechanisms that place the consumer at risk as an avenue for reducing health care costs and utilization without risking potential adverse health consequences down the road. Most such mechanisms are not sensitive enough to discriminate adequately in the consumer decision-making process. Very high out-of-pocket costs clearly inhibit utilization, but whether this effect leads to lower long-term costs while improving health care outcomes is a complex issue.

Other avenues for reducing costs that focus on consumer behavior also have value. These include promoting healthy behaviors and certain select clinical preventive procedures and tests. The ability of health services providers to influence patient behaviors is somewhat limited, as accidents, smoking, and obesity demonstrate. Even such benign issues as patient compliance with medical regimens lack an impressive success rate. Other long-term preventive interventions such as maintenance dosages of statins and anti-hypertensives, while likely effective, are costly.

In recent years, various payers and governmental entities have increasingly supported the provision of cost and quality information to consumers with the expectation that such knowledge will enhance their ability to be more effective purchasers or purchasing agents in the health care system. The provision and use of this kind of information is somewhat controversial and certainly not an easy sell to the consumer and policy analyst alike.

Consumer capacity for interpretation of complex cost and quality data may be somewhat limited, even for sophisticated individuals. The quality of the data itself is subject to numerous questions with regard to accuracy, consistency, biases, and many other factors. The implementation of so-called consumer-driven health plans and other efforts to utilize risk, consumer discretion, and knowledge is, by any measure, in an early stage of development. Reliance on the consumer for discretionary decision making itself conflicts with the purchasing mechanisms for much of health care, which is largely dictated by physicians and other professionals. How well consumers can interpret the data and ask questions about the quality and usefulness of those data are key issues that has not been adequately addressed as yet.

Measures that target providers have had equally questionable track records. Utilization controls, financial incentives and disincentives, and even direct employment of providers to maximize control have all had limited success in containing costs and simultaneously maintaining client health and population outcome measures. Some incentives such as insurance reimbursement pools raise questionable ethical concerns as well. More recently, such creative approaches as pay for performance, in which providers are financially rewarded for better quality care using predetermined parameters, have yet to be proven effective over large numbers of providers, services, and patients. And, even if effective, these approaches raise the fundamental question of why providers should have to be paid to provide good quality care.

Insurance companies are captive of their clients, typically the employers who contract for employee health insurance benefits and pay the majority of the bill. Ultimately, the payer determines the product. Enlightened employers have been justifiably critical of insurance industry successes in containing costs and promoting quality and outcomes. However, clear-cut successes are few and far between. Clearly employers must continue to step up to the plate and show an interest in achieving national health policy goals by protecting their own employees. In today's economy, most employers are facing highly competitive markets and may not have the time, energy, and knowledge to contribute to the formulation of appropriate health insurance plans that benefit all involved parties.

Health Insurance and the Evolution of Managed Care

The continued evolution of health insurance plans and the development of new forms of managed care have largely been evolutionary rather than revolutionary processes. Health maintenance organizations were in large measure a reformulation and relabeling of prepaid group practice while independent practice associations were in some measure a reincarnation of traditional service plans. The tremendously popular preferred provider organization is a cross between traditional indemnity and service insurance, providing for discounts and for protection of consumers though contractual arrangements with provider networks. As mentioned above, the creation of so-called consumer-driven health care plans is essentially a combination of various types of service plans with high deductibles and health savings accounts attached.

True revolution in this industry will require a much more radical reformulation of health insurance, the development of a national health insurance plan, or some other even more radical concept. Continued tweaking of the insurance programs available to most consumers through individual and group contracts has ultimately provided a venue for cost shifting to consumers and providers, rather than a more fundamental reorganization of the nation's health care system.

Further evolution of managed-care mechanisms is likely to accrue as a result of the implementation of more sophisticated information systems and monitoring capabilities. The criteria for improved managed care systems include the following:

- Liberal access to needed health services
- Cost-efficient care
- Consumer and provider satisfaction

Improvements in the structure of health care plans are needed to ensure that these goals are met in an affordable framework. Until this objective is achieved, the evolution of health care plans will fail to meet our expectations for high-quality, affordable, and accessible care.

THE UNINSURED AND DISENFRANCHISED

Among the many complex and long-standing issues facing the nation's health care system are the uninsured and underinsured populations. Individuals without any health insurance whatsoever are a heterogeneous population comprising a range of situations including those chronically unemployed, underemployed, employed without

benefits, and people between jobs; dependents without access to employer-sponsored health insurance plans; individuals and families losing insurance coverage due to divorce, death, and other unfortunate and unforeseen circumstances; and individuals who effectively self-insure by knowingly not enrolling in insurance plans, usually to save premium costs.

In addition to the uninsured, estimated at about 50 million people in 2007 including children, there is also a significant number of individuals who are underinsured by virtue of carrying inadequate coverage for prudent protection. The underinsured may lack comprehensive benefits or have significant exclusions or policy limits such that their coverage is inadequate to protect against catastrophic illnesses. The very purpose of insurance is often turned upside down in these populations with individuals protecting against lesser risks and having inadequate coverage for the more substantial risks. The underinsured also include many Medicare beneficiaries who lack adequate coverage for prescription drug needs, even with the Medicare drug benefit, and who are also sorely underinsured for long-term-care services.

Many uninsured and underinsured individuals will eventually find their way into state and local safety-net programs by virtue of becoming financially eligible for such coverage after incurring significant health care service needs. Others may gain eligibility for such programs due to their economic status. Some individuals will only partially pay incurred service obligations or will default on payments and be forced to establish long-term repayment schedules, or to file for bankruptcy protection, now more difficult under the new federal law. Historically, many of these debts are written off by health care providers or are cross subsidized through cost shifting.

Absent a national health care system with comprehensive benefits and few limitations and exclusions, coverage for the uninsured and underinsured is a relatively intractable problem. The high cost of coverage, the relative ease of not paying or only partially paying for care, and the availability of a variety of safety-net programs discourage individuals from assuming full responsibility for their own health insurance coverage, particularly in the absence of employer-sponsored plans. Mandatory population-based coverage under Medicare and voluntary employer-sponsored health insurance for current employees and some retirees and dependents are examples of relatively successful efforts to ensure coverage and financial access to health care. But even in these instances, significant gaps exist, such as for comprehensive mental health and long-term care.

Among the uninsured, a significant percentage of individuals are between jobs, losing eligibility for employer-sponsored health insurance. Federal legislation mandates the availability of continuing coverage for many of these individuals for a reasonable length of time, generally 18 months. Some dependent coverage is also available through these channels. However, individuals must pay full premium charges for such coverage, a significant burden, especially for those individuals laid off from employment.

PUBLIC HEALTH SERVICES

A fundamental reassessment of the role of public health services and their organization in communities occurred after September 11, 2001. The need to provide enhanced surveillance and preventive services, particularly to protect against the ramifications of a terrorist attack, empowered a partial revitalization of public health in the United States. Some, but not all, of the potential initiatives arising from this revitalization have been achieved. Realistically, the more complete integration of public health services into the health care system and a leadership role for public health in organizing and prioritizing health care needs in communities have not occurred in most jurisdictions.

Many public health challenges remain. Funding for public health services represents only approximately 3 percent of our national health care expenditures, a relatively modest investment given the tremendous payoff in improved health and the avoidance of disease. New initiatives and expansion of existing efforts are needed to address primary prevention, screening of populations, protection of the environment, more rapid interventions for heart attacks and strokes, better public awareness and education programs, enhanced terrorism preparedness and preparation, further protection of the food, water, and milk supplies, and other traditional public health priorities.

The public-health-related systems, as the sometimes provider of last resort, need enhancements and funding in many communities throughout the nation. Programs such as Medicaid, state children's health insurance programs, other safety-net programs, and social welfare programs all need better funding, improved coordination and management, and greater integration. Entire areas of public health concern such as long-term care and mental health services still have significant deficiencies, particularly for minorities, low-income individuals, and the disenfranchised. Unfortunately, the poorest of the poor include single women with dependent children, the aged, and other vulnerable population groups for whom service needs are still not matched by service availability.

Numerous legislative and legal challenges remain to be adequately addressed with regard to public health services and programs as well. Ultimately, the role of government and the extent of the safety net are fundamental public health issues that must be defined in the legislatures and courts of the nation.

In the broad expanse of public health issues, enhancement of the environment is a key concern and priority. Among the environmental issues facing our nation there continues to be concern over indoor and outdoor air quality and the implications of air quality for disease processes; exposure to environmental toxic substances such as asbestos, lead, and radon; the relationship between the environment and child and maternal health, particularly as pertains to lung diseases such as asthma; and implications for the environment from agricultural processes and pesticides in the distribution channels.

Health and the environment are intertwined. As has been well demonstrated, numerous costly illnesses and disease patterns are attributable to environmental exposures, nutrition, and other aspects of the larger world in which we live. A comprehensive approach to health and public health requires attention to these broader issues. Indeed, addressing the challenges of global warming, population, international migration, worldwide disparities in health and wealth, and other major issues is essential to the long-term well-being of our nation's population.

AMBULATORY CARE SERVICES

Ambulatory care services form the network for the distribution of what has become the core of health care services in the United States. Increasing reliance on ambulatory services for both the provision of care and the management of patients will continue. With the hospital's inpatient role increasingly focusing on tertiary and other complex services, and with improvements in technology combined with cost and efficiency pressures in the system, ambulatory services will increasingly be relied upon as the principal source of health care for the nation's population. These services are the gateway and control mechanism for specialized and institutionally based services as well. The next phase of control is to utilize increasingly sophisticated information systems to monitor the delivery of health care by primary care and specialized providers to observe their resource utilization and their decision-making processes in the referral of patients for more complex care.

Cost pressures in the ambulatory sector will continue to escalate, yielding an increasing emphasis on efficient management of practices and careful use of resources, particularly for capital investment and health care personnel. Physician productivity enhancements will continue to be a focus of this sector. The provision of still more care, particularly specialized surgical services on an ambulatory basis, will also continue.

The infusion of newer technologies—including dissemination of information and instructions to patients; use of computerized medical records to allow for greater monitoring and less duplication; improvements in the monitoring and enforcement of quality techniques, particularly with regard to appropriate use of technologies, including drugs, and assurance of proper clinical practice, particularly for patients with chronic disease—will be major foci throughout the next few decades.

The organization of physician and other professional service practices may continue to evolve. Structural changes and legal arrangements that are responses to contractual pressures from managed-care organizations and other financial aspects of these practices are changing the organization of medical groups. As in the past, some aspects of federal and state tax law may artificially induce corporate changes in professional practices as well. Governance is also likely to be a concern, particularly among health care professionals. The increasing complexity of the legal and regulatory environment, especially as it pertains to federal and state financing programs, is a continued source of concern to the management of ambulatory practices. The best that can be hoped for at this point is simplification and clarification of appropriate rules and regulations to allow adequate decision-making freedom to effectively manage practices.

The ambulatory care arena has seen tremendous change over the past few decades and has assumed an essential role in the health care system. Pressures for more efficient and effective management in this sector will continue and the expectations of health care professionals, patients, and payers will continue to force more response from managers.

HOSPITAL AND HEALTH SYSTEMS

The hospital sector has always known change. The fundamental drivers of health care are technology and financing, and these issues cut to the core of the operation of the hospital industry. Changing technology, in and of itself, has wrought huge change in the hospital industry, ranging from the tremendous growth of ambulatory surgery to the increasing sophistication and complexity of tertiary care services.

At the same time, changes in the financing of the hospital industry, particularly the shift from retrospective to prospective reimbursement and the emergence of managed-care contracting, have radically altered the financial parameters of the industry. The expectations of providers, consumers, and payers have changed dramatically over the years, increasing the pressure on hospitals to provide an extremely high quality product and to do so efficiently. Other financial pressures on both the for-profit and not-for-profit sectors in the hospital industry have led to huge changes with regard to both horizontal and vertical integration. The dramatic and nearly complete shift from individual hospitals to for-profit and not-for-profit systems of care, and other affiliation arrangements, has radically altered the management and financing of the industry. For the for-profit sector, the past few decades have seen extreme turbulence in the financial markets and continuing realignment of the industry.

Ultimately, it is the financial pressures from payers, who recognize that the hospital sector is extremely cost intensive, that has led to the recognition that almost desperate attempts are necessary to rein in these costs. At the same time, the promise of dramatically expanding technological capabilities and the increasing successes of our interventions, as illustrated by the example of coronary artery disease, have encouraged the expansion of these services.

The priorities for hospital and health systems include further development and implementation of management information systems incorporating computerized medical records that will allow for comprehensive tracking of patients, utilization patterns, and fiscal flows as well as aid in quality assurance; contractual reporting requirements; and other legal, regulatory, managerial, and financial activities and requirements. Continued formation of appropriate alliances, affiliations, and networks for the improvement of the quality and efficiency of care is also essential.

Coping with the demands for the implementation of new technology and the control and dissemination of innovation will continue to be a critical challenge. Leadership among the medical staff, administration, and boards is yet another area of challenge and opportunity that must be addressed. Ultimately, the hospital sector must define its role in the larger system. This means determining appropriate contractual relationships, ownership arrangements, and the extent to which hospital and health systems should provide integrated delivery solutions or specialize in complex secondary and tertiary care.

Other issues also challenge this sector of the health care industry. Accountability and the role of the hospital industry in providing care to uninsured and underinsured individuals cannot be left in limbo. Patient expectations for cures and technology, professional staff expectations of pay and perks, and payer expectations of cost containment and quality enhancements often present conflicting challenges. The threat of federal government regulatory intervention, medical malpractice challenges, and other external forces further buffet the industry. The hospital and health systems industry is a moving target facing an increasingly complex and challenging environment.

THE FUTURE OF LONG-TERM CARE

The aging of the United States population will eventually peak with approximately 20 percent of the population aged 65 and above. This notable achievement in the population pyramid has already approximately been reached in Japan and Germany and portends an increasingly key role for long-term care services worldwide in the future. And, even in Asia, and particularly China, economic development has raised havoc with the traditional role of the nuclear family.

Although the nursing home has historically represented the most common modality for providing long-term care services, the reality of improved overall health status for the elderly population combined with alternative delivery mechanisms for social, health, and supportive services suggests a much wider range of living arrangements will be utilized in the future. The increasing scope of the continuum of care, encompassing an array of settings from home health services to various at-home and alternative living situations, already exemplifies the explosion in creativity for this sector.

The need to address the integration of social and health services as the population ages will require creative approaches to providing financing for these services and for a more information-systems-based answer. Challenging the historical separation of social and health services and accepting innovative perspectives to meet the needs of an increasingly mature population will be significant challenges for the future.

The increasing application of technological innovation to facilitate individuals' lifestyles will also accelerate the ability of the population to cope with limitations of functional status and to meet health and social needs. These types of changes tend to occur rather slowly as our social and economic systems adapt to changing needs in the population.

Increasingly sophisticated consumers and a new generation of healthier, more adaptable, and more knowledgeable seniors will demand better responses from our social and health services systems. Over time, these demands and expectations will produce market responses and governmental action. In addition, individual initiative and the use of patients' own resources will greatly enhance the environment for long-term care services.

Individual health care providers within the long-term care environment will also need to respond to changing expectations as new generations of seniors raise the bar and demand higher quality services with more efficiency and greater ambiance. The continuing care retirement communities and assisted living facilities that have been developed over the past 30 years are beginning to reflect this higher level of expectation and service. Better use of technology, information systems, improved architecture and design, and other innovations will contribute to enhance the delivery of services in this arena.

Among the most significant challenges in the area of long-term-care services are issues of financing and health care personnel. From a financial perspective, among the key policy decisions to be faced in the future is the role of government in paying for long-term care services. Expansion of the Medicare program into a greater role in this area is fraught with the potential for huge liability and adverse risk selection. The past attempt to expand Medicare with greater coverage for catastrophic illness was a political and policy failure due to the attempt to pass along some of the increased costs to beneficiaries.

Identifying additional sources of revenue that can be utilized for long-term care services is a very tough challenge for our nation. Today's reliance on a consumer's own resources, particularly for those in nursing homes through the spend down provision, may still represent the most financially and politically viable alternative for the future. For those who can afford to protect their asset base, long-term care insurance today does offer a private alternative. However, long-term care insurance is expensive, and, while feasible, a mandatory insurance program for all Americans is unlikely. Private sector long-term care insurance may also not appeal to those who are willing to accept the implications, if necessary, of coverage under state Medicaid programs for nursing home and related services.

The increasing health of successive generations may also provide some protection for our nation in the future. Data confirm that individuals are living longer and healthier lives, and ultimately, keeping people out of the long-term care system is the ideal solution to this conundrum. Better functional status, improvements in mental capacity, technological applications to facilitate living in one's home, and perhaps even increased family support may eventually lead to a lessening of the need for the use of long-term care services, particularly those that are more expensive. Rationing may result in care being allocated to those in greatest need, with others in the population adjusting to these new expectations.

Ultimately, addressing the issues of long-term care and our aging population is really a social, political, and economic rather than technological challenge. As a nation, we need to prioritize how we want to care for those in need of these services, whether they are younger or older, and define the level of support that we are willing to provide. The challenges that we face in the longer term with regard to social security and Medicare, and to a large extent, Medicaid, are integral to addressing the long-term care needs of our society.

MENTAL HEALTH SERVICES

Mental health services in the United States have progressed into a new era of progress and promise. The introduction of psychotropic drugs facilitated the process of deinstitutionalization and community-based care, ushering in the first phases of modernization in the treatment of mental illness. The early recognition of the social and economic implications of mental health problems and their interaction with the larger society was a national wakeup call, which focused attention on the needs of individuals with mental health problems. Although funding for these services has often been inadequate, only by opening the hearts and minds of Americans during these early years of change were we able to come out of the darkness as a nation and improve prospects for all people in need of care.

Over the past 30 years, the application of scientific and biomedical knowledge to the mental health field and advances in neuroscience and pharmacology have freed mental health services from the shackles of misconceptions and miscommunications. A scientific-based recognition of the etiologies of mental illness, and the identification of biomedical pathways for cures have brought mental health closer to the medical, economic, and political mainstream. While some of the messages of the old days remain, future prospects are finally much brighter.

Above all, the continued elucidation of the physiological causes of mental health problems, combined with a better understanding of social and psychological bases for less complex emotional illnesses, will promote these key trends. The biomedical research pipeline currently in place in pharmaceutical and biotechnology companies as well as in government research laboratories around the world will continue to produce interventions that will moderate, if not cure, many of these diseases and, perhaps more important, facilitate human functioning and improve health status. The social context of mental health problems as they pertain to families, the workplace, and other environments will also benefit greatly from this progress.

Further enlightenment on the part of payers, particularly third-party insurance companies and government programs, to support the provision of mental health services is also critical. Federal legislation pertaining to inclusion of mental health benefits in insurance programs and plans, while not practically effective at the present time, has established our national recognition that mental health services should be considered in a manner similar to somatic health care. Increasing attention to mental health services, insurance provisions that further and fairly define coverage levels, deductibles, exclusions, and limitations will be key to assuring that these services are provided in an appropriate and adequate manner. At the same time, improvements in governmental programs and private treatment alternatives that can adequately address the needs of more severely ill individuals are also critical to our long-term success.

Mental health services still face significant limitations. In the public arena, and in the political environment, mental health is still not a key national priority. Advocacy for mental health services and for patients, while having improved substantially, still lacks many of the commitments found elsewhere in our health care system. Mental health services continue to lack adequate support for financing in both public and private arenas. Mental health services are especially challenging for the elderly, individuals with more serious and long-term difficulties, the homeless, and those for whom mental health issues cause significant workplace or home dislocations.

Public perception of mental health issues lags reality. Mental health services are quite uneven across geographic regions and between various population groups. Many mental health diagnoses still are difficult to define, treat, and control, and many significant clinical delivery challenges remain. The widespread adoption of managed mental health care has led to an increased emphasis on shorter term and drug-based interventions and less attention directed to psychotherapy, direct clinical one-on-one interventions with practitioners, and longer term continuous care. Evaluating the quality of mental health services is also still a substantial challenge, particularly with regard to outcome measures.

Perhaps of equal concern are increased rates of mental illness, a result of many trends in our society including increased crowding, workplace stress, and home pressures. Living longer itself provides extra exposure to mental health risks. Comorbidity between mental health and various somatic illnesses including most infectious and chronic diseases is also a concern for the future, as it has been in the past.

Ultimately, progress in the field of mental health services over the past couple of decades has been tremendous. The picture is likely to continue to improve in the future. Overdiagnosis and overapplication of pharmacological agents, shortages of adequate funding in a variety of settings, and historical

biases and prejudices will continue to plague the field. But a snapshot taken two or three decades ago, when compared to today's environment, produces startling contrasts. Another snapshot taken 20 or 30 years from now will produce even more dramatic comparisons to today.

FUTURE OF THE PHARMACEUTICAL INDUSTRY

The pharmaceutical industry, which also encompasses biotechnology and medical device companies, faces numerous challenges for the future. Among the most serious threats to this industry are issues related to the product development pipeline: product pre- and postapproval processes in the United States and around the world; efficacy and safety reviews and standards; pricing pressures and cost considerations related to marketing, production, and research; regulatory compliance and product distribution restrictions; worldwide concerns regarding policy and public relations; and the role of the industry in the evolution of health care systems.

Concurrent with increasing success with pharmaceutical products for diagnostic and therapeutic interventions and successes in fighting many diseases has been an increased exposure for the industry as the target of public frustration and anger and political attacks. How the industry copes with its serious ongoing business challenges while at the same time effectively answering its very public critics will help determine the future direction for this sector of the health care system.

Product Pricing

Many pharmaceutical products face complex pricing issues that will fundamentally affect the profitability of pharmaceutical and biotechnology companies. Pricing of pharmaceutical products by manufacturers reflects extensive research and development, marketing, and administrative costs; development and operation of production facilities; quality assurance; and certain other factors. Pricing of products is such that many of these costs, particularly for marketing and distribution, lead to substantially higher prices for products than public and political perceptions may feel are justified. Furthermore, overhead costs and downstream distribution costs further increase product pricing, in both retail and institutional settings.

Other factors further complicate product pricing issues. Because many pharmaceutical products are marketed and distributed nationally and internationally based on local pricing to the market and the ability to pay, there is tremendous variation in the pricing of individual products across the country and around the globe. Even domestic pricing can vary considerably depending on the purchasing power of the organization buying the product, negotiated prices and contractual arrangements, and price constraints built into various governmental and managed-care programs. International pricing differentials are often huge as well. In general, from an international perspective, products are priced highest in the United States since the United States marketplace is viewed as the least price sensitive and the market of greatest financial opportunity.

Price differentials, both in the United States and internationally, lead to the perception of price gouging for those paying at the higher end of the pricing structure. Importation of drugs from other countries, such as from Canada and Mexico, occurs as a result of pricing differentials. There are complex issues involved in this issue, such as country laws limiting import or export of drugs, adequacy of medical prescription review, quality control concerns, and, alarmingly, different products sold under the same or similar names in different countries.

The public perception is that Americans are being overcharged for products in this arena. The reality is that prices reflect what the market will bear in each individual market, and for each purchaser, rather than a generalized conspiracy to rip off American consumers. Companies seek to maximize overall product revenue by charging a core

audience market rates and selling additional product, where feasible, to clients who cannot pay as much at lower price points. However, this pricing model may not hold up in the long term due to public perception and to the political implications inherent in such an approach.

International Needs

Another complex issue is the role of U.S. pharmaceutical research and production in the international arena, especially as it pertains to developing countries. The United States, Western Europe, select Asian nations (an expanding membership group), and other countries that conduct most of the research that produces new drugs invest in these efforts with the expectation of being paid back through product sales, and profits. But a key international issue arises as to how to fairly distribute technology that we have paid for to countries and peoples in the world who cannot afford to pay for those technologies. An excellent example of this issue is the development and distribution of drugs to deal with the AIDS epidemic. Ultimately, wealthier developed nations simply have to share their technology with the poor nations and peoples of the world. Improvement of health and economic well-being in these regions will ultimately lead to greater purchasing power and an improved standard of living.

Blockbuster Drugs

The Holy Grail for many pharmaceutical firms is the blockbuster product that generates huge cash flow and, ultimately, huge profits. However, many products are not blockbusters. The profitability of blockbuster drugs helps fund additional research. About half of the U.S. biomedical research funding derives from pharmaceutical and biotech companies. The other half is funded by the federal government, primarily through the National Institutes of Health. An alternative model would provide greater funding from governmental sources. The reduction of product development costs could lead to lower pricing levels for drugs and related products. However, empirical evidence would have to support such a thesis. And even today, much of the federally funded biomedical research leads to, directly or indirectly, products refined and sold by private enterprise.

Perhaps an even bigger issue facing the pharmaceutical industry is the question of where future products will come from. There are limits to the successes of company laboratories in producing marketable drugs, as has become evident over the past few years. Furthermore, some drugs with anticipated substantial long-term market opportunity have been associated with serious adverse consequences when approved for marketing and utilized by larger numbers of patients. The recent problems with Bextra, Celebrex, and other nonsteroid anti-inflammatory drugs are an excellent example of this situation. Other drugs have failed in mid- or late-stage clinical trials after the investment of hundreds of millions of dollars. But, drug discovery is a complex, high-risk proposition and pharmaceutical manufacturers expect significant payoffs when products are brought to market.

Drug Industry Advertising

The issue of advertising, marketing, and distribution expense is another area subject to public debate. For many drugs, about one-third of revenue is spent on advertising and promotion. It is well known that ethical drug companies spend huge amounts of money on advertising to physicians and to other providers. In addition, during the last decade there has been an explosion in pharmaceutical company expenditures for direct-to-consumer advertising for products that consumers cannot even purchase without a prescription. All these costs are included in the pricing model for prescription drugs and medical devices. Instituting a legislative ban or substantial reduction in such expenditures might curb some health care costs, but such an approach is not typically consistent with our capitalist system and may have other untoward side effects that are as yet unknown. Certainly the industry has a degree of susceptibility on this issue.

Other Issues

Numerous other issues of product development, distribution, innovation, quality, financing, intellectual property, and more confront this complex and increasingly important segment of the health care industry. These include the future role of retail pharmacies; the roles, regulations, and interactions and health effects of herbs, foods, and natural products; drug use, and misuse, in the elderly; the relation of prescription and over-the-counter products; and the increasing role of consumers in this arena.

HEALTH CARE PERSONNEL

Health care personnel face many challenges. The increasing sophistication and complexity of health care technology demand ever-more highly trained and expensive technical personnel. Increasing specialization and quality enhancement pressures have induced institutions and professionals to enhance employee training, monitoring, and staffing levels. The often significant adverse consequences of poor personnel performance reduce the allowable margin of error in this sector of the economy.

Shortages of adequately trained personnel, particularly for nursing, have already reached crisis proportions in many areas of the nation. The need to train, attract, motivate, and retain high-performing health care professionals has been a constant theme throughout the industry. Whether it be medical staff, technicians, personnel, or support individuals, creating a motivating workplace in the face of the challenges of patient care and cost pressures is a constant issue for virtually all areas of the health care industry. With personnel costs accounting for a high percentage of health care expenditures, managing these costs is a particularly acute concern for the operation of health care institutions.

The absence of clear national planning for health care personnel needs presents a variety of problems. Not since the efforts of federal and state governments in the 1960s and 1970s has the nation presented a coherent policy for the development of health care personnel needs. Medical education, postgraduate training, and many other areas of specialized need are particularly notable for the lack of national direction from government. Long-term strategic planning to deal with personnel needs for the future would help. Voluntary organizations have attempted to fill the void by conducting planning assessments and using other mechanisms. But the absence of national political and policy leadership is clearly evident.

The need to develop leadership among the nation's physicians, nurses, and other health care personnel should also be a high national priority. Clinical and administrative leaders are essential to ensuring the success of the health care system. Numerous examples of the payoff from excellence in leadership exist. Excellent leaders have harnessed the power of information systems, employee motivation, fiscal discipline, and patient outreach to substantially improve health care delivery in many health care organizations and institutions. Leadership makes the difference.

The personnel sector of the nation's health care delivery system has always been in flux, responding to changes in technology, population-based demand for services, specialization, and financing. The challenges will continue to grow in the future. Many sectors such as mental health, long-term care, nursing, and some physician specialties face particularly challenging situations as the nation's population ages. These challenges will best be met when the nation accepts a strategic and long-term perspective on these needs.

HEALTH CARE POLICY AND POLITICS

The design and operation of the nation's health care system is intertwined with the nation's economic and political environments. The political environment defines the broad spectrum of government involvement in health care, ranging from financing to regulatory intervention. The ultimate government intervention would be a national health care system, highly unlikely given our nation's commitment to free markets. At the other extreme, a totally market-driven system has obviously failed to meet the expectations of all consumers and providers and has pressured payers into difficult situations as well. Managed care, once seen as the ultimate solution, primarily by shifting risk to the providers, has also clearly failed to live up to its expectations. The increasing cost of health services, the increasing burden of the uninsured and the underinsured, the aging of the population, pressures on salaries and competitiveness in the industrial and commercial sectors, and other factors portend an increasingly difficult future.

Voluntary planning and subsequent government supported efforts to influence health services through the CHP (Comprehensive Health Planning) and the HSAs (Health System Agencies) combined with certificate of need regulations, mandatory budget regulations, rate setting commissions, and other interventions demonstrated the market distorting and often counterproductive nature of external regulation of health care systems. Throwing in a dose of democratic representation to keep all constituencies happy further muddied the waters. Clearly partial and voluntary approaches do not result in comprehensive solutions.

The realities of our political system will limit the degree of reform that can be implemented in the health care system. Government at all levels has limited control over the operation of the health care system and can utilize its regulatory and financial power only to a point to implement change. Truly radical change can alienate many constituencies whether justified or not by social and national goals. These constituencies, such as organized medicine, the pharmaceutical industry, employers, insurers, and even consumer groups, have a tremendous amount of power to block change or to substantially modify its implementation. The result of these processes is often that when changes do occur, their form and function are far from ideal or as originally envisioned. Rational analysts may develop outstanding strategic plans, but the implementation of those plans must go through complex political processes and face a variety of economic realities. If enough special interests find that their objectives are protected and promoted through change, then things can happen. Otherwise, there is a limited basis for optimism.

The politics of health care were muddied by a plethora of broader issues culminating in the national elections of 2008. The divisive war in Iraq, the mounting costs of that war and various other governmental spending initiatives, and the early stages of the financial burdens accruing from the aging of the baby boom population have certainly raised the stakes in any consensus on addressing health care needs from a more global perspective. Frustration with federal gridlock and uncertainty has led to state-based experimentation and initiatives, most of them not providing convincing role models for broader implementation. The mounting fiscal challenge limits the ability to commit funds to new initiatives in health care no matter how useful. And lack of effective leadership results in paralysis rather than action in the policy arena. These larger concerns, combined with very public episodes of failure within the health care system, and the immense challenges involved in successfully reforming health care systems, suggest that the health policy bar has been raised higher than ever before.

Ultimately, the future of health policy and politics in the United States will be determined by the political will of the people in combination with economic, political, ethical, and practical forces. Where all these currents will lead us is at this point, as always, uncertain.

QUALITY OF CARE

Assessing and ensuring the quality of care of health services in the United States are tremendous challenges. Providers, consumers, and payers are increasingly demanding not only improvements in the quality of care, but also institutionalized safeguards to protect against adverse consequences during the care process. Increasingly sophisticated computerized information systems and other technologies for assessing quality of care and for providing protective interventions and feedback to those in the system are slowly enhancing the quality of care that patients receive. Barriers to implementation of these systems include costs, provider opposition, and a myriad of practical considerations. Knowledge about quality improvement and enhanced operating systems is spreading throughout the system, but at a slower pace than many observers would prefer.

Lessons learned from the industrial sector are also infiltrating the health care system to enhance quality of care and to protect consumers and providers alike against adverse consequences. Well-documented failures in the system have led to costly mistakes in patient care with associated death and injury, added cost from unnecessary duplicated services, inappropriate care, and other errors. However, widespread consensus of the need to improve in all these areas has been achieved and the system is moving in the right direction.

The coming years should see enhanced quality assurance within the health care system. Increasing computerization of information will greatly facilitate this movement. Further enhancement of clinical pathways, quality improvement techniques, and other methodology will support the movement. Demands from payers and consumers will provide financial incentives, and providers themselves will increasingly seek to protect their own positions though enhanced quality efforts. While these efforts are most strongly implemented in the institutional setting, larger and midsize ambulatory practices will increasingly adopt various versions of them to promote quality further down the line. Improved training of health care personnel will promote this movement. Increasing consumer awareness and other external entities such as government and voluntary organizations will further reinforce the need for quality enhancement. Litigation, including medical malpractice concerns and regulatory interventions, also serves to provide an incentive for better quality of care.

All players in the health care system seek improvements in quality, efficiency, and operational integrity. The technology for institutionalizing these improvements is increasingly coming online. Financial, political, and legal pressures will coalesce to promote the quality improvement movement as well. Improving the quality of care is an evolutionary rather than revolutionary movement that requires continuous effort and proselytizing. The effort is well underway at this point in time, and all participants in the health care system will benefit.

INTERNATIONAL HEALTH

Although the focus of this book is on health care services in the United States, a strategic perspective on the international scene is certainly worth keeping in mind. Health care systems internationally vary dramatically in terms of levels of funding, funding mechanisms, organization and delivery systems, and managerial approaches. Many Western European countries and some countries in other parts of the world follow a model for health services delivery that is at least analogous to that of the United States in terms of the prevalence of technology and the medical community. Some countries have national care systems, such as the United Kingdom, with its British National Health Service, while others have national or regional financing systems such as the Canadian system in which each province runs a separate governmentally sponsored health program.

Some countries have combinations of governmental systems of one type or another and a significant private sector for those who can pay. Many developing countries have a very small private sector and a relatively large, but severely underfunded public system that is focused on the provision of a limited array of services and on some public health efforts. There are many emerging models for health care delivery throughout the world as most nations struggle to come to grips with the complex realities of attempting to provide an array of services to their citizens while recognizing significant costs and political pressures. There is no one universal solution nor is there any model in the world that is clearly superior and without problems of one sort or another.

The changing dynamics in world population, economic growth, trade, and control of resources are drawing attention to Asia and other regions. There is a fundamental shift under way whereby the economic and political attention of the world's leaders and populations has been shifting from North America and Europe to these new growth regions. Health care, too, is experiencing the early stages of a shifting focus with much more attention to service needs, and profit opportunities, in Asia and other expanding markets. Biomedical research is also shifting its focus to these regions, as exemplified by the initiatives undertaken is Singapore. The future holds many opportunities in health care for these newer economic powerhouses, both as markets for services and as producers of health care products and services for the rest of the world.

For developed nations, the fundamental question is whether to have a government-owned, -operated, and -funded health care system or to provide governmental funding to an array of privately managed services. Few governments can realistically elect to provide no funding whatsoever, since in that case, the lower socioeconomic strata would literally be left to die. And, the increasing costs of health services are a worldwide phenomenon that effectively precludes any simple, universal solution. Furthermore, many of the fundamental demographic trends, such as the aging of the population in more developed countries, the challenges of large numbers of uninsured or unfunded patients, the accumulation of a variety of diseases, such as the AIDS epidemic, place tremendous burdens on any nation.

It is peculiar in some respects that the percentage of gross domestic product allocated to the health care system varies so dramatically across the nations of the world. Even among somewhat analogous developed countries, the differences are dramatic. And these differences certainly do not account for differentials in outcome measures such as length of life, mortality, and morbidity. Ultimately, fundamental questions must be raised as to why, in the aggregate, one country can buy equal or more health at a much lower cost per person, or as a percentage of gross domestic product, than another country.

Also from an international perspective, of course, all nations must face the inequities that exist in availability and access to health care throughout the world. Because health care is such a fundamental need among all peoples, the disparities in access, funding, and availability of services really relate to inequity in the distribution of income and wealth worldwide. Redistribution of the wealth in the world, of course, is a complex issue, certainly beyond the scope of this book, but one worthy of careful debate and consideration. Improving economic development and opportunity, and thus raising the quality of life and of health care worldwide, is clearly a worthwhile goal.

Another important aspect of global health certainly involves the spread of disease, particularly infectious diseases worldwide. Although at one point we might have felt that the global spread of infectious disease was under control and not a major threat, we can now appreciate that this was a premature conclusion. All nations must work together to combat the spread of infectious disease as well as other threats to health on a global scale as evidenced by the efforts to combat SARS, bird flu, and even biological and chemical terrorism.

Global health requires a global commitment. Whether or not there are adequate resources in the world to address the health care needs of all people, consistent and comprehensive efforts to improve the health of nations across the globe will benefit everyone.

THE FUTURE OF HEALTH CARE

Pulling together all the disparate content of this book is not easy. The nation's health care system is exceedingly complex and is delivering a product that is probably the most sophisticated and most challenging collection of services ever assembled in the history of mankind. Reaching the moon was a relatively straightforward and discrete achievement in comparison to improving the health of over 300 million people.

Innovation in Health Care

It is critical to the nation's future health that innovative practices and biomedical and clinical research be promoted and incentivized. Innovation is the key to improving health and health care services. Fundamentally, the health care system is the delivery mechanism for the technology that is developed in the nation's biological research laboratories and in clinical practice. Innovation in health care delivery that promotes more efficient and effective services is also critical.

Leadership of the health care system is dependent on creative and dynamic individuals who can force appropriate change. Consumers must demand better quality and more user-friendly health care. Above all, payers must provide incentives within the reimbursement structures for health care organizations to provide better care to more consumers more efficiently. The entire national structure of health care services must move in unison toward these objectives, even if significant deficiencies exist within the system. Innovation and technological advancement are the keys to our future, a future of continuing improvements in health outcomes.

Technology

Technology is the driving force of health care. The development, testing, and distribution of technological advances are fundamental to improving the nation's health. Our nation must encourage these efforts through tax and reimbursement policy and other initiatives to enhance the armament of clinical practitioners.

At the same time, it is also essential that technological innovations be thoroughly vetted, proven in clinical trials and other forums, and held to high standards of safety, efficiency, efficacy, and financial feasibility. Cost-benefit analysis and other analytical techniques must be utilized along with clinical evaluations to keep technology in proper perspective.

The technological imperative that has driven health care for so many years must now be matched with critical assessments of the limits to which technologies we can afford. Increasingly, the blank check of the past is facing the economic reality of the present and future. As a nation, we must ask these critical questions and decide where to draw the line, while at the same time assuring that there is adequate access to appropriate and successful technologies to the extent possible.

The Most Radical Changes

Not likely, but at the extreme, truly radical changes would fundamentally transform the delivery of health care in the United States. These changes could include a nationalization of the system with centralized management and some local governance, along the lines of the national health care systems in the United Kingdom and elsewhere. As has been demonstrated, direct control over resources may (or may not) result in less utilization and lower costs. The existing system could be transformed by radical reductions in reimbursement rates forcing much lower salaries and benefits for personnel, much more rationing of services and capital investment, and other extreme measures. Some would suggest that this has already been done through managed care and lowered government reimbursement levels. Even more radical would be to go beyond existing levels of rationing and severely limit care to older individuals,

as well as reduce levels of service to those with serious illnesses and injuries. This approach would make Dr. Kevorkian seem kind. Or, at the other end of the spectrum, we could figure out how to effect a truly comprehensive and health promoting approach to each person's life incorporating prevention, early detection of disease and early intervention, screening, treatment, and on-going follow-up and assessment, along with education, behavioral change, dietary monitoring, and reversal of global warming thrown in as well! Of course most radical changes are untested and would likely have innumerable unintended consequences, some good and some bad.

SUMMARY

Through all the challenges, the health of our nation has continued to improve by most measurable standards. Very significant deficiencies still exist, yet we at least recognize and are trying to deal with them. The spread of disease continues, yet we continue to fight back. The technological changes that have occurred in recent years recognize our greatest biological achievements in finally understanding the molecular basis of illness and disease and designing clinical interventions based on that knowledge. The future indeed is challenging, but bright, and the nation's health in all likelihood will continue its slow, but steady progression in the right direction.

REVIEW QUESTIONS

1. List the most difficult issues facing health care in America today.
2. List the incremental changes that have occurred within the U.S. health insurance industry.
3. How does technology drive health care?
4. Describe changes that have taken place within the hospital sector.
5. Describe health care systems at the international level.

REFERENCES & ADDITIONAL READINGS

Bodenheimer, T. S., Grumbach, K. (2002). *Understanding health policy: A clinical approach,* 3rd ed. Stamford, CT: Appleton & Lange.

Herzlinger, R. E., & Parasa-Parisi, R. (2004). Consumer-driven health care: Lessons from Switzerland. *292*(10), 1213–1220.

Marquis, M. S., Rogowski, J. A., *Journal of the American Medical Association,* Escarce, J. J. (2004). Recent trends and geographic variation in the safety net. *Medical Care, 52*(5), 408–415.

U.S. Department of Health and Human Services. (2000). *Healthy people 2010: Understanding and improving health and objectives for improving health,* 2nd ed., Vol. 1. Washington, DC: U.S. Government Printing Office.

World Health Organization. (2002). *The world health report 2002: Reducing risks, promoting healthy life.* Geneva: World Health Organization.

INDEX